Global Health Governance and the Fight Against HIV/AIDS

Also by Wolfgang Hein and Lars Kohlmorgen

Globalisation, Global Health Governance and National Health Politics in Developing Countries: An Exploration Into the Dynamics of Interfaces (Wolfgang Hein and Lars Kohlmorgen, eds), 2003

Tourism and Sustainable Development (Wolfgang Hein, ed.) 1997

Global Health Governance and the Fight Against HIV/AIDS

Edited by

Wolfgang Hein
Head of Research Programme, German Institute of Global and Area Studies, Germany

Sonja Bartsch
Senior Research Fellow, German Institute of Global and Area Studies, Germany

Lars Kohlmorgen
Senior Research Fellow, German Institute of Global and Area Studies, Germany

palgrave
macmillan

First published 2007 by
PALGRAVE MACMILLAN
Houndmills, Basingstoke, Hampshire RG21 6XS and
175 Fifth Avenue, New York, N.Y. 10010
Companies and representatives throughout the world

PALGRAVE MACMILLAN is the global academic imprint of the Palgrave Macmillan division of St. Martin's Press, LLC and of Palgrave Macmillan Ltd. Macmillan® is a registered trademark in the United States, United Kingdom and other countries. Palgrave is a registered trademark in the European Union and other countries.

ISBN-13: 978-0-230-51727-1 hardback
ISBN-10: 0-230-51727-7 hardback

This book is printed on paper suitable for recycling and made from fully managed and sustained forest sources. Logging, pulping and manufacturing processes are expected to conform to the environmental regulations of the country of origin.

A catalogue record for this book is available from the British Library.

A catalog record for this book is available from the Library of Congress.

10 9 8 7 6 5 4 3 2 1
16 15 14 13 12 11 10 09 08 07

Printed and bound in Great Britain by
Antony Rowe Ltd, Chippenham and Eastbourne

To Brigitte, Werner and Sabine
and all those who are fighting for a healthier world.

Contents

List of Figures and Tables

Foreword: Governing Interdependence

The neglect of health in international relations

Health has for too long been faced with serious neglect by scholars of international relations. Possibly a major reason for this has been that in the post-industrial societies of the developed world health policy is considered first and foremost a national policy arena, anxiously protected against outside influence and meddling, be it by regional organizations such as the European Union or global agencies such as the World Health Organization. Political scientists have long analysed health through a purely national lens, also due to the erroneous equation of health with the health systems. In consequence it was the 'comparative policy analysis' of incomparable systems that carried the day. This thinking has also informed the analysis of health systems in developing countries, which to some extent emerged as a subfield of development studies. Health therefore was particularly subject to what Ulrich Beck und Christoph Lau (2004) have called 'methodological nationalism'. In contrast the environment has been most attractive to the analysts of global governance – and indeed has helped establish this field of academic endeavour (Young 1997). From the beginning of its entry as a new functional policy arena it was considered inherently global; indeed its most famous advocacy slogan stated 'Think global – act local'. It was self-evident that pollution and global warming transcended borders and needed global policy responses. From this followed stimulating academic debates on regimes, risk society, governance without government and the like.

But while academia was concentrating on the new environmental agreements that were being negotiated with great publicity, a new killer was silently spreading in the world of health. In the 1980s a new disease was identified which seemed to have originated in the developing world but hit most brutally in some of the richest countries. It did not – at first instance – seek out the weak and the poor but men in their prime, some of them beautiful, rich and famous like Rock Hudson and Freddy Mercury. Its nature did not allow simple solutions; its prevention was possible but also required the control of one of the most basic human drives: sexuality. While researchers were working full steam to find the cause and the pattern of distribution of the new disease society engaged in a culture war around health that had not been as vehemently fought since the nineteenth century equated immorality and sloth with death and disease.

The role of HIV/AIDS in making public health global

The story of HIV/AIDS has been told many times; suffice it to say here that it radically changed the face of public health. Above all – and this is particularly relevant in the context of this book – it established three features that are the sine qua non of a new public health:

- *It transformed public health into a global endeavour.* No longer was there a clear separation between diseases of the rich and poor; the simple division between a developed world with chronic conditions only and a developing world with infectious diseases no longer applied.
- *It highlighted the key role of politics in public health* and drew attention to the many different sectors and organizations that needed to cooperate in order to fight the disease. People died because politicians were not willing to take action, because religious groups were not ready to face sexual facts, and because organizations competed rather than cooperated (Engel 2006).
- It brought the *voice of people 'living with HIV AIDS' and their human rights* into the centre of the dispute. New national and global civil society organizations emerged and found their focus (and their enemy) when medicines to treat the disease started to become available.

As in the course of the 1990s the disease changed its face to become a disease of the poor, of women and of developing countries it became abundantly clear that these three features would define public health at the end of the twentieth century: no longer could public health be pursued just at the national level, no longer could the health sector deal with these challenges on its own and no longer could health be considered as a purely professional endeavour. Health had moved outside of all the classical constraints.

HIV/AIDS shapes global health approaches

As HIV/AIDS began to increase at an extraordinary rate throughout the world other dimensions of concern emerged: the rapid spread of HIV/AIDS was no longer considered just a health risk, it was defined as a security concern of global dimensions. National intelligence reports were written on the threat that could emerge from states that collapsed into anarchy due to high rates of the disease and HIV/AIDS was taken to the United

Nations Security Council as the first ever health issue. The intention was to generate willingness for disclosure of disease rates and joint global action – but particularly the large developing nations, India and China, were not yet willing to follow this line of thinking. Indeed China was still putting AIDS activists into prison.

In parallel a series of newly emerging diseases caught the attention of policy-makers. Laurie Garrett (1994) in her ground-breaking book *The Coming Plague* stated: 'What is new, however, is the increased potential that at least some of these diseases will generate large-scale, even world wide epidemics. The global epidemic of human immunodeficiency virus is the most powerful and recent example. Yet AIDS does not stand alone; it may well be just the first of the modern, large scale epidemics of infectious disease' (preface, p. xv). She was right and today we are concerned with avian flu, SARS, drug resistant malaria and tuberculosis and the fear of a global pandemic of influenza. The World Health Organization had warned for many years that the world was not well prepared for this new spread of disease and had proposed a revision of the International Health Regulations to ensure surveillance, early warnings and rapid response to the new (and re-emerging old) threats but, just as in the discussions at the UN Security Council, its member states were not yet willing to take the step. In addition, the concern for national security overtook the interest in global collective action in the wake of 9/11.

HIV/AIDS continued to be centre stage, particularly when the first treatment regimes became available. HIV/AIDS became the symbolic issue around which the neglect of the developing world – the poor South – by the rich North was articulated. Global health became a synonym for getting more money for health into developing countries. Like Laurie Garrett (2007), I would argue that the enormous increase in funds for global health was a 'direct consequence of the HIV/AIDS epidemic'. She dates this to the International AIDS Conference in Vancouver, Canada in 1996. The very extent of the epidemic together with the moral outrage by civil society groups in the developed countries turned the development paradigm on its head. Why should an AIDS patient in Zimbabwe die sooner than one in New York? No longer was the issue to wait for development to proceed in order to gain more health – it was investment in health that was to both generate development and to address issues of social justice and fight poverty. And indeed a groundswell of financial aid has been generated from foundations, charities, overseas development assistance and special programmes. New organizations and funding mechanisms have emerged and the private sector, in particular the pharmaceutical companies, began to play a major role in the new alliances and partnerships that have sprung up at all levels of governance – analysed in detail in this book. HIV/AIDS has since eclipsed every other health issue in the developing world.

Recognizing interdependence

But in 2003 with SARS a new agenda entered the global health arena – again the scare was initially felt in the more developed parts of the world – among the Asian banking centres, and rapidly developing areas of China and Canada. The outbreak is blamed for a drop in stock prices and revenues for airlines, tourism and retailers in several Asian countries, according to the OECD. It is assumed that the economic losses associated with SARS were in the region of perhaps 2 per cent of East Asian regional GDP in the second quarter of 2003, even though only about 800 people ultimately died from this disease. Following the avian flu outbreak similar calculations were undertaken in relation to the loss of global GDP during a global influenza pandemic, at a 2 per cent loss this would represent around US$200 billion in just one quarter (or US$800 billion over a whole year), and it is fair to assume the immediate shock during a flu epidemic could be even larger and last longer than SARS. The 1918 epidemic, for example, came in three waves, spread over two years (World Bank 2007).

The recognition that global health did not consist mainly of support to poor countries but required frameworks within which the global community would work jointly to solve common problems finally hit home. Countries were now willing to move forward with revising the International Health Regulations and to include restraints to their sovereignty that would have been deemed impossible only a few years back. Not only were the new IHR adopted in a record period of time (2000–5), faced with a new avian flu outbreak countries even agreed to implement them more rapidly than originally conceived. And as if this speedy action was not enough, during more or less the same period the World Health Organization was able to get the agreement of its member states to another critical global public health issue: the Framework Convention on Tobacco Control (2003–6). Global health was moving out of the era of charity into recognizing that interdependence needs global governance agreements – and indeed, much of the process that was used to reach an agreement on tobacco was modelled after the experiences gained in environmental global governance.

Health moves into foreign policy

In the course of this development both approaches to global health – charity and interdependence – have become part of the foreign policy agenda. In the larger realm of international relations the objectives of foreign policy were already undergoing significant redefinitions since the end of the Cold War. 'In the past it was enough for a nation to look after itself. Today it is no longer sufficient' (Cooper 2003). The concept of security is expanded to include non-military threats, economic risks, illegal activities, environment, migration and infectious diseases with a perspective on the security of the individual rather than the state, as reflected in the UN proposals on human security. Ministries of Foreign Affairs are shifting with regard to issues of 'hard power': initially war and peace and then – as countries compete economically – economics and trade. In recent years there has been an augmentation in international agreements on 'soft issues' – such as the environment and health – some of which are now recognized to have significant 'hard' ramifications on national economies.

The unstructured plurality of global health

This book illustrates the extent to which global health has become an exemplary area of challenges, problems and innovations in global governance – many of them emerging from the fight to prevent and control HIV/AIDS and to treat its victims. The authors introduce a logic – the interface – with which to analyse this complex system of an increasing number of actors, at different levels and from both the public and the private sectors. They show how the traditional state-centric system of international politics both runs in parallel to and interfaces with a system of global governance which tries to bundle and coordinate lobbies, interest groups, policy networks, advocacy groups, alliances, partnerships, foundations, international organizations and states – all of which in turn come together in different hybrid forms of organization (Willke 2007). Additionally, the familiar processes of state-based multilateral governance are increasingly challenged both by market multilateralism (Bull and McNeill 2007), for example the World Economic Forum, and by 'charitainment' as personified by Bono. No longer do diplomats just talk to other diplomats – everyone talks to everyone else. Access to and legitimacy within this system are no longer gained through status as a nation-state but through a range of other mechanisms: expertise, moral standing and increasingly the demonstrated ability to achieve results. The logic of the interface and its various levels can help make analytical sense of the unstructured pluralism and its mix of cooperation and competition.

The global health arena abounds with examples to study global governance in the making, ranging from treaties between member states to a wide range of new approaches and mechanisms. Global health is not only about disease, it also means taking joint responsibility for the determinants of health in new ways. Health is part of other policies that try to manage globalization: trade policy, security policy and foreign affairs. Global health is also about people – about solidarity and global citizenship (Kickbusch and Lister 2006). Health, I would argue, is an exemplary area to study not only the governance of independence but also the failure of the charity model of development. The academic study of global health governance can help overcome 'methodological nationalism' and it can sharpen our understanding of how to govern interdependence in a world where relations flow 24 hours a day, 7 days a week, 365 days a year.

The revolution eats its children

The field of HIV/AIDS which was the revolutionary starting point of global health development has now become part of the problem. The data on HIV/AIDS prove those wrong who thought it could work to fight a single disease with significant resources. But even more tragically the stand alone fight against AIDS has reduced the investment in other areas of public health with severe consequences, in particular for mothers and children (Garrett 2007). At this point it is abundantly clear that the crisis of public health must be defined not as a disease but as a governance crisis (Kickbusch 2005). This is also the major conclusion of this book. It convincingly argues that the way back to a simple system of international relations for health is now impossible – hopefully the emerging system of global governance will develop into a stable and sustainable architecture that will help ensure the health of many and not just the few.

Professor Dr Ilona Kickbusch

Preface

This book analyses the emerging system of global health governance, exemplified by the conflicts and institutional changes related to HIV/AIDS. It is based on a two-year research project on 'Institutional Changes in Global Health Governance', conducted at the GIGA German Institute of Global and Area Studies and financed by the Volkswagen Foundation. In addition to the three editors of the book, the research group comprised two GIGA staff members, Gilberto Calcagnotto and Christian von Soest, as well as Jan Peter Wogart and Martin Weinel. This volume is a collaborative effort by these authors, though each takes full responsibility for the chapters they have written.

In quite different ways many people made significant contributions to the production of this book. Many thanks to all those to whom we refer in the following paragraphs, but also to many other people who supported our project.

First of all we think of our cooperation partners in Brazil – Renato Barboza, Luiza Heimann and Umberto Pessato in São Paulo, Breno Augusto Fontes in Recife, Paulo Teixeira in São Paulo and Mônica Viegas Andrade in Belo Horizonte; in South Africa – Mandisa Mbali in Durban, Per Strand in Cape Town and the Human Sciences Research Council in Pretoria (in particular Adam Habib, Olive Shisana and Roger Southall); the London School of Hygiene and Tropical Medicine, in particular Kent Buse; and the Globalization, Trade and Health Team at the World Health Organization (Nick Drager, Jens Gobrecht and Benedikte Dal). Furthermore, our empirical research would not have been possible without the cooperation and the patience of a large number of interview partners; thanks to all of them.

At GIGA thanks go in particular to the President of the Institute, Robert Kappel, for continuous critical support of the research project. We also thank Gero Erdmann for helping design the case study on South Africa, facilitating many contacts, and conducting a number of interviews important for our research work. Furthermore, support from people not directly involved in the research process has also been important, particularly by Monika Jamborek, Ingo Luplow and Karin Putzer who carried out the necessary administrative work, Wilma Willers and Ingrid Zieger who assisted us in many practical problems, Judy Smith-Hoehn who did the language editing, and Enno Blanke who assisted us in the last phase of putting together the manuscript. Furthermore, we have to thank those interns at GIGA who helped us a lot at different stages of the project: Corinna Seemann, Michael Murphy, Tomasz Bielecki, Kathinka Burkhardt, Eric Njoya, Janine Heibl and Oliver Liegel.

Last, but certainly not least, we would like to thank the Volkswagen Foundation, which supplied us with the necessary financial support to conduct this research. They also generously financed two international workshops: one on 'Interfaces of Developing Countries' National Strategies with Global Governance. Conflicts and Cooperation in the Health Sector' (June 2002, Hamburg), which was important for us to develop our research concept, and one together with WHO (Globalization, Trade and Health Department), GTZ and the German Health Ministry on 'Defining and Shaping the Architecture for Global Health Governance. Current Issues and Future Perspectives' (February 2006, Hamburg), during which most of the results from this research project could be presented and discussed with many international experts in this field. We thank the participants of these two workshops for their valuable contributions to our work and the Volkswagen Foundation for their financial support of these events.

Wolfgang Hein, Sonja Bartsch and Lars Kohlmorgen

Notes on the Authors

Sonja Bartsch is Senior Research Fellow at GIGA German Institute of Global and Area Studies. Prior to joining GIGA she worked as research fellow at the Institute of Political Science at the University of Hamburg. Her areas of interest include global governance, development cooperation, civil society organizations and public–private partnerships.

Gilberto Calcagnotto, a Brazilian sociologist, is Senior Research Fellow at the GIGA Institute of Latin American Studies, specializing in sociological and political studies on economic and social development, democratization, civil society, and transformation processes, mainly in Brazil and Mercosur.

Wolfgang Hein is Head of the Research Programme 'Transformation in the Process of Globalization' at GIGA German Institute of Global and Area Studies and Professor at the Institute for Political Science at the University of Hamburg. His main research interests are in the fields of globalization, sustainability and development and global governance with a focus of health.

Ilona Kickbusch has had a distinguished career with the World Health Organization and Yale University. She has published widely on matters of global health with a focus on global health governance. She is presently establishing a new programme on 'Global Health Diplomacy' at the Graduate Institute of International Studies, Geneva, with a focus on the interface between foreign policy and health.

Lars Kohlmorgen is Senior Research Fellow at GIGA German Institute of Global and Area Studies and Lecturer at the Institute for Political Science at the University of Hamburg. His main research interests are in the fields of international relations, globalization, global governance and civil society.

Christian von Soest is Research Fellow at the GIGA Institute of African Affairs. His areas of research include development policy, state and public administration in southern Africa (South Africa, Botswana and Zambia) as well as African states' relationships with global actors.

Martin Weinel is Research Fellow at the Centre for the Study of Knowledge, Expertise and Science (KES), School of Social Sciences, Cardiff University and Lecturer at the Institute of African Affairs at the University of Leipzig. His research interests are in the fields of HIV/AIDS policy, particularly in South Africa, and knowledge production.

Jan Peter Wogart is Senior Research Associate at GIGA and lecturer at the University of Applied Sciences in Bremen. From 1976 to 2000, he worked for the World Bank and the International Finance Corporation. His main research interests are in the fields of global health governance, the private sector and intellectual property rights.

Abbreviations

ABIA	Associação Brasileira Interdisciplinar de AIDS (Brazilian Interdisciplinary AIDS Association)
ACT-UP	AIDS Coalition to Unleash Power (United States)
ACWL	Advisory Centre on WTO Law
AIDS	acquired immune deficiency syndrome
ANC	African National Congress
ART	antiretroviral therapy
ARVs	antiretrovirals (antiretroviral drugs)
AZT	Azidothymidine resp. Zidovudine
BHAP	Brazilian STD-HIV/AIDS Programme
CCM	country coordinating mechanism
CDC	Centre for Disease Control
CEN/CENAIDS	Conselho Empresarial Nacional de AIDS (National Business Aids Council, Brazil)
CESCR	Committee on Economic, Social and Cultural Rights
CIPIH	Commission on Intellectual Property Rights, Innovation and Public Health
CLs	compulsory licences
CMH	Commission on Macroeconomics and Health
CNAIDS	Comissão Nacional de AIDS (National AIDS Commission) (Brazil)
COSATU	Congress of South African Trade Unions
CPTtech	Consumer Project on Technology (United States)
CSO	civil society organization
DC	developing countries
DFID	United Kingdom Department for International Development
DHHS	United States Department of Health and Human Services
DNDi	Drugs for Neglected Diseases Initiative
DSB	dispute settlement body
DSP	dispute settlement procedures
ECI	Enhancing Care Initiative
ECOSOC	Economic and Social Council
ESCR	economic, social and cultural rights
EU	European Union

FCTC	Framework Convention on Tobacco Control
FTA	Free Trade Agreement
GAPA	Grupo de Apoio à Prevenção à AIDS (AIDS Prevention Support Group – Brazil)
GATS	General Agreement on Trade in Services
GATT	General Agreement on Tariffs and Trade
GEG	global economic governance
GF (GFATM)	Global Fund to Fight AIDS, Tuberculosis and Malaria
GHG	global health governance
GNI	gross national income
GNP	gross national product
GPA	Global Programme on AIDS
GPP	global public policy
GPPP	global public–private partnership
Grupo Pela VIDDA	Grupo Pela Valorização, Integração e Dignidade do Doente de Aids (Group for Appreciation, Integration and Dignity of AIDS Patients) (Brazil)
GSK	GlaxoSmithKline
GTZ	Deutsche Gesellschaft für Technische Zusammenarbeit (German Technical Cooperation)
HAI	Health Action International
HDR	Health Development Report
HIV	human immunodeficiency virus
HST	Health Systems Trust
IAVI	International AIDS Vaccine Initiative
ICASO	International Council of AIDS Service Organizations
ICTSD	International Centre for Trade and Sustainable Development
IDU	injecting drug user(s)
IFP	Inkatha Freedom Party
IFPMA	International Federation of Pharmaceutical Manufacturers and Associations
IGO	intergovernmental organization(s)/international governmental organization(s)
IHR	International Health Regulations
ILO	International Labour Organization
IMF	International Monetary Fund
IPRs	intellectual property rights

JHTTT	Joint Health and Treasury Task Team
LACCASO	Latin American and Caribbean Council of AIDS Service Organizations
LDCs	least developed countries
LFA	Lupus Foundation of America
M&E	monitoring and evaluation
MAP	Multi-Country AIDS Program (World Bank)
MDGs	Millennium Development Goals (UN)
MSF	Médecins Sans Frontières
MSM	men who have sex with men
MTCT	mother-to-child transmission
NAC	National HIV/AIDS Council
NGO	non-governmental organization
NHG	national health governance
NICs	newly industrializing countries
ODA	Official Development Assistance
OECD	Organization for Economic Cooperation and Development
OPAS	Organização Pan-Americana da Saúde
Oxfam	Oxford Committee for Famine Relief
PAHO	Pan-American Health Organization
PhRMA	Pharmaceutical Research and Manufacturers of America
PLWHA	people living with HIV/AIDS
PMA	Pharmaceutical Manufacturers Association
PMTCT	prevention of mother-to-child transmission
PPP	public–private partnership
PR	Principal Recipient
R&D	research and development
SACP	South African Communist Party
SANAC	South African National Aids Council
SAP	Structural Adjustment Programme
SARS	severe acute respiratory syndrome
SPS	Sanitary & Phytosanitary Measures
SPT	Sustained Patent Treaty
STD	sexually transmitted/transmissible disease(s)
Sub-PR	sub-principal recipient
SUS	Sistema Único de Saúde/Unified Health System (Brazil)
TAC	Treatment Action Campaign
TB	tuberculosis

TNC	transnational corporation
TNPC	Transnational Pharmaceutical Corporation
TRIMS	(Agreement on) Trade-Related Investment Measures
TRIPS	(Agreement on) Trade-Related Aspects of Intellectual Property Rights
TWG	Transitional Working Group
UN	United Nations
UNAIDS	Joint United Nations Programme on HIV/AIDS
UNCTAD	United Nations Conference on Trade and Development
UNDP	United Nations Development Programme
UNESCO	United Nations Educational, Scientific and Cultural Organization
UNHCHR	United Nations High Commissioner for Human Rights
UNHCR	United Nations High Commissioner for Refugees
UNICEF	United Nations Children's Emergency Fund
USAID	United States Agency for International Development
WB	World Bank
WDR	World Development Report
WHA	World Health Assembly
WHO	World Health Organization
WIPO	World Intellectual Property Organization
WTO	World Trade Organization

Introduction: Globalization, HIV/AIDS and the Rise of Global Health Governance

Wolfgang, Hein, Sonja Bartsch and Lars Kohlmorgen

After around fifteen years in which North–South relations have focused on the debt crisis, structural adjustment and global economic governance, issues of social development and, in particular, health-related concerns have emerged as central themes in the dialogue. Two issues have been at the forefront of public attention. On the one hand, infectious diseases not only constitute a threat for global public health, but also threaten the social and economic stability in the developing world (with HIV/AIDS at the centre of attention), whilst on the other hand, significant institutional changes are currently taking place, leading towards the emergence of an increasingly complex system of global governance. The prominence of these two issues reflects the fundamental changes that have occurred in global health since the Alma Ata Declaration of 'Health for All' and the establishment of primary health care systems under the leadership of the World Health Organization (WHO) were at the centre of international health politics.

This book analyses the transformation of the traditional system of international politics into a system of global governance, focusing on the conflicts and institutional changes related to HIV/AIDS. In this regard, it should contribute to a better understanding of the prospects of fighting the most dramatic pandemic of present times. After summarizing the epidemiological, economic and socio-political impacts of globalization on global health in general and the HIV/AIDS crisis in particular, we then sketch the basic concepts of global governance and global health governance, present our propositions and research questions, and conclude with an outline of the chapters of this book.

Global health challenges and shifting responses

Processes of economic, political and communicative globalization have fundamentally changed the conditions for achieving progress in global health (Lee 2003; Lee and Collin 2005), most notably the political changes brought about by the neo-liberal dominance in global politics in the 1980s and 1990s as well as the densification of social relations in a globalizing society that has had an increasing impact due to the rapid spread of diseases and the social and economic consequences of ill-health. We can identify a number of aspects which indicate that health has increasingly become a key global issue:

- We observe a more rapid spread of health problems as a consequence of (1) an expanding worldwide mobility (for example, infectious diseases) as well as (2) the globalization of consumption habits as a result of global advertising and cultural densification (for example, smoking, changing patterns of food consumption). HIV/AIDS is seen as a global threat that is comparable to epidemics such as the plague and cholera in the nineteenth century; and new, hitherto unknown diseases like Ebola and SARS are interpreted as examples of new global challenges to health. One reaction to these relatively new threats through infectious diseases is the renegotiation of the International Health Regulations, which coordinate restrictions on travel and the exchange of goods, cooperation in surveillance, and research in emergency situations (Fidler 2005).
- The defence mechanisms of antimicrobials (antibiotics and antiviral, antiparasitic and antifungal drugs) are weakening due to overuse by the middle and upper classes and incomplete therapies by the poorer segments of the population, as well as by widespread use of antibiotics in animal feed. The development of multi-drug resistant strains has become a serious problem in the treatment of tuberculosis and malaria, in particular as research on antimicrobials has slowed down considerably since the 1970s (WHO 2001b).
- The more rapid spread of drugs and medical technology from rich countries to – in principle – all corners of the earth has the potential to improve global health in general, but also leads increasingly to ethical problems as it makes the selectivity of health care related to income more and more obvious.
- In the face of the debt crisis and structural adjustment programmes, 'health', like other social programmes, was no longer seen as a primary focus of development cooperation. In most countries, resources were insufficient for the health needs of the poor, and many developing country governments were desperately seeking funds to uphold a minimum of social services.[1] The crisis of the primary health care strategy became visible in the 1980s, when even the most fundamental services

(preventive measures, vaccines, pregnancy) were increasingly underfunded. This can be seen as an element of the crisis of state-dominated cooperation in international health.

- Linked to these processes, the supporters of comprehensive systems of primary health care also lost ground within the WHO in the 1980s and 1990s, with the organization refusing to take a strong position in support of grassroots strategies to develop local health care (which were frequently backed by civil society organizations (CSOs)) (Werner and Sanders 1997).
- The liberalization of international trade and the reduced scope of national regulatory tools decreased the control of national societies over the production of and access to medical drugs, health equipment, and – with the General Agreement on Trade in Services (GATS) – to some degree also over the supply of health services (WHO/WTO 2002; Koivusalo 2003; Mackintosh and Koivusalo 2005).
- Since the mid-1990s, there has been a mounting preoccupation with the vicious circle of rising poverty and growing vulnerability to health problems in large parts of what is becoming an increasingly global society. Social exclusion is also a health concern and a starting-point for the spread of epidemics beyond the limits of slums and marginalized societies as well as a serious problem for the provision of health-related services (for example Diaz-Bonilla et al. 2003).
- Governments of OECD countries show growing concerns because of the increased transborder spread of health problems and infectious diseases in addition to the possible political and economic instabilities related to the high prevalence of poverty-related diseases (like HIV/AIDS in some world regions). Thus, in the 1990s, health played an increasingly important role at the G7/G8 meetings.

These developments highlight the significant change that has been taking place in the global health arena during the last twenty-five years. During the 1980s and the first half of the 1990s, the neo-liberal economic and development paradigm resulted in a move away from the Alma Ata norm of 'health for all'. In the 1980s, based on the assumption that the Alma Ata model of Primary Health Care was too idealistic and unfeasible in most low-income countries, the concept of Selective Primary Health Care dominated discourses and health activities. This strategy focused on specific diseases in developing countries and on the lack of immunization and also defined so-called attainable goals. Many donors, international organizations and scholars favoured this new concept. This orientation corresponded well with liberal health sector reforms, demanding a more important role for private health care providers and a contribution even from the poor to paying the costs of health services (World Bank 1993). Resource transfer would then be targeted to situations of specific urgency, that is, where epidemics of infectious diseases have broken out.

Structural Adjustment Programmes (SAPs), which often demanded cuts in public spending as a means of macroeconomic stabilization, affected fragile attempts to develop primary health care systems in poor countries. A targeted health care provision, based on selective help and on a stronger private component, corresponded with the hegemony of neo-liberal concepts.

Although empirical studies have produced mixed results and the impact of SAPs on health remains a controversial issue (for an overview: Breman and Shelton 2001), one can maintain that the relation between SAPs and health provision is at least problematic, as both the supply of and the demand for health services are put under pressure when budget cuts weaken state authorities while private household incomes remain stagnant. Certainly, the failure of political elites in many developing countries to fully support the implementation of the Primary Health Care strategy has also contributed to reducing the importance of this approach in current global health policies,[2] although it remains part of declarations and speeches and of the agenda of health policy objectives (Werner and Sanders 1997; Gwatkin 2000; Cueto 2004; Thomas and Weber 2004).

The developments in the last quarter of the twentieth century reflect the fact that the globalization discourse has first and foremost centred on the dynamics of economic globalization,[3] in particular on the role of global finance and transnational corporations (TNCs), which have capitalized on technological breakthroughs and reorganized production, sales and influence on a global scale. Against these economic forces of neo-liberal globalization, which tend to increase social inequalities on the global and the national scale (Stiglitz 2006), nation-states, and particularly the poor in the less developed regions of the world, seemed more and more powerless. However, one could observe a strengthening of political forces – in the form of global social movements as well as in established political institutions – that demanded that the better-off North should become more involved in tackling the root causes of poverty in the South.

In the second half of the 1990s, these demands began to meet with more sympathy among those who realized that social inequality was not just a by-product of structural adjustment as a short-term shock therapy, which would/could be overcome by more economic growth effected by successful adjustment to the global economy. The World Bank and other powerful supporters of neo-liberalism – as demonstrated by a similar change of orientation in G7/G8 meetings – experienced a new paradigmatic turn. Joseph Stiglitz, at that time the World Bank's chief economist, spoke of a 'post-Washington Consensus', demanding 'to go beyond the now well-documented failures of the Washington consensus' (Stiglitz 1998), and World Bank President James Wolfensohn's speech to the Annual Meeting of the World Bank and IWF in 1997 bore the title 'The Challenge of Inclusion', alluding to the threats global problems constitute to the world as a whole:

> Whether you broach it from the social or the economic or the moral perspective, this is a challenge we cannot afford to ignore. There are not two worlds, there is one world. We breathe the same air. We degrade the same environment. We share the same financial system. We have the same health problems. AIDS is not a problem that stops at borders. Crime does not stop at borders. Drugs do not stop at borders. Terrorism, wars, and famine do not stop at borders. (Annual Meeting address, 23 September 1997)

The development of poverty reduction strategies, whatever their limited results so far, certainly was solidly based in that paradigm change within the World Bank, but also went beyond the Bank, as revealed by the broad discussion on the Millennium Development Goals. International attention towards health issues in developing countries was propelled by this renewed focus on poverty reduction, which came with the Post-Washington Consensus (World Bank 2000, 2004a; UNDP 1997, 2003a), as well as by studies on the relationship between health and macroeconomic development (CMH 2001) and an increasing notion of health as a global public good (Kaul et al. 1999, 2003; Kaul and Conceição 2006). The latter developed in the context of the above-mentioned densification of global social relations and the discussion on global governance. Concerning the field of health, a 'healthy society' with a low incidence of infectious diseases (and, in fact, also a high consciousness with respect to the need to prevent chronic diseases) can be considered a *public* good, since no one – at least within a given territory with unrestricted mobility – can be excluded from enjoying this good and there is also no rivalry in consumption. Health is increasingly being considered a '*global* public good' since diseases and the resistance of pathogenous agents to antibiotics are ever more difficult to control within a local or national area, the development of effective drugs has basically become part of a global market and, furthermore, improving health is now considered a precondition for reducing poverty as a global phenomenon (Chen et al. 1999; Mills

2001). This implies that the material interests of the 'rich' concerning global health far exceed health risks per se and also include many other aspects of the development of global society from which they cannot isolate themselves (for example political instability and insecurity, economic crises and so on). 'Health' becomes part of increasingly dense global social relations and, as such, an ethical as well as a material issue.[4]

The high prominence of health, however, can only be partly explained by these perspectives on poverty reduction, the role of health for macroeconomic development (see CMH 2001), and health as a global public good (Chen et al. 1999; Smith et al. 2003). Its significance was also a result of the perception that ill-health in developing countries and the spread of infectious diseases like HIV/AIDS, SARS or tuberculosis could pose a dual threat to global security: one that results from the global spread of these diseases and that affects the global population directly, and one that is linked to political instability resulting from ill-health, poverty and underdevelopment and that has an indirect effect on national and international security (Peterson 2002; Youde 2005; Fidler 2004).

This new perception of health risks is related to a broadening of the security concept since the end of the Cold War. While security was traditionally perceived as military protection against external threats to one's own territory and population, the concept has been expanded since the 1990s to include non-military threats, emanating from economic risks (oil dependency, financial volatility), illegal activities (drug trafficking, organized crime), environmental changes (global warming, conflicts over water), and social problems (migration, infectious diseases). In July 2000, the UN Security Council convened its first-ever session on health and acknowledged 'that the HIV/AIDS pandemic, if unchecked, may pose a risk to stability and security' (SC Resolution 1308: 2). The report of the UN 'High Level Panel on Threats, Challenges and Change' stresses that 'any event or process that leads to large-scale death or lessening of life chances and undermines States as the basic unit of the international system is a threat to international security', listing infectious diseases and other social threats like poverty as one of six clusters of threats (UN 2004: 23).

The social, economic and political implications of the HIV/AIDS pandemic in sub-Saharan Africa particularly, had thus become a factor that put health higher than ever on the global political agenda. First of all, HIV/AIDS is seen as an obstacle to social and economic development at the national level. The high prevalence rates, especially among young adults, have devastating effects not only on those directly affected, as they reduce their life expectancy, educational perspectives and job productivity, but also affect their families and children, who have to cope with the loss of breadwinners and parents. Besides these impacts of HIV/AIDS on individual lives, there is a relationship between macroeconomic development and health in general, and between economic growth and HIV/AIDS in particular, as examined in various studies (CMH 2001; Greener 2002; Gaffei 2003; Haacker 2004). It is estimated that per capita growth in half of the countries in sub-Saharan Africa is reduced by 0.5–1.2 per cent each year as a direct result of AIDS and that by 2010, per capita GDP in some of the hardest-hit countries may drop by 8 per cent (GF 2005b). Apart from these monetary effects on national income and economic growth, diseases and ill-health also have a profound impact on the development of the human capital and the social fabric of a society. The report of the CMH points to the negative intergenerational and societal spillovers of disease. Other studies also highlight the serious long-term consequences of high morbidity and mortality rates, especially in the case of HIV/AIDS (Greener 2002; Gaffei 2003; Bell et al. 2003).

Besides these social and economic consequences, HIV/AIDS also has a negative effect on the stability of political and economic institutions and – many argue – on the national security in some countries of the developing world. HIV/AIDS and infectious diseases strike hardest at the productive parts of the population, at the pool of experienced individuals that would qualify for leading positions in society, leading to economic decline. Many countries, especially in sub-Saharan Africa, already have to cope with a lack of teachers, civil servants, police and military forces, as well as healthcare professionals, or will have to do so in the near future. This has serious repercussions for social and economic institutions at the national level – the public administration, the legal system, the military – and limits the state's ability to deliver public services, provide social cohesion and guarantee national security (Ostergard 2002; Haacker 2004; Youde 2005).

Moreover, HIV/AIDS has increasingly been perceived as a problem with international and global repercussions. For example, if a country's military capacity is weakened because of HIV/AIDS or other diseases, this could shift the balance of power and contribute to growing regional instability or violent conflict. Civil war and civil-military conflicts which result from economic, political and social instability that are linked to health problems at country level may contribute to international instability (Peterson 2002). In addition to these indirect HIV/AIDS-related threats to international security there are possibly direct threats that result from the transnational spread of this pandemic that might reach countries with – currently – low prevalence rates.

The rise of global health governance

The rapid technological, economic, financial and social developments in the process of globalization and the above-mentioned new perceptions of global health have had a significant impact on national and international political processes and led to profound transformations in the architecture of international health politics from a nation-state-based structure towards a complex system of global health-related institutions.

For most of the second half of the twentieth century, international policy-making in health can be characterized as a matter of state-dominated cooperation (with the WHO playing a prominent role since its establishment in 1948) and a comparatively loose net of non-state actors (Loughlin and Berridge 2002). International cooperation in the health sector concentrated on issues such as the support of national health systems, vaccination campaigns and so on. Also, the establishment of primary health care systems following the call for 'health for all' at the 1978 Alma Ata Conference, basically corresponded to the logic of international state cooperation for the support of public policies in poor countries.

In the 1990s, the field of international health politics changed due to the stronger realization of the equity problems of globalization and the need for a global welfare component to counteract the destabilizing forces of global markets and the security risks as pointed out above. Irrespective of whether globalization was perceived as a threat or a challenge, supporters and opponents started to acknowledge the need for international and transnational coordination, which would make it possible to 'govern' the process in the absence of a central political authority. In this post-Westphalian[5] system of global governance, traditional forms of state regulation through nation-states and international governmental organizations (IGOs) are both complemented by and competing with new forms of private regulation through non-state actors and hybrid regulation through public–private interactions. Today, a large number of different actors interact with each other at various spatial levels in the fight against the HIV/AIDS pandemic, including UN organizations, bilateral agencies, national governments in the South, transnational and national companies, global and local CSOs, as well as public–private partnerships. All of these actors have their own agendas, are guided by specific interests and dispose of different power resources. Their ability to influence politics in the global health architecture varies depending on the actors' properties and the specific types of interfaces that structure their interactions.

Thus, political globalization can be seen as an expression of a new configuration of actors, summarized by the term 'governance'. Governance includes regulation by the state (nation-states, intergovernmental organizations), by private regulation (the private sector and civil society) and forms of hybrid regulation (cooperation between states/IGOs, private sector, and/or civil society). Modifying a definition by Renate Mayntz (2005), we can speak of global governance as the totality of collective regulations to deal with international and transnational interdependence problems (Bartsch and Kohlmorgen 2005b).

The reference to an increasingly complex structure of different types of actors in global health is commonplace (Dodgson et al. 2002; Lee et al. 2002; Kickbusch 2003; Hein and Kohlmorgen 2003). An analysis based on the process of globalization and the development of a global society stresses the following relationship: the rising importance of transnational actors and processes supported by a liberalization of global trade rules meant, on the one hand, that intergovernmental regulations based on the aggregation of interests at the level of national governments were increasingly biased towards national economic interests and were not flexible enough to incorporate transnational social problems. On the other hand, this same process of transnationalization strengthened the capacity of non-state actors to raise issues and influence decision-making in international politics and to introduce their own resources (knowledge and finance) into global social policies. The threat of increasing global insecurity and instability and the difficulties faced in developing new, effective and politically legitimized political institutions finally led wealthy country governments to at least partially support new governance arrangements. With reference to the more general phenomenon of similar developments in other fields of inter- and transnational relations and the development of global politics in general, this new institutional structure of global health politics has frequently been called *global health governance* (GHG).[6]

Thus, we can summarize that during the last twenty-five years, the political landscape in the field of health as well as in global politics in general has been transformed considerably. We have witnessed an institutional change from a structure that consisted primarily of independent national health politics and some international efforts to control cross-border effects of ill-health towards a system of global health governance. The latter is explicitly concerned with transborder issues that may affect populations worldwide either directly (for example through the global spread of infectious diseases) or indirectly (for example through political instability and global insecurity due to a vicious circle of ill-health, poverty and underdevelopment). In this book, we will analyse the rise of GHG starting from the following propositions, which we will further elaborate in Chapter 1.

- The development of GHG is closely related to a strengthened integration of global society. Quite different types of actors all over the world are becoming increasingly dependent on each other, indicating a growing need for global norms (like human rights, including economic, social and cultural rights (ESCR)) and a growing risk of infectious diseases and related instabilities in certain parts of the world that have an impact on the lives of people in other parts of the world.
- Globalization has been accompanied by increasingly powerful global trade institutions. At the same time, many UN organizations in the field of social development, such as the WHO and ILO, have been weakened through an 'ideologization' of conflicts ('effectivity' vs. 'equity') and a tendency towards non-acceptance of majority decisions by the major financial contributors of those institutions.
- The new institutional configuration of an evolving GHG structure (like hybrid regulations and networks between different types of actors) functions as a mode of integration and building compromises at the global level. Social rights are moving to the forefront as formerly weak actors and new actors pursuing social rights are strengthened.
- GHG is a typical product of the combination of moral values and material interests that characterize the development of political institutions in an integrating social system. It accompanies the densification of social interactions on the global scale, and the development of a global society.
- The fight against HIV/AIDS has raised issues around which many of the new features of GHG have developed. Though this disease is, of course, quite specific in its medical as well as social characteristics, the conflicts about prevention versus treatment and about the affordability of and access to antiretroviral therapies, present a field which allows insights into important characteristics of global health governance.

Overview of the book

The chapters of this book concentrate on the major issues discussed above and highlight key actors and their interactions in the fight against HIV/AIDS in the context of the emerging global health architecture. They will include an analysis of international governmental organizations concerned directly or indirectly with health (the WHO, World Bank, UNAIDS, WTO), powerful private sector participants (pharmaceuticals), civil society organizations, hybrid organizations such as the Global Fund and GPPPs as well as country studies of nations directly involved in the

HIV/AIDS battle (Brazil, South Africa). Although we analyse and discuss several other actors in the various chapters, such as the US government's actions and reactions to HIV/AIDS or the important role of foundations (such as the Bill and Melinda Gates Foundation), future research should include further country studies in both the North and the South, and more research on major private sector participants, foundations, bilateral programmes of industrialized countries and the role of the World Bank as well as on the whole field of the development of AIDS vaccines, in which an initiative incorporating a large number of GHG actors has now been started (the Global HIV Vaccine Enterprise).

Chapter 1 lays out the theoretical foundations for the empirical studies that form the core of this book. We will discuss the emergence of the current structures of global health governance as a consequence of the transformation from a Westphalian system of nation-states to a post-Westphalian system of global governance for health policy-making both at global and national level. While most of the studies on global health governance have taken an international public health and international law perspective, our book mainly uses an International Relations approach to analyse the characteristics of global governance processes, in particular the relationship between state, private and hybrid actors in GHG and the role of different types of power (resource-based, legal, discoursive and decision-making power) in pursuing actors' interests. We will refer especially to the conflict between 'market creation' and 'welfare', which influences both the interactions between the actors and the outcomes of the global governance processes in the field of health.

For a more systematic analysis of the interactions between the various actors at global, national and local level, we propose the concept of *interfaces in global governance*. Norman Long's (2001) concept of social interfaces serves as a starting-point and will be adjusted to the analysis of global governance processes in general, and to the field of global health governance in particular. The interface concept will serve as a tool to analyse global governance and to understand the political dynamics that might help to break the deadlock caused by the inflexibility of traditional governmental organizations. We distinguish between organizational, legal, resource-based and discoursive interfaces and argue that the type of interface not only influences the relative weight of the different actors, but also the patterns of conflict or cooperation between them and thus the results of the global governance processes. This approach focuses on a specific problem that has been largely neglected in global governance and International Relations theory: the problem of interactions between different *types of actors* (horizontal interfaces) and between actors at the global, national and local *levels of politics* (vertical interfaces). Using the interface concept will allow us to develop a better understanding of the institutional changes that took place with the emergence of GHG and – looking at the dialectics between self-interests and ethical principles in health politics – of the impacts of these institutional developments on the fight against poverty, of which the target of universal treatment of people living with HIV/AIDS in developing countries is an important expression. From this perspective we scrutinize the multiple political conflicts involved in the intensification of the fight against HIV/AIDS since the late 1990s and the movement towards making universal treatment of infected people a generally accepted norm in global public health.

The concept of interfaces links the individual chapters of this book and functions as a framework of reference for the main research questions that can be summarized as follows:

- What are the current characteristics of the main actors and institutions of global health governance and how have they evolved in light of the HIV/AIDS crisis?
- What kind of interfaces between actors of different types and from different policy levels can we identify, describe and analyse?
- How do processes at these interfaces link the whole structure and dynamics of GHG?
- How do the structures of GHG influence the poverty-oriented fight against diseases (with a focus on HIV/AIDS)?
- How does the institutional change from international health politics to global health governance fit into overall changes in global politics that result from the challenges of globalization?

The introduction of the interface concept leads us to propose a framework of analysis which takes the reaction of various actors to new challenges as a starting-point. They use different types of interfaces with other actors to push for solutions that conform to their interests; the results of these conflicts force existing organizations of GHG to adapt to new requirements (or otherwise lose influence) and/or might lead to the development of new organizations.

The globalization of markets as a result of technological progress and an extended system of global economic governance (in particular the TRIPS agreement) has had a significant impact on the issue of access to medicines and other aspects of GHG. This new challenge played an important role in mobilizing and strengthening CSO activities in the field of health and it led to strong interfaces between GHG and global economic governance (GEG) on the one hand, and between GHG, GEG and the field of human rights on the other. This meant that the conflict between global market creation and health care as a component of human rights has in fact considerably widened the scope of GHG. The constellation that allowed the attainment of a substantial reduction in the prices for antiretroviral medicines (ARVs) between 1999 and 2004 – an essential step to allow a general treatment of HIV/AIDS patients in developing countries – therefore sets the starting-point for our analysis of GHG.

Chapter 2 gives an overview of the conflicts concerning access to medicines (availability, affordability) at the interfaces between the international system of intellectual property rights (in particular: TRIPS) and public health-oriented actors that are supposed to make medicines available to those in need of them, or that aim at maximizing impact to that purpose through advocative action (CSOs). The chapter sets out by outlining the institutional set-up of WTO and TRIPS, including the references to welfare in these agreements. This is followed by an analysis of the strategies and interests of various groups of actors in these conflicts and the various intermediate outcomes from the 2001 Doha Declaration on the TRIPS Agreement and Public Health up until the signing of the TRIPS amendment in December 2005 and the beginning of negotiations on new ways to support essential health R&D.

Chapter 3 examines the role of transnational pharmaceutical corporations (TNPCs) and their reactions to the challenge of being held accountable for the lack of access to essential medicines. The interests of TNPCs focus on strong, internationally guaranteed intellectual property rights (IPRs), and their strategies to secure and defend them are outlined. After having shifted their main focus from the World Intellectual Property Organization (WIPO) to the TRIPS agreement in order to use the WTO dispute settlement mechanism for securing IPRs, the issue of access to medicines, for them, meant the defence of their strong position at the legal interfaces between international and national law, while at the same time upholding an image of socially responsible actors at discoursive interfaces. This was also crucial to ensure the support of major industrialized countries in IGOs. This can be seen as the basic rationale behind their readiness to make compromises in the conflict on prices of ARVs and to withdraw their legal action against the South African government. Finally, the involvement in public–private partnerships, which means focusing their organizational and resource-transfer interfaces in the field of GHG on institutions of hybrid governance, demonstrates how TNPCs interpret their role in GHG: assuring investments in innovation through strong IPRs and supporting selected public health goals through voluntary engagements.

Chapter 4 examines the role of CSOs – including faith-based organizations as special cases – in GHG. The different types and functions of CSOs and their interfaces with other actors in GHG are examined. CSOs are analysed as the main actors who brought up the issue of access to ARVs in the global conflict arena by linking the needs of people, whose interests are not adequately represented in global politics (advocative action), with accepted global norms (human rights). By creating an expanding policy network and by mobilizing public opinion, they transformed the general challenge of improved access to medicines into a concrete challenge for TNPCs and governments both from developing and industrialized countries. The advocative role of CSOs has also been strengthened through concrete cooperation in the field, which raised their importance as contractual partners to governmental organizations and in PPPs, as well as through their role in processes of self-empowerment (here, in particular, of people living with HIV/AIDS).

While the most important IGOs in global health remained at the sidelines during the early stage of the conflict on access to ARVs by promoting prevention as the more 'cost-effective' way to combat HIV/AIDS, two reasons forced them to enter the arena when these conflicts gained momentum. On the one hand, the conflicts had become so prominent and the demand for treatment so strong that they had to take a position in order to reaffirm their role in international health politics. On the other hand, though comparatively low-priced ARVs constitute a necessary precondition for the treatment of most patients in poor countries, this is in no way sufficient. Additional resources are needed to pay for medicines in very poor countries, but moreover, treatment requires a medical infrastructure for diagnosis, surveillance and accompanying measures – and, of course, further measures in the field of prevention are necessary. In order to explore the changing conditions in this field, we need to analyse inter- and transnational cooperation in the development of financing mechanisms and also consider institutional support for the improvement of health systems in developing countries and of norm-setting.

Chapter 5 concentrates on the role of traditional international governmental organizations in GHG (the WHO, the World Bank and UNAIDS). In 2001, the WHO began to take an increasingly strong pro-treatment position by also stressing the need to guarantee a universal access to treatment (promoting '3 by 5'[7] as an intermediate strategy) and also reacted to the challenge of organizing the institutional field of expanding treatment. This, however, now implies acting in a field of GHG with more complex interfaces, developing functions as interface manager and avoiding the typical dilemma related to organizational interfaces in IGOs, which in the past created deadlocks in the decision-making processes among groups of states. Furthermore, this chapter briefly analyses the power and role of the World Bank in the GHG system and examines UNAIDS with regard to its internal interfaces and functions as well as its external interfaces in the global fight against HIV/AIDS.

Chapter 6 looks at the Global Fund to Fight AIDS, Tuberculosis and Malaria (GF) as a new hybrid institutional form which links governmental and private forms of governance. The GF was founded as an organization to raise significant amounts of funding outside the UN system. This was a further step towards developing strong interfaces – essentially organizational and resource-based interfaces which incorporated different groups of private actors – on an unprecedented scale outside traditional IGOs, which not only strengthened the position of private actors but also that of strong nation-states in the field of global health politics. In order to meet the challenge of fighting HIV/AIDS more effectively, however, it had to rely on interfaces with existing governmental organizations, in particular the WHO, UNAIDS and organizations at the nation-state level.

The following two chapters then focus on the vertical interfaces between the previously analysed global actors of GHG and national HIV/AIDS politics, taking Brazil (Chapter 7) and South Africa (Chapter 8) as examples. South Africa and Brazil can be seen as important cases of more advanced developing countries not only being largely passive recipients of the goods and bads of GHG, but being in a position to exert an impact on global policy-making. Here the interactions between politics at the national level and the developing global governance system become clearly visible. We will show that national politics in no way loses importance in GHG. In a complex system of interfaces, different actors increase their room to navigate. Instead of the duality between IGOs and nation-states with a reduced flexibility to react to challenges, national society can now link up with a rather broad set of global actors and is also affected by these actors. In principle, national governments can decide to become involved in GHG or attempt to stay out, as South Africa did in order to defend political autonomy against various demands and pressures from a complex field of actors beyond their control. The conflicts around access to treatment showed, however, that countries are not able to position themselves completely outside the global governance field.

On the other hand, in middle-income countries like Brazil and South Africa, poverty remains an important social characteristic of large parts of the population and the general access of the population to treatment (and thus the achievement of a level of medical care comparable to that of industrialized countries) has been dependent upon the decrease of the prices for ARVs. The HIV/AIDS politics of both countries and their cooperation with GHG institutions proved to be very different. While Brazil is usually seen as a model case, guaranteeing overall free access to ARVs as early as November 1996 – based in part on local production and also on a tough negotiating strategy on licences with pharmaceutical corporations – the South African government had to be pressured by civil society to finally take this step in 2003. Brazil plays an important role in the global move towards treatment, pushing 'treatment' in intergovernmental interfaces as well as in interfaces with CSOs; while South Africa, with its policy to reaffirm national control, is linked to the global system more through interactions with TNPCs and CSOs.

Regardless of the low priority South Africa has been giving to the treatment of HIV/AIDS for a long time, the country took a strong position in using TRIPS safeguards to circumvent patent rights claimed by TNPCs. The two court cases concerning the right to compulsory licensing and cheaper parallel imports of ARVs in South Africa, in fact, played an important role in the campaign for access to medicines. While Brazil profited from an intensive cooperation with the World Bank and was quite willing to cooperate with other governmental and non-governmental international organizations, South Africa has been trying to minimize the influence of international and transnational organizations. Basically, GHG affected the country through the cooperation between CSOs and their use of discoursive interfaces (besides the general effects of globalized conditions for fighting diseases).

In the concluding Chapter 9, we synthesize the results from the case studies in light of our main research questions, stressing the role of various types of interfaces in the emerging system of global health governance within an incomplete transformation from a Westphalian system of *international* politics to a post-Westphalian system of *global* politics. Whereas the empirical work presented in Chapters 2–8 focuses on governance processes in the fight against HIV/AIDS, the theoretical and conceptual discourse on global governance and the role of interfaces between the various spatial levels of policy-making will facilitate an application to other aspects of global conflict and cooperation in health and beyond. The rise of global health governance can be seen as a dialectical answer to the challenges posed by Alma Ata as well as by neo-liberalism: it transcends the limits of state-based international health politics and is characterized by competition and cooperation between various types of actors, allowing for an incorporation of new actors. While creating a coordination problem, it also reaffirms the values of global responsibility and advocacy, as it opens up global politics to global civil society. The current shape of global health governance makes room for a broad discourse on global norms – a discourse which is, of course, moulded by very unequal power relations, but is more inclusive than an international system shaped by national governments alone.

Notes

1. See for example Suárez-Berenguela (2000) for Latin America; Lachenmann (2003) for Africa; World Bank (2001) and Betz (2003) for India.
2. Nevertheless, countries like Cuba and Costa Rica, and the Indian state of Kerala, in realizing the Primary Health Care concept at least in some of its aspects, show good results in health provision (for example low infant mortality), as stated by the World Bank (World Bank 2004a).
3. It makes little sense to offer a list of references on which our conceptions of globalization are based. Most of our general conceptions of globalization are broadly accepted (see the standard texts by Held et al. 1999 and Held and McGrew 2002); in fact, our analysis starts with a critical reading of the global governance discourse.
4. In this study we will not enter more deeply into the discussion on 'health as a global good' and 'global public goods for health' (Kaul et al. 1999; Smith et al. 2003). We basically accept Smith's definition of a 'global public good for health' as 'a good for which it is rational, from the perspective of a group of nations collectively, to produce for universal consumption, and for which it is irrational to exclude an individual nation from its consumption, irrespective of whether that nation contributes to its financing' (Smith et al. 2003. 270). One could argue, however, over whether it might be more appropriate to refer to 'individuals' and the 'global community' instead of 'nations' and 'group of nations'.
5. This refers to the role of the Westphalian Peace in 1648 in the development of a system of international relations between sovereign nation-states. Hence 'post-Westphalian' means a system of global politics, including actors beyond the nation-state (non-state actors, but also local and provincial governments as well as international organizations acting independently in transnational affairs).
6. For further research, concepts and discussion on global health governance see: McKee et al. (2001); Dodgson et al. (2002); Lee et al. (2002); Loughlin and Berridge (2002); Hein and Kohlmorgen (2003); Kickbusch (2003); Beaglehole (2003); Beigbeder (2004); Thomas and Weber (2004). There are also a number of publications which deal with specific global health issues, for example the relationship between international trade and health (Blouin et al. 2006), global health jurisprudence (Aginam 2005; Fidler 1999), or global governance processes in the case of HIV/AIDS (Poku and Whiteside 2004; Barnett and Whiteside 2002a).
7. '3 by 5' means the target to treat 3 million people by the end of 2005 – which was not achieved – but which then led to the target of 'universal treatment by 2020'.

1
Interfaces: a Concept for the Analysis of Global Health Governance

Sonja Bartsch, Wolfgang Hein and Lars Kohlmorgen

From the Westphalian system of nation-states to post-Westphalian global governance

In the introduction we summarized the basic aspects of the relationship between globalization, poverty and health and briefly referred to the developments that led to the emergence of the current structures of global health governance (GHG). In this chapter we will develop an analytical approach towards a better understanding of this GHG architecture, which combines International Relations theory with a concept to analyse the linkages between global governance actors.

We will first take a closer look at the impact of the transformation from a Westphalian[1] system of nation-states to a post-Westphalian system of global governance on global and national politics. Subsequently, we will consider the characteristics of global governance processes in more detail. This entails an introduction of different modes of regulation (state, private, hybrid regulation) and a distinction between different types of power (resource-based, legal, discoursive and decision-making power) and competing interests (market creation vs. welfare), which influence both the interactions of actors and the outcomes of the global governance processes. For a more systematic analysis of the interactions which link the various actors at global, national and local level, we introduce the concept of *interfaces in global governance*. Norman Long's (2001) concept of social interfaces serves as a starting-point and will be adjusted to the analysis of global governance processes. This will lead us to a *concept of 'interfaces and change in global governance'* and a number of hypotheses which further specify the propositions made in the introduction.

The architecture of global (health) governance, of course, is not fully developed yet: GHG must be seen as an ongoing process of institutional change. It is part of the transitional process from a Westphalian structure of international relations between sovereign nation-states to a post-Westphalian global political system. David Fidler (2004, 2005) has thoroughly analysed 'post-Westphalian Public Health' with respect to the global reaction to SARS and the revision of the International Health Regulations (IHR); he concludes that the new IHR constitute a shift towards 'an expanded governance strategy that integrates multiple threats, actors and objectives in a flexible, forward-looking and universal manner' (2005: 68). The discussion on global governance has contributed many elements towards an understanding of this transformation, but we are still quite far from understanding the newly emerging, incomplete system.

Figure 1.1 illustrates this transformation of *international* relations into a system of *global* politics. It is not intended as a model of global governance but rather as a scheme to characterize the dissolution of the 'old' structure of international relations in the process of a rapidly increasing density of transborder social, economic and political relations. The traditional system was based on *an aggregation of interests at the national level* (with A_1, A_2 and A_3 representing the various interest groups – business, unions, CSO – in nation A, and so on). Thus, negotiations at the international level were led by governments on the basis of these nationally aggregated positions, which, in the first instance, reflected power relations within nation-states. The outcome of these negotiations was a result of power relations between nation-states, either mediated by decision-making procedures within international governmental organizations (IGOs) or various characteristics of specific countries (or group of countries) within the international system. In Figure 1.1, the larger circle around country B reflects its central position within the system and points to its hegemony.

The intensification of international economic and social relations has produced a situation in which the Westphalian system was transformed by international negotiations that increasingly limit the power of national societies towards a sovereign formation of their internal political and economic order and of their external relations (in particular the GATT-WTO process). Globalization, the liberalization of markets, and the increasing need to deal with transnational/global problems created the opportunity for the direct interaction of non-state actors, thus establishing new transnational spaces of interests and power that prevent a full aggregation of interests on the national level but produce dynamics and opportunities through a transnational cooperation of non-state actors, which increasingly limit the political options of nation-states.

Figure 1.1 shows that simply by designing the structure of hypothetical relationships for three different non-state actors in three national

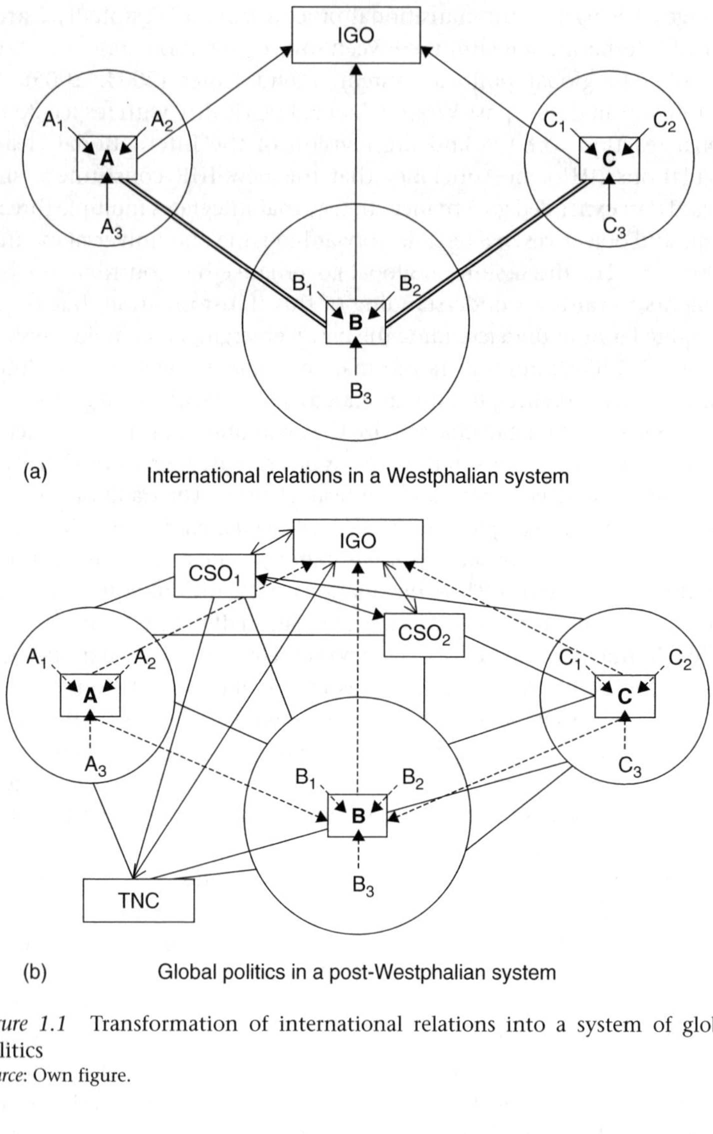

Figure 1.1 Transformation of international relations into a system of global politics
Source: Own figure.

societies we arrive at quite a complex structure of relations. Whereas in the ideal Westphalian system there are basically the two alternatives between cooperation in an IGO or a bilateral cooperation between states, in the post-Westphalian structure there are many possibilities for cooperation and conflicts among nation-states, IGOs, CSOs and transnational corporations, in other words including the 'old' actors of the Westphalian systems, but transforming their roles by challenging their political monopoly through the emergence of new, genuinely transnational actors.

In the organization of protests against unequal social development, national borders play a decreasing role, just as social and political risks are more and more globalized. The *rise of a global polity* (Ougaard 1999; Ougaard and Higgott 2002) relates to this dialectic of inequality and the reactions of wealthier actors to the risks as well as to problems of global equity inherent in problems of global health. Structures of conflict and compromise, that is the aggregation of political interests, are also increasingly globalized, which implies the additional importance given to the reaction to global risks. These developments, of course, also have their impacts back on the national level of health politics. Though on the one hand, nation-states, in organizing their health systems, have become more and more dependent on conditions they cannot control, global markets and global political cooperation, on the other hand, have a huge potential for improving health care. Global health governance is about how to realize this potential.

Characteristics of global governance processes

Thus far, we have used the term 'global governance' without specifying our understanding of the term more precisely. It is useful to start looking separately at the two components 'global' and 'governance'. Addressing the spatial aspects of political globalization we realize that politics in general are characterized by shifts of political authority. Capacities to regulate and conduct policies are transferred upwards and downwards from the nation-state to international actors on the one hand (internationalization), and local actors on the other hand (regionalization, localization), as well as sideways from state actors in general to a wide range of non-state actors (privatization, transnationalization) (Rosenau 1997; Jessop 1999).

Multilevel governance and modes of regulation

In order to capture these developments the term 'multilevel governance' was introduced by Gary Marks (1993). It was originally used as a concept to analyse political relations in the European Union ('type I multilevel governance'; Marks and Hooghe 2004). However, since then it has been broadened to describe related aspects of global governance, as summarized by Bob Jessop (2004: 57): 'The key question becomes how state and non-state actors manage, if at all, to organize their common interests across several territorial levels and/or across a range of functional domains.' This relates to what Marks and Hooghe (2004) call 'type II multilevel governance' – characterized by task-specific power sharing between different types of actors and task-specific responsibilities, a multiplicity of levels, and a flexible institutional design – although Bob Jessop does not take it for granted that power sharing and responsibilities are necessarily task-specific. Comprehensive research and conceptual considerations on this second type of multilevel governance are available only in a few policy fields (for international environmental regimes see Young 1999). James Rosenau refers to some of these aspects when he analyses the 'domestic-foreign frontier' (Rosenau 1997) and develops a typology of six governance modes which can be used to describe modalities of 'type II multilevel governance' (Rosenau 2004), but does not apply them to any specific policy fields.

Globalization, however, is not only a process of creating a new spatial order of multilevel politics (with greater relevance of the global and local level), but also an expression of a new configuration of actors (with greater relevance of civil society and private actors). These two developments fostered the emergence of new forms of politics and regulation (like networks of private actors or partnerships between state and non-state actors), supplementing the traditional modes of public regulation. The interaction of these different processes is usually called *governance*. Our understanding of governance refers to Mayntz (2005), Kooiman (2003) and Rosenau (2002, 2004). Governance is the interplay of different institutional forms – *regulation by state* (through nation-states, IGOs), *private regulation* (through private sector and civil society actors) and *hybrid regulation* (through cooperation by states/IGOs, private sector and/or civil society) – and comprises the interactions of various actors (with different power resources and interests) at different spatial levels of politics.

Whereas in a national society, state governance produces binding rules and a legal system which constitute a limiting framework for other modes of governance (social organization 'in the shadow of hierarchy'), global governance is characterized by the lack of a central government authority at the global scale. As a result, international (state) governance depends on fragile compromises and variable power relations between sovereign national states (even if institutionalized in the form of IGOs) and finds itself on a more equal footing with forms of private and hybrid governance, which are based on a more truly global constituency. International governmental cooperation and organization may produce international law, but only in a very limited number of cases has this led to agreements close to hard law with clearly defined specifications and clear-cut sanctions on violators – the WTO being the prime example. Thus, global governance gives relatively more weight to private organization and hybrid forms, which try to overcome the inherent limits of state organization.

Consequently, we propose a notion of global governance that is broad for two reasons: First, it focuses neither on hierarchical nor on non-hierarchical modes of regulation and thus includes all actors that contribute to the processes of governance. Second, it does not only refer to the global or international and transnational level of governance but also to the national level. The national level can be considered part of global governance if it influences or is influenced by the global level. Referring to a definition by Renate Mayntz (2005), we define global governance as the totality of collective regulations to deal with international and transnational interdependence problems (Bartsch and Kohlmorgen 2005a).

Global governance can thus be understood as a process of dealing with problems and – if possible – of problem-solving. However, it is important to stress that the acknowledgement of problems and the willingness to tackle them are not self-evident. Problems have to be identified and put on the agenda, and the related discourses have to be framed. Oftentimes, problems are only tackled if powerful actors have an interest in solving them. Moreover, when a problem is acknowledged we have to ask whether appropriate structures of governance are in place and which strategies prevail to solve – or shift, or neglect – the problem. The institutional setting in which problems can be addressed is always the result of historical traditions and structures as well as deliberate decisions made by involved actors based on interests, power and resources (Mayntz 2005). Thus, if we want to capture who influences global policy-making we cannot just focus on the effectiveness of problem-solving, but have to analyse the interactions in global governance in light of the different types of power resources and interests of the respective actors.

Power, interests and policy areas

The actors and their activities are shaped by structural economic, political and socio-cultural conditions. This implies that actors – by virtue of their structural position and role – have certain features, tasks and resources that affect their capabilities to exercise power. The structural balance of power, for example the world market with its disparities as well as the global political and military field of power relations, are regarded as frameworks of the actors' interactions and as the origin of their resources of power. A more detailed analysis, however, requires a differentiation into different types of powers that are more closely linked to the properties of the actors themselves. In order to integrate power relations and the sources of power into our analysis of interfaces in GHG, we refer to Barnett and Duvall (2005b), who introduce multiple forms of power and investigate their influence on processes of global governance, and to Bas Arts (2003), who focuses on the power of non-state actors. Based on these studies, we differentiate between four types of power:

- *discoursive power* (the ability to frame and influence discourses);
- *decision-making power* (the ability to be involved in decision-making and in formal norm-setting);
- *legal power* (the ability to exercise power based on legal structures and laws);
- *resource-based power* (refers to the actors' disposal over material resources (for example finances, staff) and immaterial resources (for example knowledge, information) and their ability to provide these resources).

The other important component that has to be taken into account when analysing processes of global governance are the interests of the actors involved. Many authors presume the existence of collective interests in dealing with specific challenges. However, this obstructs the observers' view of the fact that precisely the actors' self-interests play a significant role in terms of the preference for specific governance structures, strategies to redesign them, and the cooperative or conflictive character of the interaction process. The self-interests of actors involved define the spectrum of feasible policy outcomes under given circumstances. Partisans of Rational Institutionalism (Keohane and Martin 1999) rightly point out that institutions are more than just short-lived entities, which emerge because of rapid combinations of power and interests. They argue that actors and their interest-oriented actions that follow an instrumental rationality are an essential factor in expounding the emergence and function of international institutions. This creates different combinations of common, complementary or conflictive interests depending on the position of actors in global and national societies.

Especially the differentiation between *market-creation interests* and *welfare-oriented interests* is of crucial importance in global governance processes. To a certain degree, 'market creation', in the sense of establishing conditions for a sustained liberalization of international trade, has been a central feature of the post-Second World War system of IGOs, in particular the IMF and the GATT. The process of globalization has been accompanied and to a considerable extent made possible by a further step towards the creation of a global economy with the liberalizing elements of the structural adjustment strategies of the IMF and the World Bank and the establishment of WTO with its various agreements, among others the Agreement on Trade-Related Aspects of Intellectual Property Rights (TRIPS).

Similarly, from the very beginning, the UN system has comprised welfare-oriented institutions like WHO, UNICEF and, to a certain extent, the ILO, but only later did the whole system of multilateral development institutions arise as a basically welfare-oriented institutional complex.[2] It has, however, been a persistent topic in development theory that development cooperation has a rather limited impact compared to the dynamics of international economic relations. Globalization and the respective strengthening of international economic institutions has furthermore reinforced the impact of inter- and transnational economic forces, and thus also the need for welfare-oriented institutions, which counteract the effects of uneven development and support processes of global cohesion.

The new rise of welfare-oriented policy areas in global governance occurred after a period when welfare-oriented actors had lost power due to a neo-liberal hegemony that pushed the global political framework for globalization and gave a strong position to actors in the area of market creation. Hence, in order to make an accurate analysis of the institutional forms in which the strengthening of global welfare politics and also the rise of GHG took place, we have to look carefully at the constellations between different actors, the modes of regulation in which they operate, their interests, and their power resources. The expected positions of the various actors of global health governance with respect to the dimensions global/national/local and market-creation/welfare are indicated in Table 1.1.

Concerning the interaction between the national and the global level, the distinctions between the three governance modes on the one hand, and the policy areas of market creation versus welfare on the other hand, are crucial. The increasing interconnectedness of global society and the ensuing virulence of conflicts between market creation and welfare make it more and more difficult to react swiftly to the increasing global challenges in the framework of the state governance mode: IGOs do not have sufficient authority to pursue the politics of securing the supply of global public goods against the diverging interests of nation-states and market-oriented actors. The increasing importance of private

Table 1.1 Actors with respect to level and area of dominant activity

	Market creation	Mixed strategies	Welfare
Global	WTO; TNCs (pharmaceuticals, medical appliances, insurances and so on)	G7/G8; CSOs, GPPPs	WHO, UNAIDS, UNICEF, CSOs
National	Trade interests, world market-oriented corporations, Gvmt. finance and trade departments, large ind. countries' governments in general	CSOs, government	Gvmt. welfare departments, most developing country gvmts, CSOs
Local	Trade/consumer interests; competitive local companies	CSOs, local governments	Local governments, local CSOs; health activities of global CSOs/IOs

and hybrid modes of regulation reflects the need for more flexibility to react to these challenges. This concerns primarily the welfare side of the global game, as the dominance of economic forces pushing global market creation has led to a rather strong state-led institutionalization of that interest at the global level (IMF, WTO).

Interfaces in global governance

The concepts of 'governance modes', 'power' and 'policy areas' constitute important starting-points for conceptualizing the relationship between different levels of governance within the post-Westphalian system. To better understand the changes in global governance, however, we need an instrument that allows us a more systematic analysis of the interactions and linkages between the different actors, which in fact make up the core of global governance processes. In short: we have to ask what constitutes the binding forces among the multitude of actors in global governance in general and in a specific field like global health governance.

In global politics, political programmes are seldom developed and implemented by one actor alone without interference from others. This refers to global governance processes in general, but in particular to governance at different levels and the intersections between these levels. Therefore, in order to understand the impact of the global on the national level – and vice versa – we have to analyse the interplay of international/transnational and national actors. This can also improve the understanding of how institutions structure the interaction processes between actors at these levels, including the role of transnational actors as being directly linked to both levels and therefore cutting across the global–national frontier.

While there is some research on single types of actors,[3] the linkages between these actors are not well covered. Moreover, only a few theoretical approaches explicitly deal with interactions in (global) governance. Oran R. Young (1996; see also Stokke 2001; Stokke and Vidas 1996; Koenig-Archibughi 2002) scrutinizes the 'institutional interplay' of regimes and the relation of regimes to their institutional environment. However, as Young focuses less on single actors but more on regimes and their scopes, the concept of institutional interplay is only to a lesser extent applicable for an actor-oriented approach. Our approach is closer to Mayntz and Scharpf (1995) and Jan Kooiman (2003), who focus more on the interactions between individual and/or collective actors. Kooiman defines interactions as 'mutually influencing relations between two or more actors or entities' (2003: 13) and differentiates between a structural and an intentional level of interaction. At the intentional level, Kooiman looks at the actors and their objectives and interests, whereas the structural level refers to the 'material, social and cultural context' (that is institutions, social constructs, forms of communication, technological development, power relations) in which interactions take place. Moreover, Kooiman distinguishes three forms of interaction: 'interferences' (relatively open, flexible and spontaneous interactions such as self-organization in private governance), 'interplays' (horizontal, semi-formalized interaction, mostly found in hybrid forms of co-governance) and 'interventions' (vertical and formalized interaction as in hierarchical governance).

In an attempt to develop a concept which allows an integration of Kooiman's structural and intentional levels and at the same time opens up the term 'institutional interplay' for a more actor-oriented analysis, we propose taking up Norman Long's concept of 'interfaces' and discussing its potential (and its usefulness as a base for further elaboration) to analyse interactive processes of institutional change in global health governance.

Norman Long's concept of interfaces

Norman Long developed the concept of 'social interface' for his approach towards an actor-centred development sociology. Long defines a social interface 'as a critical point of interaction or linkage between different social systems, fields or levels of social order where structural discontinuities based upon differences of normative value and social interest, are most likely to be found' (Long 1989: 1–2).

In a more recent text Long demands a 'thorough deconstruction of the notion of structure' (Long 2001: 62), which leads him to conclude:

> In more substantive terms, structure can be characterized as an extremely fluid set of emergent properties that, on the one hand, are a product of the interlocking and/or the distantiation of various actors' projects, while on the other, they constitute an important set of reference points and constraining/enabling properties that feed into the further elaboration, negotiation and confrontation of actors' projects.

Thus, while the second part of the quote refers to 'structural discontinuities', that is to different structures in which the interfacing actors are embedded, the first part refers to properties of changing structures that emerge through the process of interfacing. Although an interface as defined by Long can link actors with common interests, he stresses the dynamic and conflictive nature of interfaces arising from different interests, resources and power. Mostly, interfaces imply the clash of cultural paradigms and different worldviews (Long 2001: 70), but the conflicts could also be due to differences in the constraining or enabling properties defined by different governance modes to which actors are related.

Long explains that 'studies of social interfaces should aim to bring out the dynamic and emergent character of the interactions taking place and to show how the goals, perceptions, interests, and relationships of the various parties may be reshaped as a result of their interaction' (Long 1989: 1–2). Thus, interfacing influences and changes the actors' original strategies. There is always an interplay and a mutual influence on the actors' behaviour even if they are in an antagonistic relationship and have great disparities in power, resources and interests. This reciprocity may lead to a harmonization of conflicting strategies. If interactions continue, the development of boundaries and shared expectations is likely, which shape the interaction and may constitute 'an organized entity of interlocking relationships and intentionalities' (Long 2001: 69). Interfaces are not only two-sided forms of articulation but are more complex, as they include a variety of different interests, relationships and modes of rationality. Moreover, Long stresses that it is important to focus not only on one single interface and the related actors and institutions – in a kind of micro-perspective – but also to include the actors and institutions beyond this concrete interface – in a macro-perspective. Interface analysis should be based on broader institutional frameworks and fields of power (Long 1993: 217ff.; 2001: 66) and should not be understood as a mechanical point where two actors, programmes, or similar meet, but instead as a complex social field of interactions and conflicting or merging cultural and political habits and behaviours, which normally consists of related sets of specific interfaces.

Long applies his social interface approach to the field of sociology of development primarily concerning the interaction of international and national/local actors in the concrete development of projects and programmes. Thus he concentrates on the influence of vertical external activities on local actors and the changing strategies of the external actors in these programmes due to their interaction with local actors. Most of the elements of Long's approach can be used for our approach to the analysis of global governance, which goes beyond the field of development cooperation and includes the analysis of horizontal interfaces between different types of actors on the global level as well as on the other levels of global governance. We will modify Long's approach by concentrating less on cultural practices and sociological aspects (though not denying their importance) but focusing more strongly on the political processes and dynamics, that is adapting it to institutionalist approaches in International Relations. The following characteristics of this concept seem to make it particularly useful for the analysis of global governance:

(1) The term 'interface' refers to a specific space, where two different *social systems* or *fields of social order* interact (here: global/national systems; institutional systems related to modes of regulation), which are characterized by specific institutions and specific backgrounds.
(2) On the other hand, the term 'interface' leaves a high degree of flexibility with regard to the interacting systems: (a) it does not only refer to the 'interplay' of existing institutions but also to spaces of interaction which include new types of actors; (b) it can refer to quite different forms of interactions (discoursive, financial transfers and so on).
(3) An interface is a place where recurrent interactions between specific types of actors take place, which might lead to new institutional developments in the transnational (that is, also 'translevel') space.[4]

Types of interfaces in global governance

Taking these considerations into account, we adapt Long's definition of interfaces to the analysis of global governance as follows:

> We define interfaces in global governance as socio-political spaces of recurrent interactions of collective actors in the handling of transnational and international affairs. This relates to more institutionalized policy fields as well as to specific challenges.

Analysing interfaces thus implies describing and examining the actors involved in the interactions of global governance in their original structural contexts, that is, their sets 'of reference points and constraining/enabling properties' (Long 2001: 62). Interfaces represent the intersections of modes of life, worldviews, interests and strategies in which power relations are important for the emergence of new institutional contexts. Our proposition is that politics at the interfaces is influenced both by the constellation of actors defined by those factors and by the different modes of governance involved (regulation by state, private regulation, hybrid regulation, see above).

To understand how global governance is influenced by particular actors and the interaction of these with other actors, it is necessary to take into account that interfaces can assume quite different forms and can be classified according to various criteria. As we are particularly interested in the impact different actors have on shaping institutional change and policy outcomes in GHG, we propose a typology of interfaces in relation to the types of power. Above, we distinguished between decision-making, legal, resource-based and discoursive power. There is a certain congruence between types of power and specific types of interfaces. Certainly, it makes sense to talk of *discoursive interfaces* when considering the role of mass media, but also the importance of expert commissions that produce reports which intend to shape the perspectives of influential persons on important political issues (thus the use of discoursive power). In addition there are *resource-transfer interfaces* involving the relationships between donors (countries, foundations) and IGOs on the one hand, as well as the latter and receiving countries or other actors on the other hand. With respect to decision-making power, it seems useful to distinguish between *organizational interfaces*, that is, decision-making structures in relevant organizations and institutions. *Legal interfaces* are not only created by international law (and a specific outcome of processes at organizational interfaces), which consist of international bodies monitoring the compliance with international law (like WTO dispute resolution), but also by national courts when dealing with international law incorporated into national law (for example, patent law following TRIPS rules). We define discoursive, organizational, legal and resource-transfer interfaces as follows:

- *Discoursive interfaces* are related to communications about a basic understanding of, but also on strategies to deal with, the issues that arise at interactions between different levels of politics and different types of actors. These might imply programmatic aspects, if longer-ranging concepts of cooperation and problem-solving are developed.
- If these programmes are related to existing or newly created organizations, *organizational interfaces* appear, which in the case of international/global organizations typically comprise actors from the international and national levels of politics (partnerships, participation in organization and/or decision-making bodies, operational cooperation, consolidated programmatic cooperation).
- Organizational interfaces, depending on the nature of the organization, might also include *legal interfaces*, which are structured through international and national law (actors attempting to influence legislative processes and negotiations, the implementation of law, legal conflicts and international agreements).
- *Resource-transfer interfaces* play an important role particularly in the transfer of finances to poor countries but, of course, also from rich countries to multilateral organizations in various fields of social politics. Resource-based interfaces also arise as a strategy to defend specific regulations (or the prevalence of specific political regimes) against irrefutable criticism, for instance from a human rights perspective. Transfer of resources occurs between different levels of politics (typically: national > international > national) but also between different policy areas and types of actors (for example, nation-states > CSOs, or IGOs > CSOs). Resource-transfer interfaces can relate both to material resources (for example, funding) and immaterial resources (for example, labour force, technical assistance, knowledge).

Of course, there are interdependencies between different types of interfaces as between the use of different types of power. A resource-transfer interface (such as development assistance given to a developing country) implies a disparity in the power relation between the involved actors, as the actor providing the resource (the donor country) is definitely in a more powerful position than the receiving actor (recipient country). Although resource-based power also structures discourses and is crucial for discoursive interfaces, on the other hand, discoursive interfaces provide the opportunity for economically weaker actors to influence the governance process.

Interfaces and institutional change

Quite obviously, actors dispose of different degrees of access to different forms of power, and according to their objectives (that is, specific interests and logics of action), the actors' diverse motivations lead them to make use of the various forms of interfaces. For example, it is important for the interaction of two actors to know whether the interface is based on resource exchange or if it is characterized by a discourse. Moreover, it is obvious that the logic of action differs if actors interact, for example, in a legal conflict, in negotiations at an international conference, in an official decision-making body of an IGO, in the implementation of a bilateral programme, or in discussions/discourses on specific issues.

Figure 1.2 illustrates schematically how global governance at the interfaces 'works' on a new challenge that appears and contributes to institutional change. Various concerned actors (governments, IGOs, CSOs, transnational corporations and so on) react to challenges by raising their issues through the different types of interfaces in organizations related to various modes of regulation.

With regard to the character of organizational interfaces we have to take into account that every organization develops specific internal interfaces between the organization and its members and among the single members (general assemblies, executive councils, local offices and so on), as well as external interfaces with other organizations. This leads to the situation that an organization can be regarded both as a forum, in which specific conflicts are addressed, and as an actor that interacts with other organizations in global governance.[5] In the first case, actors try to influence decision-making processes at the organizational interfaces of the global governance institutions concerned. Having won the support of existing institutions for one's position will generally strengthen the position of that actor in specific conflicts. If the results are mostly satisfactory, the institutions will normally be strengthened, too.

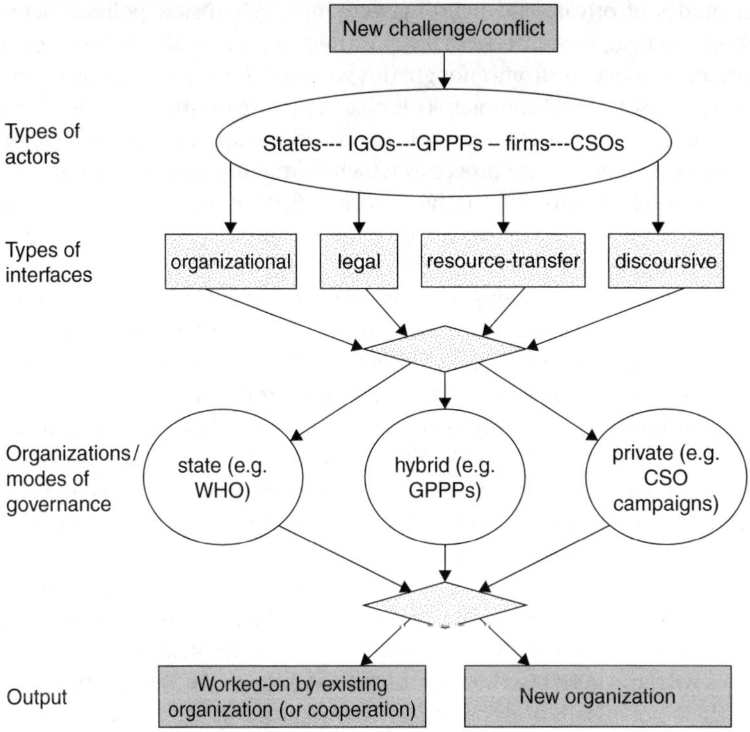

Figure 1.2 Interfaces and change in global governance

However, due to the complexity of interactions on the global scale, other institutions will be brought into the process in most cases. Frequently, the organizational settings have produced situations where conflicts blocked the working of the organizational interfaces between the IGO and the nation-states as their constituency. If certain actors do not succeed in pushing through their favoured strategy, they might turn to other institutions in order to reach compromises by forms of cooperation, or they might try to win the support of other actors to create new institutions and shift the activities to a new forum.[6] This forum shifting is not only a result of the intentional action of single – normally powerful – actors, but can also occur if the majority of actors no longer considers the existing institutions to be effective.

This institutionalization of new structures – both at the global and the national level – is encouraged by a governance situation that is already characterized by a growing number of actors, which are increasingly acting in modes of private and hybrid governance. When new political actors enter the field, new interfaces arise. If their impact on the previous complex of interfaces is strong enough, this will probably lead to changes of the existing institutional complex. This means that we mostly find a process of consecutive (re-)structuration of the relationship between the actors involved in governance processes which frequently leads to new institutional developments, be it rather informal institutions that structure, for example, a continuous exchange of information, or the origin of new organizations.

This institutional change is even more complicated due to the multilevel character of governance. In terms of vertical interfaces, the institutional change affects the constellation of actors at the global level as well as at the national level of countries involved and will mobilize processes of coordination and conflicts at specific interfaces between the two policy levels observed. The modes of governance dominate the processes at the interfaces. In conjunction with this, the influence of actors of different types and levels varies considerably, depending on the type of interface and its location in the multilevel system.

Of course, actors dispose of a varying capacity to access power resources and will try to use interfaces accordingly. Actors like national governments, but also IGOs, might have access to organizational interfaces with the WHO or the World Bank. Members of CSOs can use those of their organization according to their statutes and practices, but are often excluded from formal policy-making processes through state-based regulation. Most actors can use resource-transfer interfaces (though disposing of quite different levels of resources and being subject to different restrictions) and discoursive interfaces (but may be dependent on decisions and restrictions set by their authoritative bodies and on the degree of access to specific media). Legal interfaces are created by legislative bodies (diplomatic conferences in international politics) and can then be accessed by affected legal subjects. When analysing the involvement of different types of actors at the interfaces it is important to consider that various conflicts might affect overlapping sets of interfaces. These frequently constitute an important element inducing institutional change through establishing new kinds of linkages between actors.

In order to capture changing constellations at specific interfaces that reflect institutional change we will have to look at sequences of interfacing processes. New institutions might then create new sets of interfaces bridging (at some points) the structural discontinuities between the interfacing actors and thus provide means of governance in the context of an undefined global authority.

Combining these considerations with the characteristics of multilevel governance (focusing on the global–national relationship), we propose the following hypotheses:

(1) Multilateral institutions, in which the state governance mode is dominant, experience difficulties in adapting in a flexible way to the needs of managing a complex field of organizations and interfaces – basically due to their organizational interfaces with national governments.
(2) The growing importance of the private and hybrid regulation modes allows the development of new forms of resource-based and organizational interfaces and favours in particular an increasing importance of discoursive interfaces. Pathways to bridge the gaps between different fields of global governance are created.
(3) Strengthening welfare issues in global governance through state-based international institutions might succeed in specific areas where there is an overarching interest in authoritative decisions with which national governments have to comply (like the International Health Regulations to prevent the international spread of health emergencies). In general, new institutional forms of private and hybrid governance are more flexible and have a greater likelihood of producing results in the short run (GPPPs, mobilizing new financial resources).
(4) On the other hand, as Rosenau highlighted in his term 'fragmegration', the integration of ever new actors representing institutional forms of private and hybrid governance also implies processes of fragmentation of governance structures, which will have to be countered by agreeing on the establishment of interface managers – a function which might become important in the future of WHO work.

The processes to be analysed are complex and do not lend themselves easily to rigorous tests of hypotheses. Our research has to be seen, basically, as a heuristic enterprise using theoretical concepts and confronting them with the unfolding of governance processes in the case of fighting HIV/AIDS. This will demonstrate that they give plausible explanations of the structures of institutions and conflicts which are developing.

Conclusion

In this chapter, we presented an approach for the analysis of interfaces in a multilevel system of complex governance structures. The concept of interfaces as developed by Norman Long refers to socio-political situations in which established social systems interact with each other. In a multilevel system, factors such as the specific national constellations (including typical attitudes towards specific external actors), their path dependency, or institutional strength will play an important role. On the other hand, the concept of multilevel governance refers to the effects of globalization, stressing the importance of the global level and the structuring of inter-level relations. This means that the large number of interfaces links actors which operate in very different settings, that is, the linkages are characterized by very different structural discontinuities. The most important of these discontinuities, implying 'different sets of reference points and constraining/enabling properties that feed into the further elaboration, negotiation and confrontation of actors' projects' (Long 2001: 62), is constituted by the links of actors to different and often conflicting interests. We can maintain that the current central challenges to global health governance (access to medicines, lack of finance, lack of technical knowledge, problems of coordinating aid in poor countries and so on) concern actors in a field of conflict between global market creation and global welfare politics. These structural discontinuities characterize the most important interfaces in GHG: on the one hand, between groups of developing countries dependent upon improved global welfare and most industrialized countries interested in an ongoing liberalization, and, on the other hand, between IGOs and transnational actors linked either to 'market creation' or to 'welfare' (Table 1.1). This produces a fundamental conflict which permeates many of the conflicts at the interfaces of GHG and which is only partially bridged by the increasing interdependence of global society and the resulting extended understanding of global security.

The constellation of actors in the fight against HIV/AIDS – as in the field of global health governance in general – is very heterogeneous, with actors differing not only with regard to their character (public, non-public), their institutional structure (formalized, informal), or their level of activity (global, national, local), but also with regard to their interests, their logic of action and their power resources.

Our concept proposes that the manifold interfaces function not only as points of mediation between the particular interests of these actors (for example, pooling of funds and knowledge at the resource-based interfaces; coordinated activities through organizational interfaces), but also as arenas of global conflicts (for instance, conflicts between market- and welfare-oriented interests at the legal interfaces; conflicts on prevention versus treatment at the discoursive interfaces).

An elaborated approach to interfaces in systems of multilevel governance should help to identify conflicts and forms of cooperation in the system of global health governance. It suggests that the multiplicity of actors interacting at a large number of different interfaces increases the flexibility of GHG as a self-organizing system to react to problems which might be difficult to solve in a bi-level state-dominated system, in which decision-making and resource transfer are closely related to specific alliances and power struggles. Mobilization and transfers of resources are hampered by bureaucratic requirements and forms of competition in state institutions that produce difficulties with respect to a smooth functioning of their organizational interfaces linking the organizations as a whole to their member states. A larger number of various types of actors can mobilize innovative concepts, forge flexible alliances, raise resources from groups which would object to increasing taxes, and overcome the reluctance of actors to cooperate with certain other actors for whatever reason. On the other hand, the result is quite often a fragile compromise between the particular interests of different actors, which comes along with a fragmentation of activities both at global and national level – which in fact characterizes the specific institutional setting in the fight against HIV/AIDS. This, however, seems to be an unavoidable trade-off for a larger mobilization of actors and resources. The need is not for a reconcentration of responsibilities, but for a better coordination of the resulting creative chaos and the establishment of effective, accountable and legitimate interface managers.

Notes

1. Referring to the role of the Westphalian Peace in 1648 in the development of a system of international relations between sovereign nation-states.
2. The 'development complex' is welfare-oriented insofar as it pretends to promote less developed areas. This does not preclude the fact that some organizations in this context, at least in particular periods, promoted strategies which had a primarily (global) market-creating focus, implying the assumption that welfare would be best served by an optimum adjustment to markets (Washington Consensus).
3. For research on non-state actors see for example: Kaldor (2003); Arts et al. (2001); Higgott et al. (2000); Baker and Chandler (2005); Keane (2003); Cutler et al. (1999); for research on IGOs: Rittberger (2002); Karns and Mingst (2004); Barnett and Finnemore (2004); Wolf (2005); Rittberger and Zangl (2006).
4. Interfaces might be organized by existing organizations; they become 'repeated practices' leading to informal rule systems (Rosenau 2004: 32), but they might also remain merely spaces of informal interaction between actors belonging to different social systems.
5. This is discussed in more detail in Chapter 4 by differentiating between functions of an IGO as forum or as actor.
6. Braithwaite and Drahos (2000) characterize these processes as 'forum shifting', Helfer (2004) as 'regime shifting'. See also Chapter 5.

2
Global Health Governance and WTO/TRIPS: Conflicts Between 'Global Market-Creation' and 'Global Social Rights'

Wolfgang Hein

Introduction: WTO/TRIPS: globalization and market creation

Transnational pharmaceutical corporations (TNPCs), and also producers of baby food like Nestlé, are important contributors to the production of global public goods for health. As private enterprises they do not, of course, directly produce public goods, but are primarily oriented towards maximizing profits. However, some of the goods they produce are supposed to be made available publicly for those in need of them, either through the state or through some form of publicly regulated collective scheme, mostly in the form of an insurance.

The ambiguity referred to has its basis in the different modes of governance that play a role in the interfacing between institutions politically responsible for public health (national health ministries as well as WHO) and private for-profit organizations. The former have to care for the availability and affordability of needed inputs or to prevent public damage from the marketing of harmful products or concepts. Conflicts can be observed on the introduction of the Essential Medicines concept in the 1970s or, quite prominently, with Nestlé on the marketing of baby food to substitute for breastfeeding – a conflict in which CSOs marked their first major worldwide success on a health issue.

Technical progress and international negotiations interacted to reduce barriers to a globalization of trade in goods and services. The creation of global markets implied a widening of the transnational space for TNCs and the development of international law, which is changing the legal interfaces between institutions responsible for access to public goods and private producers of these goods. The effective international implementation of intellectual property rights (IPRs) constitutes the one area of international law where these two modes of governance – the state to guarantee the delivery of public goods and the market to use the incentive to maximize private benefits for optimizing the offer of goods – have clashed concerning essential health issues.

In short, this problem can be characterized as a problem of the global organization of private activities that produce 'global public goods for health'.[1] A medicine that yields improvements in health should be accessible to everyone, that is, there should be non-excludability in access to this good. Certainly, there is a rivalry in consumption, but if one refers to the pure production costs after research and development (R&D) has been financed, these are, in general, comparatively insignificant. So, if basic human rights are accepted,[2] *it should be rational for the global community to provide basic medicines as global public goods.*

This chapter will focus on the impact of the TRIPS agreement on access to drugs and on new forms of interfacing between public and private actors in global health. It provides an analysis of the interests and the strategies of the various groups of actors which are involved in these conflicts and examines their impact on the various intermediate outcomes from the 2001 Doha Declaration on the TRIPS Agreement and Public Health up to the TRIPS amendment in December 2005 and the beginning of negotiations on new ways to support essential health R&D in 2006. In doing so, it offers an overview of the conflicts about access to medicines and treatment of HIV/AIDS, which will be analysed from the perspective of specific actors and countries in the following chapters. The first section will look at the institutional structures of WTO and TRIPS and the legal and organizational interfaces created by them. Then, the role of intellectual property rights for pharmaceutical companies and the constitution of country positions in WTO negotiations is summarized, followed by an analysis of the effects of TRIPS concerning the human right to (the enjoyment of the highest attainable standard of) health[3] and the increasing strength of advocacy activities for the access to affordable medicines. The section ends with a presentation of the adjustment of TRIPS in response to these demands. The chapter concludes with an analysis of central interfaces in conflicts where market-creating rules might be challenged successfully by welfare-related actors and examines the contribution of these conflicts to the development of GHG.

International economic law: a system of global governance competing with global public health

WTO/TRIPS: characterizing the organization

The WTO constitutes the central institution for market-creation on the global scale and has thus far developed an extended corpus of international law regulating the development of world trade. Various parts of the 1994 Marrakesh Agreements establishing the WTO are closely related to the provision of health services in developing countries.[4] In recent years the Agreement on Trade-Related Intellectual Property Rights (TRIPS) has been at the centre of conflicts, but the General Agreement on Trade in Services (GATS) and the Agreement on Sanitary and Phytosanitary Measures (SPS) also have potentially important impacts on global health.

All the agreements are managed by WTO bodies in most of which all member states are represented. This holds for the Ministerial Conference as the governing body which meets at least every two years and decides on important current affairs and on the course of negotiations on new agreements. It is also the case for the General Council, which handles the day-to-day work of WTO between the Ministerial Conferences, the Dispute Settlement Body, the Trade Policy Review Body, the three councils for each broad area of trade (Goods, Services and TRIPS Council) and their subsidiary bodies ('Committees'). This broad representation of members can mislead the observer with regard to existing inequalities as many poor members are not in a position to send delegates to all meetings. Another critique refers to informal meetings of a smaller number of 'interested' delegations and the so-called Green-Room[5] meetings, called by a committee chairperson or the Director General. These should facilitate package deals which allow complex compromises. The WTO stresses (on its website) that these negotiations are nevertheless 'transparent', as every member is kept informed about what is going on and has an opportunity to provide inputs; an assumption that, however, needs to be questioned.

The existence of a strong dispute-settlement process (DSP) is a powerful instrument to implement WTO rules:[6] If *consultation and mediation* processes do not lead to a dispute settlement, the DSB establishes a *panel*[7] which is expected to produce a *final report* after half a year of examination of facts and arguments as well as meetings with the parties and other interested states. Each party has the right to appeal the panel findings; appeals are dealt with by the *Appellate Body* composed of seven persons broadly representative of WTO membership. Within 90 days a definite report is produced, which either rejects the complaint or allows the imposition of trade sanctions against the member that has violated trade rules. The creation of an Advisory Centre on WTO Law (ACWL) in 2001 helped to compensate inequalities concerning legal expertise (see: www.acwl.ch/e/about/about_e.aspx). The uneven potentials and effects of trade sanctions, however, constitute a problem. In fact, a developing country suspending tariff concessions to an industrialized country might create more problems to its own economy, it being dependent on particular imports, than doing harm to big industrialized countries, which do not depend on markets in those countries (Hoekman and Kostecki 2001: 90).

The Secretariat (including the Director General) basically plays a facilitating role – for example by trying to propose compromise solutions in the case of deadlocks. Besides that, members of the Secretariat play an important role in the delivery of technical cooperation to developing countries (helping them to actively participate in WTO affairs) – which is part of their official mission – in addition to, and this is much more difficult to assess, participating in what I call the 'Geneva connection', a network of communications about issues important for the IGOs and CSOs present in Geneva (see section at the end of this chapter).

Implementing TRIPS: basic issues

The final goal of the TRIPS agreement[8] is to reach a global harmonization of IPR rules defining rather high minimum standards with which all member states have to comply. All member countries have to introduce a corresponding legislation on IPRs (for example twenty years' minimum protection of IPRs; rules on copyrights, trademarks, geographical indications and industrial design; rules on enforcement).

To understand the current situation on access to medicines, the provisions for transitory periods for implementation are important. While, in general, the TRIPS agreement only grants a one-year period to adjust national legislation to TRIPS provisions, developing countries were entitled to delay the date of application for a further period of four years (until 1 January 2000). In cases where a developing country already had a system of patent protection in place, but is obliged 'to extend product patent protection to areas of technology not so protectable in its territory on the general date of application of this Agreement for that Member' (TRIPS Art. 65.4), there would be an additional transitional period of five years until 2005. This was the case in India, which had introduced a Patents Act in 1972 protecting only production *processes* but not products as such. Least developed countries (LDCs) also have a transitional period of ten years (in 2002 this was extended until 2016 with respect to patents for pharmaceutical products). Besides monitoring implementation, the TRIPS Council is the first addressee for taking up new issues, such as those arising in the context of access to medicines.

Thus far, none of the conflicts which were finally settled by the DSP directly affected the issues around access to ARVs, though in the US versus Brazil case on local working requirements (patent protection DS 199/4) the issue of the production of ARVs was raised (but the case was withdrawn by the US). Another case with repercussions on the access question was the so-called India Mailbox case where the US complained that India had failed to provide an adequate mailbox facility[9] to receive and preserve applications during the transition period (WT/DS 50/AB/R, 19 December 1997; see: UNCTAD/ICTSD 2005: 776f.).

As the TRIPS agreement demands changes in national legislation, there is, however, another field of legal procedures. Pharmaceutical companies can use national judicial systems to complain against an infringement of political decisions against an allegedly TRIPS-consistent patent right. Such a court case, of course, implies an interpretation of TRIPS which will have an impact on the further development of TRIPS law. The two South African court cases in which TNPCs sued the government of South Africa are the most famous of such cases (see Chapter 8). These conflicts reflected the fact that many TRIPS provisions are rather vague, so that legal interpretations play an important role for defining the rights and obligations of member states (UNCTAD/ICTSD 2005: 703f.).

WTO/TRIPS and welfare

The objective of WTO is to regulate and facilitate world trade; it is not a welfare-oriented (or multi-purpose) organization. Nevertheless, free trade has always been promoted with the promise that it will create a win-win situation for all participants. Thus, in a number of ways, it is normatively related to global welfare: the WTO is based on the assumption that expanding trade has a generally positive impact on welfare. The preamble to the agreement establishing the World Trade Organization includes goals supporting 'development' and improving standards of living. Furthermore, safeguard mechanisms can be used in situations of social and economic crisis, and specific WTO committees deal with welfare-related problems. In the case of TRIPS, the following clauses can be seen as 'entry points' for social concerns:

(a) The preamble recognizes 'developmental and technological objectives' of national IPR systems and 'special needs of the least-developed country Members in respect of maximum flexibility in the domestic implementation of laws and regulations in order to enable them to create a sound and viable technological base'.

(b) Article 7 stresses that IPRs 'should contribute to the promotion of technological innovation . . . in a manner conducive to social and economic welfare'; Article 8.1 highlights that: 'Members may . . . adopt measures necessary to protect public health and nutrition, and to promote the public interest in sectors of vital importance to their socio-economic and technological development.'

(c) Furthermore, there are safeguard mechanisms. Article 30 allows 'limited exceptions to the exclusive rights conferred by a patent, provided that such exceptions do not unreasonably conflict with a normal exploitation of the patent'.[10] Article 31 deals with the authorization of compulsory licensing, which 'in the case of a national emergency or other circumstances of extreme urgency' can be used without authorization of the right holder. Parallel importing, that is imports of products supplied by the patent owner or a licensee at a lower price in another country, is also permitted, if not excluded by national patent law.[11]

In the case of an international agreement with 'teeth' like the WTO, however, making a broad use of these general clauses is not without risks: interpretations can be challenged by opposing positions, and in the case of a negative panel decision there is a threat of sanctions. The difficulties in effectively using the existing options in a complex legal framework constitutes one of the central weaknesses of most developing countries in this system; they played a role in the South African court cases (see Chapter 8) as well as in the Brazilian poker about licences (see Chapters 3 and 7).

Thus, issues of social development constitute normative points of reference to interpret and readjust provisions of the agreements – depending, of course, on relations of interests and power in global politics. In general, however, in the current world order, the problem of systematically relating trade order to social order is unresolved. The global governance system consists of a multiplicity of structures, as nation-states still constitute *barriers* to the development of a unified legal system to organize politics and resource transfers. Nevertheless, in the ongoing process of globalization, the need for coordination and conflict resolution is increasing. This can explain the rise of *new forms of interfaces which link organizations of global economic and global social governance*. Social forces which are not locked into the 'old' system of state-oriented institutions seem to be best situated to propel these links. As IGOs are by definition tied to nation-states, their existing organizational interfaces are much less flexible than civil society organizations to deal with global social problems (see also Chapter 4). We will discuss these developments in detail after having looked at the triangular relationship between IPRs, TNPCs and nation-states.

Intellectual property rights: TNPCs, the prices of pharmaceuticals and the constitution of country positions in WTO negotiations

The World Trade Organization is based on *an intergovernmental agreement to reduce state intervention* concerning the global movement of goods and services basically organized by private actors. Thus, these private actors – in this context primarily pharmaceutical companies – are immediately affected by its regulations, but national governments are the formal actors in the WTO. In this section, we will look at the interface triangle between WTO, states, and the private for-profit sector, which is at the centre of the role of WTO as a global market-creating organization. As TNPCs will be analysed in more detail in Chapter 3, only the most basic features will be summarized here.

Pharmaceutical industry and R&D for required medicines: the rationale for intellectual property rights

TNPCs are prone to be in the midst of conflict, as they are clearly profit-oriented private firms, but are producing a good which, from a normative perspective, ought to be a global public good for health. The problem, obviously, is twofold. On the one hand, the global community (which in this context can be translated as 'global health governance') has to agree on guaranteeing production and access – which we will discuss later – and on the other hand, on how to stimulate and finance research and development.

If we take it for granted that the most cost-effective way to produce the medicines needed for the best possible care for global health is by having R&D for drugs carried out by large TNPCs – which is certainly not universally accepted – then the problem is how to attain the most adequate incentives for stimulating R&D for those medicines. This implies the question of how to allow TNPCs to amortize the R&D outlays for developing a specific drug, including costs of failure. The firm must be profitable as a whole, globally. Over a long period in capitalist societies, IPRs, and patent rights in particular, have developed as the central mechanism to give firms a temporary monopoly on the products they developed, in order to prevent competitors from copying the products and selling them for a price not reflecting development costs, thus enabling them to recover the capital invested in R&D. One research project arrived at an estimate of US$802 million for the development costs for a new medicine.[12] Therefore, it is not surprising that the industry is strongly opposed to any form of weakening the patent system even if they might accept that this system has its flaws.

A discussion of the history of international standard setting in the field of intellectual property rights, dating back to the nineteenth century, goes beyond the scope of this study (see Drahos 2002). In 1967, the Stockholm Convention Establishing the World Intellectual Property Organization (WIPO) was signed. In WIPO, however, the industrialized countries faced the same situation as in UNCTAD or UNESCO: developing country blocs could defeat Northern proposals and push their own concepts (Drahos 2002a: 8). Reacting to pressures from the industry (Drahos 2002a, 2002b; Sell and Prakash 2004), the US insisted on negotiating an agreement on trade-related intellectual property rights in the context of the WTO negotiations. Shifting the emphasis on international IPR rules from WIPO to TRIPS has been characterized as a strategy of forum or regime shifting (Helfer 2004, also in more detail Chapter 3).

The technologically leading industrialized countries were interested in strengthening international rules on IPRs due to new technological developments (in computer and information technology, biotechnology, and the patentability of life organisms) but also – and this is of particular importance in the field of medicines – due to the increasing capacity of the more advanced developing countries to copy patented drugs. Globalization and the reduction of trade barriers meant that the competition for exports by the producers of generics could have a growing impact on the market for patented drugs. This is the background for the considerable lobbying of R&D-oriented corporations to include IPRs into the Uruguay Round negotiations.

While the principal aim of a legal market-creating framework – in the course of globalization as well as in the historical constitution of national markets – has been to create the same formal conditions for all participating actors, this does not, of course, mean that everyone will benefit equally from these rules: though an opposition of developing countries to stronger IPRs is also related to the target of catching up technologically, the consumer perspective is of primary importance with respect to access to health care. Two aspects related to TNPCs have to be considered: (a) the availability of effective medicines to treat specific diseases and (b) the accessibility of these medicines (basically related to price levels).

In fact, the lack of access to ARVs for the majority of HIV-infected people in developing countries constituted the real scandal that mobilized a broad political opposition. Millions of people were facing death because they (and their governments) could not afford patent-protected medicines at prices demanded by TNPCs. Parallel to this circumstance, the fact that the lack of profitable markets had also been a central factor preventing pharmaceutical corporations from undertaking any serious efforts to develop medicines for the treatment of tropical ('neglected') diseases became an important political issue.

The Commission on Intellectual Property Rights, Innovation and Public Health (CIPIH), established by WHO in 2004, published its final report in 2006 which discusses these problems at length. The report distinguishes between the status of the availability of treatment for three types of interventions (Type I: diseases with large numbers of vulnerable people in rich and poor countries; Type II: substantial proportion of cases in poor countries; Type III: overwhelming or exclusive incidence in poor countries). It refers to the lack of affordability in poor countries of existing interventions against Type I and II diseases, and the general non-existence of effective interventions for diseases occurring only in developing countries (CIPIH/WHO 2006: 27ff.).

Constitution of country positions: the aggregation of political interests at the country level

The Westphalian system of international relations is based on a primary aggregation of interests at the national level. Basically, two types of actors play a central role in influencing the position of national governments on the issue of access to medical treatment: the pharmaceutical industry (and, of course, other producers of medical implements which are not in the foreground of our research) and the 'development community', which in itself is quite heterogeneous. The following political forces and conflicts will have to be taken into account to analyse country positions:

- lobbying of interested actors in specific government institutions (pharmaceutical associations; actors of the 'development community');
- (perceived) impacts of WTO regulations on public health and public health-related issues as well as possible conflicts with other trade and/or investment interests (local pharmaceutical firms, health ministries, other economic actors);
- impacts of CSOs and other actors on country positions through public pressure;
- external pressures;
- political processes within administration and national political institutions.

As regards IGOs, the power of private actors depends on their ability to exert significant influence on the positions of powerful states. In this respect, the pharmaceutical industry basically uses the means of lobbying, which implies the use of resource-based power (if not for corruption, it will usually refer to the economic weight of the industry) to influence the decision-making power of government members and (where necessary) also of legislators.

The most important stronghold of pharmaceutical corporations has been the US government. Lobbying of pharmaceutical companies has played a decisive role in making the US push for the TRIPS agreement. Since then, the US government has always been a strong defender of IPRs – during both the Clinton and the Bush administrations. Throughout the negotiations on the Doha Declaration and afterwards, US positions only moved when intense public pressure, both from within and beyond the country's borders, rose against them. The EU position in the negotiations of the agreement was basically similar (UNCTAD/ICTSD 2005: 4f.), but later on, the EU seemed to be more open to compromises. The EU Commission appears to be under more pressure to accommodate industrial interests to other actors' concerns, like those of civil society or the development community.

It was certainly not in the interest of developing countries to create a strong international system of IPRs which would hamper technological learning through processes of product copying and re-engineering. In the TRIPS Negotiating Group, India's demands that '[a]ny principle or standard relating to IPRs should be carefully tested against these needs of developing countries' (UNCTAD/ICTSD 2005: 6), did not achieve much more than a reference in the preamble of the agreement (see above). One should assume that developing countries try to defend and make use of the flexibilities TRIPS has left to them, as was the case concerning the Doha Declaration and the ensuing TRIPS amendment. In the process of interest aggregation at the national level, however, in many developing countries health considerations do not play a central role, and flexibilities in the field of IPRs are frequently sacrificed in favour of short-term economic interests like improving access to northern markets, as has been demonstrated in negotiations on bilateral and multilateral free trade agreements (FTAs).

In general, a situation of competing national systems striving for economic growth and economic development, where the most competitive economic actors and other elites have a better opportunity to influence the strategies of national governments than the poor, tends to relegate social issues to the second line of priorities (trickle-down argument). If economic growth is accompanied by increasing inequalities (as is the case in many countries), the hopes for trickle-down effects seem to be rather empty promises. The actors that might throw in their weight to improve the situation of the poor appear to have more power in the context of global politics: these are (a) a technocratic elite contemplating the costs and benefits in the long run and organizing reactions to threats on a global scale and (b) a host of advocatory movements and organizations thinking in terms of a global society ('solidarity', 'global community').

TRIPS and social development: basic aspects

Human rights

During much of the 1990s, 'health as a human right' has not been very much at the forefront of the global discourse on poverty. Health was basically seen as one aspect of global inequalities. It was precisely the lack of access of HIV/AIDS patients in developing countries to available, life-saving medicines that became a global scandal and succeeded in mobilizing extended networks of CSOs and, quite rapidly, wider public opinion around the issue of the 'human right to health' (Fischer-Lescano and Liste 2005).

Article 25 of the Universal Declaration of Human Rights states: 'Everyone has the right to a standard of living adequate for the health and well-being of himself and of his family, including food, clothing, housing and medical care and necessary social services'. This right was reinforced by Article 12 of the International Covenant on Economic, Social and Cultural Rights, a legally binding instrument concluded in 1966 and ratified by all OECD countries with the exception of the US: 'States Parties recognize the right of everyone to the enjoyment of the highest attainable standard of physical and mental health' (Article 12.1), which includes 'the creation of conditions which would assure to all medical service and medical attention in the event of sickness' (Article 12.2). These documents, however, are rather inconclusive with respect to the 'standard of health' that is supposed to be 'attainable'. In 2000, the Committee on Economic, Social and Cultural Rights (CESCR, a sub-committee of ECOSOC, the UN Economic and Social Council) adopted a twenty-page document entitled 'The Right to the Highest Attainable Standard of Health',[13] stating that 'a State party cannot, under any circumstances whatsoever, justify its non-compliance with the core obligations set out in paragraph 43 above, which are non-derogable'(§47). Now, §43 obliges state parties 'to provide essential drugs, as from time to time defined under the WHO Action Programme on Essential Drugs' (like ARVs since April 2002).

Most least developed countries (LDCs), which have per capita public annual health expenditures of less than US$10 (CMH 2001: 56), however, are certainly not in a position to fulfil such an obligation. Therefore, states also have the obligation to assist other states in fully realizing the right to health and to 'ensure that the right to health is given due attention in international agreements' (§39); §64 explicitly calls for a number of IGOs to 'cooperate effectively with States parties, building on their respective expertise, in relation to the implementation of the right to health at the national level'.

The right to health is codified in a number of other international agreements,[14] but it is not enforceable by any institutionalized process. If people cannot afford available life-saving treatment, this is a matter of global responsibility. As the potential for powerful health interventions increased with economic and communicative globalization, the internationalization of IPRs through TRIPS obviously constitutes an ethical problem inasmuch as it interferes with the full use of these opportunities. In fact, it is an interesting point to see whether pressure by civil society can substitute for the lack of material sanctions available to support the implementation of human rights.

TRIPS regulations and health issues in developing countries

When in 1977 the WHO first produced a list of *essential medicines,* very few of the listed drugs were patent-protected. This means that there were no legal obstacles to copying them anywhere in the world, but it also points to the fact that there were rather few newly developed medicines on the market which were particularly geared to diseases prevailing in developing countries.

IPR rules ought to favour pharmaceutical R&D and prevent the copying of products and technology – this seems improbable in countries with a low technological basis but also ignores the historical experience of industrialized countries (see Chapter 3). In general, there seem to be opportunities for those countries that already have a well-established local pharmaceutical industry, such as India, China and Brazil. In other middle-income countries the existing market and qualified labour force might attract investments from TNPCs, but the potential for developing local R&D capacities seems rather limited (MIHR 2005; Chaudhuri 2005).

It was the issue of ARVs which first led – at least for the wider public – to a discourse on the link between IPRs and the access to *affordable* medicines in the South. In fact, only after nearly another decade is the question of the affordability of medicines for the treatment of chronic diseases increasingly becoming a political issue (see for example Gelders et al. 2006). ARVs have been on the market since the early 1990s and have been used to treat HIV/AIDS patients in developed countries. Prices of medicines to treat one person for one year remained high until 2000: according to Médecins Sans Frontières (MSF), the lowest prices of the first-line antiretroviral (ARV) triple combination per patient per year was US$10 439 in October 2000.[15] At that time, IGOs active in the fight against HIV/AIDS in developing countries – basically the WHO and the World Bank – concentrated on strategies of prevention, as this was seen as the most 'cost-effective' strategy. This approach took the extremely high prices of ARVs for granted; 'treatment for all' was simply unaffordable for the international community. This situation changed since the late 1990s: the Brazilian government was determined to provide free access to ARVs to all infected people and successfully negotiated licensing agreements with pharmaceutical companies (see Chapters 3 and 8). Generic versions of ARVs entered the market in July 2000, initially at a price of US$2767 per person per annum (MSF testimony quoted above).

CSOs in global health governance: the campaign for improving access to ARVs

In the second half of the 1990s global civil society took the lead in organizing protests against the lack of access to treatment for people in developing countries which finally led to the process of renegotiating WTO rules. From 1996 onwards, Health Action International (HAI) successfully developed a campaign against the effect of TRIPS on limiting the access of poor people to patented medicines. This campaign has been supported by MSF, which after receiving the Nobel Peace Prize in 1999, gained a strong position in global public opinion. In November 1999, the MSF Campaign for Access to Essential Medicines was launched, which since then has assumed the leading role in the coordination of civil society activities in this field.

CSOs organized pressure on Northern states basically by influencing public opinion. The rising media coverage of the access issue was an important development which has increased pressure on governments and the pharmaceutical industry. Political actors of interest groups frequently talk (or complain) about the pressure they feel from the media.[16] The strong presence of the access issue in specialized information networks can easily be demonstrated (for instance in ip-health mailings, or in the kaisernetwork); it is far more difficult, however, to find comprehensive information on the mass media coverage of a specific issue.[17] At least, US opinion polls demonstrate that (a) there is a rather considerable awareness of HIV/AIDS as a general threat to global health and (b) there is a certain scepticism about governments' activities in this field which are seen as ineffective (perhaps also due to costs to taxpayers), but (c) there is support for government policies to improve 'access to affordable drugs'.[18]

Protests of CSOs against high drug prices and the impact of TRIPS can be seen in the tradition of contention of global social movements against GATT and the WTO and their schedules for international economic liberalization (see for example O'Brien et al. 2000). During the 1990s, however, CSOs became increasingly engaged as cooperating experts in policy-making processes and as actors in international negotiations. They also gained importance as advisers to developing country members of the WTO.[19] In this way, CSOs assumed an important role more or less as midwives for the development of formal global politics. There is also an increasing tendency for intergovernmental organizations and bilateral aid agencies to channel aid – in particular aid in the health sector – via CSOs, that were more and more accepted as partners of established organizations and as opinion-leaders (see Chapter 4).

Similar to the development of national civil society structures filling the public space which opened with the decay of feudal institutions, global civil society fills a space which arises with the increase of transnational social relations beyond the nation-states and the formal inter-state relations (Hein 2005). As within a nation-state, this refers to the construction of opinions, the formation of social norms, and the expression of political critique and demands as part of the process of agenda-setting in political institutions. We witness the development of a complex field of civil society activities and structures which to some degree substitute for non-existing state structures. Their hybrid character is also expressed in the fact that they are more or less recognized as legitimate representatives of underprivileged groups in a particular political field (for example Oxfam and MSF in health politics) and have a significant impact on negotiations between representatives of states in another political field that has attained a higher degree of formal organization on the international level (trade/WTO).

New types of political relations between CSOs, private corporations and IGOs are themselves embedded in a changing public understanding of specific issues. Linking global social movements to constructivist analysis, Sidney Tarrow (2005) discusses the origins of establishing a specific political issue and of constructing the perceptual field in which it has to be interpreted. This social definition of a problem feeds back into politics – among others, through the changing perception of an issue through political actors themselves. Tarrow uses the concept of 'framing': 'Proposing frames that are new and challenging but still resonate with existing cultural understandings is a delicate balancing act, especially since society's "common sense" buttresses the position of elites and defends inherited inequalities' (Tarrow 2005: 61). He stresses the need for 'convergence': 'existing political streams that combine with long-standing bundles of ideologies, practices, values, and targets' (ibid.: 62). Recently, Joshua Busby has shown the importance of AIDS advocates framing their arguments 'to tap into moral and religious attitudes' (Busby 2006: 2) and analyses the conditions for 'framing' created by culture (need for a 'cultural match') and politics (shaping the interest of 'policy entrepreneurs' to take up a specific issue, framed in a specific rhetoric).

The political conditions of 'framing' also relate to a situation in which the generally more powerful actors in a conflict feel threatened by the results of inequalities and inequities. Busby (2006) discusses the role of threats as part of the framing process of the HIV/AIDS issue. Feeling threatened by particular developments (the re-emergence of infectious diseases; political instability and so on, see Introduction) increases the readiness to reconsider the priority of one's own short-term interests in relation to an 'enlightened self-interest' in fighting the causes of these threats.

Corporate social responsibility

The global activities of CSOs, their reference to core human rights, and the successful framing of the issue in major industrialized societies – including the impact on public opinion and the reaction of politicians – have exerted a strong pressure on TNPCs. Pharmaceutical companies cannot deny that the industry as a whole is highly profitable. They had to show *corporate social responsibility* and to contribute to the fight for 'better health for all'. To offer effective cooperation to improve access, at least to ARVs, and to reach some results in the field of neglected diseases, were indispensable elements in a strategy to defend (or better re-establish) the image of the industry ('good practice in pharmaceutical industry', see DFID 2005). The Global Compact between industry, civil society and state actors, initiated by UN General Secretary Kofi Annan in 1999, was explicitly set up for this purpose. The participation in and support of global public–private partnerships (GPPPs) is obviously seen as an appropriate strategy: the voluntary character of these activities and the potential to keep control on GPPP activities are central aspects in this regard (see Chapter 3 for more details).

Another instrument which is accepted by the pharmaceutical industry is differential pricing. In 2002, the European Union proposed to add ARVs to a list of medicines with 'tiered prices' – implying either a price cut of 80 per cent or a price 10 per cent above production costs for 49 least developed and 23 other low-income countries – which would be identified by a logo in order to prevent reimportation to the EU.[20]

Whatever TNPCs were offering to cooperate in the field of access to drugs in poor countries, the basic objective has always been to prevent any weakening of internationally accepted IPR rules as a basis for securing profitability. In comments on the CIPIH report, the International Federation of Pharmaceutical Manufacturers' Associations (IFPMA) rejects all critical comments on strong patents laws (Noehrenberg 2006).

TRIPS and health: adjustments of intellectual property rights regulations

The Doha Declaration on the TRIPS Agreement and Public Health

In the conflict around IPRs and health, CSOs insisted that the problem of access to medicines is not a problem to be solved by philanthropy alone, but that it is more deeply rooted in the emerging legal basis of the global economy. Based on fundamental doubts on the rationality of IPRs in the field of medicines and public health – and reinforced by the South African and Brazilian conflicts – there has been an increasing pressure from CSOs and governments from developing countries on the WTO to clarify the relation of TRIPS to public health concerns. After the failure to launch a so-called Millennium Round of trade negotiations at the Seattle Ministerial Conference in 1999, a declaration on IPRs and access to medicines which would take up developing countries' concerns seemed to be an important precondition for the success of the following ministerial meeting in November 2001 in Doha. In early 2001, the African Group requested that the TRIPS Council deal with this problem based on documents by the WHO and UNCTAD, which stressed the flexibility of TRIPS (Correa 2002).

During the Doha Ministerial Conference (9–14 November 2001), after some controversial debates in the TRIPS Council and the WTO's General Council due to the resistance among industrialized countries (USA, Japan, Switzerland, Australia and Canada), the so-called Doha Declaration on the TRIPS Agreement and Public Health was accepted. The declaration recognizes 'the gravity of the public health problems afflicting many developing and least-developed countries, especially those resulting from HIV/AIDS, tuberculosis, malaria and other epidemics' (§1). It explicitly acknowledges concerns about the effects of intellectual property protection on prices (§3). Paragraph 4 constitutes the heart of the declaration stating (and implicitly referring to TRIPS Article 8.1):

> We agree that the TRIPS Agreement does not and should not prevent members from taking measures to protect public health. Accordingly, while reiterating our commitment to the TRIPS Agreement, we affirm that the Agreement can and should be interpreted and implemented in a manner supportive of WTO members' right to protect public health

> and, in particular, to promote access to medicines for all. In this connection, we reaffirm the right of WTO members to use, to the full, the provisions in the TRIPS Agreement, which provide flexibility for this purpose.

Paragraph 5 stresses the right of each country to make use of what I have called the 'entry points' for social concerns in TRIPS:

> In applying the customary rules of interpretation of public international law, each provision of the TRIPS Agreement shall be read in the light of the object and purpose of the Agreement as expressed, in particular, in its objectives and principles. (§5a)

Paragraph 5 (b–d) refers to the flexibilities in TRIPS which could be used for securing access to required medicines (as summarized above) and to members' sovereignty to determine 'what constitutes a national emergency or other circumstances of extreme urgency'. Finally, §6 of the Declaration recognizes an omission in the TRIPS agreement: compulsory licensing has been authorized 'predominantly for the supply of the domestic market' (Article 31(f) TRIPS), which makes it difficult for countries that have no generics industry to use this instrument. Further negotiations on compulsory licences for the supply from third countries are to be held. Finally, §7 extends the transition period for pharmaceutical patent protection in LDCs until 1 January 2016.

In general, developing countries and CSOs[21] recognized the Doha Declaration as a success for the access campaign and for strengthening the position of developing countries in conflicts with TNPCs and countries supporting strong IPRs on TRIPS matters.[22]

The WTO Medicines (§6) Decision and the TRIPS amendment

Basically, three points proved to be controversial between those countries which tried to limit the use of compulsory licences as narrowly as possible (the host countries of major TNPCs) and those that wanted to allow a broad use of them in support of 'public health':

(1) *The 'scope of diseases'*: The US used §1 of the Doha Declaration to argue that a §6 solution should be limited to the diseases specifically identified there, while developing country delegations insisted on the point that the Declaration always refers to the protection of 'public health' in general.[23]
(2) *The determination of eligible countries*: §6 refers to countries 'with insufficient or no manufacturing capacities in the pharmaceutical sector'. As capacities vary considerably according to the medicines

involved, developing countries insist that each country should be responsible for determining whether it has the capacity to produce the needed pharmaceuticals while the US and the EU wanted a more limited solution.

(3) *The question whether the agreement should be based on Article 30 or Article 31 TRIPS Agreement*: While Article 30 would have allowed a more flexible and non-bureaucratic use of the intended mechanism, it only refers to 'limited exceptions' to patent protection which would have required further specifications. Article 31 includes procedural requirements for a compulsory licence where only the reference 'basically for local consumption' had to be waived.

The final agreement allowed compulsory licensing for export to countries not capable of producing needed medicines irrespective of specific illnesses and did not include a narrow determination of eligible countries.[24] Only regarding the third point, the advocates of a more open agreement had to accept the reference to Article 31. In addition, the compromise included some requirements of notification and marking of medicines produced under this decision by 'special packaging and/or special colouring and/or shaping' and finally, the reading of a 'Chairperson's statement' which stresses the need to prevent a diversion of products from the markets for which they are intended and lists the countries which have opted out of using the system as importers.[25]

The Medicines Decision was implemented through a waiver of TRIPS Article 31 (f) and (h), which will terminate 'on the date on which an amendment to the TRIPS Agreement replacing its provisions takes effect' (§11).[26] Though somewhat cumbersome procedures related to the issuing of a compulsory licence and to preventing re-exportation into third countries had to be accepted, the §6 decision was basically seen as a success for developing countries, demonstrating, in particular, the strength of global civil society. In fact, for pharmaceutical corporations, a strategy to object strictly to any real adaptation of TRIPS proved difficult to pursue.

It was only with the Hong Kong ministerial conference that the General Council agreed on an amendment to the TRIPS agreement, finalizing the §6 decision (6 December 2005). In fact, it constitutes the first change of any of the WTO agreements. Developing countries and CSOs tried to achieve changes of the §6 decision based on the argument that the preconditions for using the mechanism have become too burdensome, as not a single country has made use of the mechanism since August 2003. The notification requirements and the Chairperson's statement should be eliminated. Most industrialized countries insisted in taking over the 2003 text (including the Chairperson's statement). Finally, the latter position prevailed, as developing countries realized that, on the whole, the §6 solution was a success for them.

Improved access to medicines

Although until today we cannot observe an increased use of compulsory licences by developing countries, experts do agree that its legal and political strengthening has given developing countries a stronger position in conflicts with TNPCs on licences and price concessions. The presence of generic ARVs on the market, the activities of CSOs, the ensuing global public debate, and the reorientation of health IGOs have led to a different framing of the access problem in the global public debate. Relatively early on, TNPCs have realized that they need to demonstrate corporate social responsibility in order to uphold the political support of their home country in international negotiations. In the end, public pressure was so strong that TNPCs did not succeed in securing the continued support of their main political alliances for preventing modifications in TRIPS.[27] When the battle on the Doha Declaration and §6 was basically lost, TNPCs themselves were increasingly ready to compromise with respect to selling drugs cheaper, licensing developing countries (particularly Brazil) to produce drugs and to withdraw from legal action in doubtful cases.

All this has led the international prices of ARVs to plummet between June 2000 and July 2001 and then decrease gradually but constantly until 2005 (see Figure 3.4, p. 80). This includes generic and originator products. According to recent information from MSF, which regularly produces 'a pricing guide for the purchase of ARVs for developing countries', originator corporations are now offering the package of drugs for the treatment of one person for one year (ARV triple-combination, lowest world prices) at US$562, while generic products are listed at around US$152.[28] When in 2004 the Clinton Foundation involved the World Bank, UNICEF and the Global Fund to negotiate with Indian generic producers on drug prices for more than 100 developing countries, a reduction to around US$140 (per person/year) was achieved.[29]

This means that, since 2001, ARV prices have been down to a level which – in combination with international aid – no longer prevents universal access, even without the explicit use of compulsory licences. Still, a number of problems prevent a very rapid extension of effective access to all people in need:

- There is still a lack of cheap drugs for the treatment of children: a treatment with the triple combination in a paediatric formulation for a child weighing 10 kg can cost US$816, while treating an adult costs only US$182 (MSF 2005: 4f.).

- For patients who need second-line ARVs because of resistance and medical incompatibilities, the sole, rather low-priced drug (lopinavir/ritonavir from Abbott Laboratories) is only available in LDCs at the reduced price of US$550, while it is sold in low middle-income countries like El Salvador and Peru for between US$4468 and 4511 (Vasan et al. 2006: 395).
- Of course, an effective treatment also needs the establishment of diagnostic capacities, the accessibility of medical personnel and thus a functioning health system.

One can assume that the direct effects of the new 2005 Indian Patent Law regarding first-line ARVs will be negligible, as generics based on drugs patented before 1995 will not be affected. Furthermore, a generic manufacturer has the right to continue producing the drugs, even if an application filed to the mailbox (see note 9) has been granted a patent (then, the generic company has to pay a 'reasonable royalty' to the patent holder). However, whether India will use the compulsory licensing provisions included in the law to allow generic production of second-line ARVs is questionable and depends on whether India will define the need for these drugs as a national emergency and risk conflicts with TNPCs (Smart 2005; Abbott 2005b, 2006).

Chapters 5 and 6 will look at the changing policies of IGOs after the fall of ARV prices and at the activities of the Global Fund which, together with national endeavours, have allowed the number of infected people on ARV therapy in low- and middle-income countries to rise from 240 000 at the end of 2002 to approximately 1.3 million three years later (UNAIDS 2006: 151). Though this number remains well below the WHO 3 by 5 target, the increase can be seen as a positive result of increased international resources to finance the import of medicines as well as an improved health infrastructure to allow sustainable treatment.

New developments: TRIPS+ versus innovative proposals on IPRs

The amendment of TRIPS and the fall of ARV prices since 2000 are intermediate results of one specific conflict. The pharmaceutical industry successively adopted a rhetoric of supporting the global endeavour to improve access of the poor to medicines. Nevertheless, they pursued their agenda of trying to secure strong international IPRs, now shifting the forum of their activities towards bilateral and multilateral trade agreements. Taking into account the possibility of a limited impact of the newly introduced patent right in India with the possible use of compulsory licences for producing second-line ARVs (and drugs for treating other diseases, for example Tamiflu), TNPCs did everything to secure TRIPS+ clauses in bilateral and multilateral trade agreements, particularly those of the US. In all the FTAs negotiated since the late 1990s they pushed the US government to include clauses which forced the trade partners to exclude the possibility of using flexibilities included in TRIPS. Most partners agreed to these demands, as their priorities were oriented towards gaining access to the US markets for their export industries.[30] Frederick Abbott talks of a TRIPS II agenda by 'strong mercantile interests[31] seeking to increase technology and expression rents'[32] as a reaction to the change of conditions since the late 1990s (Abbott 2006). These problems had been discussed at length in relation to different US trade agreements with Latin American countries and with Thailand.[33] The TRIPS II agenda is also used by the US in WTO accession negotiations, which include bilateral demands for concessions.

The Declaration of South American health ministers[34] at the 2006 World Health Assembly is an expression of conflicting interests within developing countries. Though some of these countries have accepted TRIPS+ rules in a free trade agreement with the US (Chile, Ecuador, Peru), they commit themselves to 'the successful implementation of the safeguards and flexibilities included both in the TRIPS agreement and in the Doha Declaration' (quoted from ip-health, 1 June 2006). However, they did not commit themselves to renegotiate FTAs that are in contradiction to their own declaration.

The new Indian Patent Law and the TRIPS+ agenda seem to shift the equilibrium of forces again towards IPR interests. This assumption, however, overlooks the importance of public pressures in this field. Pharmaceutical R&D and the pricing of drugs are not only at the heart of patent legislation, but are also matters of foremost public concern related to strong social and political threats, as well as strong feelings on social justice. Public sector initiatives in the context of development cooperation are now trying to take advantage of TRIPS transitory regulations for generic production in LDCs. There are some experiences in Ethiopia, Tanzania and Bangladesh as well as further plans to develop pharmaceutical production capacities in other LDCs.[35]

'Forum' or 'regime shifting' is a strategy which is not restricted to governments of the most powerful countries. New initiatives to develop alternative forms to fund research on medicines important to poor countries, like James Love's[36] proposal to negotiate a Medical R&D Treaty under the auspices of the WHO, indicate an attempt to shift the focus of setting rules on IPRs in the field of essential medicines to the WHO. The Report of the Commission on Intellectual Property Rights and Innovation in Health (CIPIH/WHO 2006) played a central role in the deliberations of the World Health Assembly in May 2006. There is a rather broad consensus on a number of proposals in this report, in particular to eliminate taxes and tariffs on medicines in developing countries and on the promotion of so-called Advance Purchase Schemes, that is, public assurances (and pre-payments) to purchase medicines on which research is conducted, which would provide a level of security to inventors regarding the income they can expect. On the other hand, a number of points which called into question the function of IPRs to set research priorities have been heavily criticized by TNPCs (see for example Noehrenberg 2006). The WHA in 2006 passed a resolution based on the Kenyan and Brazilian proposal to establish a Global Framework on Essential Health R&D, closely related to the Medical R&D Treaty concept, which means that further conceptual work will be done on a system sharing the high costs of research and development of medicines and creating obligations and incentives to invest in projects which are considered a public priority. This has to be seen in terms of the fact that the concept of IPRs and the consequences of IPR regimes are quite heavily debated in the economic discipline.[37]

Taking into account the reluctance of industrialized countries concerning these proposals, however, one must consider what will happen at the organizational interfaces of an IGO like the WHO. Again, CSOs are taking the lead to spur innovation in GHG. In 2003, MSF founded a non-profit firm to develop new drugs, which cooperates with pharmaceutical enterprises in the context of an integrated enterprise oriented exclusively to discovering new drugs for neglected diseases ('Drugs for Neglected Diseases Initiative', DNDi), which, two years after its foundation, has already developed twenty projects.

The 'Geneva connection'

When considering the results of nearly ten years of conflicts in IPRs and access to medicines, it is important to realize that CSOs not only succeeded in mobilizing support for a stronger role of social rights in global governance, but that the whole framework of perceptions on this issue – and on the importance of global health in general – has changed. What we call the 'Geneva connection' can be seen as a microcosm of the whole complex of interfaces which moved the process of global health governance: it is a 'centre of communication' producing at least elements of a common understanding of affairs which are then reintroduced into command centres of political action (WTO, WHO, powerful nation-states, but also important CSOs like MSF).

IGOs in the fields of social and economic development and human rights are concentrated in Geneva (WHO, ILO, UNCTAD, UNHCHR, UNAIDS, WIPO, WTO, to list only the most important); UNICEF has its regional office for Central and Eastern Europe in Geneva, there is a World Bank liaison office, and many countries have diplomatic missions in Geneva. Surprisingly enough, this did not guarantee a close communication and coordination between these various offices.[38]

Things seem to have changed with the strengthening of global civil society and the development of global governance structures which have created networks of cooperation and (at least) communication between various types of actors in specific policy fields and supposedly also function as catalysts for the cooperation between IGOs. Certainly, a network consisting of CSOs in the health sector (HAI, MSF, Oxfam, and the Consumer Project on Technology (CPT)), and human rights organizations like CIEL and 3D can be seen as a complex organizational interface between CSOs in the access to medicines campaign.[39]

The development of a CSO interface has not only led to a strengthening of CSO campaigns in this field. We find communication on strategies and on interpreting 'facts' between groups and organizations with opposing political positions, discussion on compromises, selective cooperation and so on, in a field of many different options for strategies, actions, and also institution-building. We find flexible relations between individuals working in different organizations (sometimes changing the workplace), constituting not a formal network, but linked into networks which facilitate access to media and to groups organizing campaigns as well as to national and international institutions in Geneva and elsewhere (with access to important information, but also people closely linked to CSOs working in IGOs as experts for specific topics).

A decisive basis for the concrete function of this 'Geneva connection'[40] is a certain common ground of norms – basically referring to human rights and certain forms of political and personal respect – beyond sizeable differences in concrete goals and strategies. We find all kinds of communication between CSOs in different fields, CSOs and delegates from industrialized and developing countries, CSOs and IGOs, market-creating IGOs and welfare-oriented IGOs, CSOs and the pharmaceutical industry, and so on.

At first glance, the resulting system of interactions looks like a 'network of networks'. But this term is not really accurate: some of them are formal IGOs, others are in fact networks (CSO networks), but in many cases the interactions are informal and the participants are frequently not specifically legitimized representatives of their respective organization. On the other hand, not all of these interactions are even interfaces in the sense of recurrent interactions; some informal meetings might become ritualized but many are just one-time occurrences. There is no network in a narrower sense of implying a certain organizational effort for the exchange of information or joint activities.

A number of interviews with Geneva-based organizations focused on this communication system.[41] Most of the organizations are members of formal networks extending beyond Geneva (like the ESCR-net, the Access Campaign, Biomedical Adviser Group or WHO Scientific Working Groups, WHO Stakeholder Meetings), but all ascribed a great importance to regular and occasional informal meetings in Geneva. These include regular coordination meetings with other CSOs, briefings, workshops, and conferences organized by many Geneva-based organizations mostly with broad-based participation from all sorts of agencies, including national delegations in Geneva. In addition, there are many personal contacts at the margins of organized events (including receptions and parties, or 'national days' organized by the country missions) or just in the form of private meetings. Certainly, in general, people meet more frequently with colleagues from similar organizations, but all of them stressed the importance of meetings 'across the board' of all Geneva-based organizations. CSOs refer to meetings with delegates from Southern countries and the role of the South Centre in this context.

Job mobility among the Geneva-based organizations can be seen as one important element intensifying communication between different organizations, also by facilitating contacts between the old and the new colleagues. There seems to be job mobility between all kind of organizations present in Geneva, but, according to some of the interviewees, the most frequently observed paths are from CSOs to IGOs and from national delegations (in particular of the South) to CSOs; quite frequently people move from IGOs to CSOs after retirement. There are also no absolute ideological barriers to job mobility; thus, in one case, a person moved from IFPMA to MSF.

Thus, the 'Geneva connection' might be seen as a 'glocal' centre for approaching a common understanding of global health problems, which certainly does not imply a change of actors' interests and ultimate goals. It confirms the importance of discoursive interfaces which can be observed in the course of conflicts between global 'market creation' and the defenders of global social rights.

Approaching a conclusion: conflicts about intellectual property rights and the dynamics of interfaces in global health governance

During the last ten years we have observed a surprising process. The powerful pharmaceutical industry retreated on conflicts in Brazil and South Africa and finally had to accept a change in TRIPS, which strengthened the instrument of compulsory licences, as their political allies could not resist the human rights-based arguments on access to medicines (see Chapters 3, 7 and 8). This coincided with an awareness of the importance of health in the context of a broader understanding of human security. Global civil society organizations have successfully used discoursive interfaces in GHG to mobilize support for a stronger public responsibility as regards medical innovation and access to essential medicines and thus to strengthen an important aspect of welfare politics on the global level.

CSOs have been successful in framing the discourses on access to medicines and on alternatives to patent rights (or at least supplementary mechanisms to strengthen the role of medicines as global public goods). This discussion has successively integrated experts from national institutions of development cooperation and IGOs. International commissions on intellectual property rights took up these issues and played an important role in opening up a new field in inter-state health politics. The IFPMA had to acknowledge the need for better access to medicines and finally publicly welcomed the TRIPS amendment (IFPMA, News Releases, 12 December 2005). Now, TNPCs are engaged in GPPPs in the fields of access to medicines and neglected diseases and praise them as the most important strategy to contribute to these goals.

Certainly, communicative consensus-seeking among actors with very different material interests can be assumed to go, at best, only half way: TNPCs accept the need for affordable medicines for poor people and the need for action on neglected diseases, but this does not imply surrendering the use of their political and economic resources to fight for strong IPRs at the level of international law. Nevertheless, in spite of fundamental conflicts between critical CSOs and TNPCs, CSOs were flexible enough to cooperate with public actors at all levels and with TNPCs, for instance in the field of neglected diseases. In Chapter 4, the role of global civil society in the development of GHG will be analysed more broadly, in particular with reference to the diversity of CSOs.

In terms of the conflicts around the TRIPS agreement and the interfaces between actors oriented towards global market creation and those oriented towards global public health, some implications on the development of GHG can be proposed:

- Through manifold processes of self-organization, the need to link different systems of governance (global health, human rights, the world trade order, the intellectual property system touching on issues such as biodiversity and genetic resources) has led to more intense communication and to the rise of new institutional forms to solve specific problems which are moving the core of global health politics from IGOs ('international health governance') to a complex system of global health governance.
- The system borders are constantly fluid; there are many 'overlappings' with other systems in global governance and the system is open to new actors at all times.
- By transcending various governance systems in the process of a successive intensification of global social relations, GHG actors have – at least in the field of access to medicines – successfully mobilized discoursive power.
- This has resulted in a reinforcement of actors fighting for global social rights in spite of the strong position the supporters of global market creation had won with the foundation of WTO and the development of hard legal interfaces.

Notes

1. See Introduction, note 4 for the definition.
2. One might also refer to the cost-benefit calculations on providing adequate health services (see for example the Report of the Commission on Macroeconomics and Health, CMH 2001), though this seems to be problematic from an ethical perspective.
3. When speaking of the 'right to health', it is always an abbreviation of this formulation used in the International Covenant on Economic, Social and Cultural Rights (Article 12.1) or the formulation used in Article 25 of the Universal Declaration of Human Rights, which refers in more detail to the circumstances affecting health.
4. See from different perspectives: Koivusalo 2003; Fink and Maskus 2005; Blouin et al. 2006; Bermann and Mavroidis 2006.
5. These types of meetings are named after the Director General's conference room even if they take place elsewhere.
6. For more details see Hoekman and Kostecki 2001, Chapter 3 (see also the explanation given on the WTO website at www.wto.org/english/thewto_e/whatis_e/tif_e/disp1_e.htm).
7. Chosen from a list of potential panelists nominated by WTO members; parties can reject proposed panelists.

8. See the summaries on TRIPS in Hoekman and Kostecki 2001, WHO/WTO 2002, UNCTAD/ICTSD 2005.
9. A 'mailbox' is a facility stipulated by Article 70.8 TRIPS: 'Where a Member does not make available as of the date of entry into force of the WTO Agreement [i.e. Jan., 1 1995] patent protection for pharmaceutical and agricultural chemical products . . . that member shall . . . provide . . . a means by which applications for patents for such inventions can be filed.'
10. Article 30 allows the so-called Bolar provision. Countries may allow manufacturers of generic drugs to use the patented invention to obtain marketing approval without the patent owner's permission and before the patent protection expires. Generic products can then be marketed as soon as the patent expires (http://www.wto.org/english/tratop_e/trips_e/factsheet_pharm02_e.htm, accessed 19 June 2006).
11. This refers to the issue of the exhaustion of patent rights, which means that the IPR embodied in a product or service is exhausted 'when a good or service is first sold or marketed in a country'. If a national patent law recognizes a doctrine of 'international exhaustion', the IPR holder's right is extinguished whenever a good is sold or marketed anywhere in the world (UNCTAD/ICTSD 2005: 93f.). TRIPS Article 6 allows a country full freedom with respect to the doctrine of exhaustion it uses in its patent law.
12. See DiMasi et al. (2003) and some more details in Chapter 3. This number, however, does not refer explicitly to drugs for neglected diseases, and many critics argue that the R&D costs for typical diseases of the poor are much lower.
13. This document is part of a series of comments by the CESCR called 'Substantive issues arising in the implementation of the International Covenant on Economic, Social and Cultural Rights' adopted since 1989, here 'General Comment No. 14' (document E/C.12/2000/4), accessible under the following URL: http://www.unhchr.ch/tbs/doc.nsf/(symbol)/E.C.12.2000.4.En?OpenDocument.
14. See the Convention on the Elimination of All Forms of Discrimination Against Women (Articles 10, 12 and 14), the Convention on the Elimination of All Forms of Racial Discrimination (Article 5) and the Convention on the Rights of the Child (Article 24). Also, Article 35 of the Charter of Fundamental Rights of the European Union demands that 'a high level of human health protection shall be ensured in the definition and implementation of all Union policies and activities'.
15. This refers to: stavudine (d4T) + lamivudine (3 TC) + nevirapine (NVP); cf. MSF testimony submitted to DHHS (Department of Health and Human Services) for the Meeting of the International Subcommittee of PACHA (Presidential Advisory Council on HIV/AIDS) on 16 December 2003.
16. This was pointed out in several interviews carried out in Geneva.
17. The growth of the number of articles in major newspapers related to AIDS and Africa, from 500 in 1997 to 1000 in 2000 (Busby 2006: 28), can be seen as an indication of a growing media attention to HIV/AIDS issues in poor countries.
18. See three polls taken since 2002: Kaiser Family Foundation Survey of Americans on HIV/AIDS (www.kff.org/kaiserpolls/7513.cfm), accessed 15 June 2006; Health News Index Poll, survey by Henry J. Kaiser Family Foundation, Harvard School of Public Health, conducted by Princeton

Survey Research Associates, 18–21 July 2002; and a Harris Poll conducted in July 2004 for the *Wall Street Journal*'s Health Industry Edition (www.harrisinteractive.com/news/printerfriend/index.asp?NewsID=831), accessed 18 May 2006.

19. The South Centre has played an important role in organizing communication between health CSOs and Southern national delegates to the WTO (interviews of the authors with representatives in Geneva on §6 negotiations).
20. *The Pulse: Health and Pharma Quarterly Check-up*, November 2002: 5f. (www.hillandknowlton.be/HK/pressoffice/thepulse/ThePulse_Vol.1.pdf). It should be noted that, in 2001, the US government informed the European Union that it would oppose the EU move towards tiered pricing. A letter by US Trade Representative Robert Zoellick stated the 'specific opposition to any international regulation of drug prices as well as to the creation of a price database', which could increase market transparency and allowed poor countries to import medicines at lower prices (Harris and Siplon 2001).
21. See Drahos (2002a) and the websites of CSOs like MSF, Oxfam, HAI; also: personal interviews with people working for CSOs in Geneva (Oxfam, 3D, CIEL, MSF).
22. See for example Abbott (2002, 2005a); Correa (2002); ITC (2003); ip-health e-mail list.
23. As Frederick Abbott stressed: 'If developing countries were facing public health problems that required access to lower-priced medicines, it was not apparent why a distinction should be made between HIV/AIDS, on the one hand, and cancer, heart disease, diabetes or asthma, on the other' (Abbott 2005a: 328).
24. Least developed countries are eligible to use the mechanism without any restrictions; any other country must submit a notification to the TRIPS Council that it has insufficient or no manufacturing capacity for the 'product(s) in question'.
25. For the 'General Council Chairperson's statement' see: WTO General Council, WT/GC/M/82, 13 November 2003). The group of developing countries that declared using the mechanism only in 'circumstances of extreme urgency' comprises Macao, Hong Kong, Taiwan, Israel, Korea, Kuwait, Mexico, Qatar, Singapore, Turkey and the United Arab Emirates.
26. See: Implementation of Paragraph 6 of the Doha Declaration on the TRIPS Agreement and Public Health (30 August 2003), Doc. WT/L/540 (1 September 2003).
27. See for example Thomas (2004: 67) on public pressures on the US government in 2000 to push for stronger IPRs in developing countries.
28. See MSF (2005: 10). The comparison of prices between originator and generic producers is a field of unlimited manipulation. Thus, the Hudson Institute (a Washington-based think thank close to the industry) produced a White Paper (*Myths and Realities on Prices of Drugs*, Adelman et al. 2004) which used MSF data to prove that the average price of patented drugs is considerably lower than that of 'copy drugs'. This paper was obviously used extensively by organizations close to pharmaceutical corporations (IFPMA, News Release, 11 May 2004; Glassman 2004). The Hudson Institute Analysis (in its short study of six pages), however, can be criticized in various respects, among others: (1) it is not the average price of ARV drugs that is important, but the prices of

the needed triple-combinations; (2) fixed-dose combinations, which are more appropriate for use in developing countries, were not included in the Hudson study; (3) while the prices of generic products have no geographical limits, prices of originator drugs vary according to the system of differential pricing (the Hudson study uses only the lower prices for the 'poorest eligible countries' (Adelman et al. 2004: 2)). MSF stresses that the latter system excludes the poor in countries which do not benefit from differential pricing.

29. See http://www.essentialdrugs.org/edrug/archive/200404/msg00014.php.
30. Agreements are in force or signed with Jordan, Singapore, Chile, the countries of the Central American Free Trade Area, Australia, Morocco, Bahrain, Oman, Peru and Colombia, and negotiations are underway with the Southern African Customs Union and Thailand (Abbott 2006: 8).
31. This concerns the copyright-dependent audio-visual industry and the pharmaceutical and agricultural chemical industry.
32. 'Expression rents': rents based on licences.
33. There are a large number of critical texts on Free Trade Agreements with TRIPS+ provisions. The UNCTAD-ICTSD Project on IPRs and Sustainable Development has presented a number of interesting studies on these negotiations (see www.iprsonline.org/resources/FTAs-htm); Oxfam produced various briefing notes and briefing papers on this subject (Oxfam 2002a, 2002b, 2002c); see also Vivas-Eugui (2003) and Abbott (2006).
34. Argentina, Bolivia, Brazil, Chile, Colombia, Ecuador, Paraguay, Peru, Uruguay and Venezuela.
35. A GTZ public–private partnership project supports the production of ARVs in Bukavu (DR Congo) in a pharmaceutical plant, erected by Boehringer Mannheim in 1972 and sold to private investors in 1999 (Grill 2005; www.gtz.de/de/themen/soziale-entwicklung/hiv-aids/12394.htm).
36. James Love is the director of the Consumer Project on Technology (CPTech), the most important US consumer protection organization.
37. See Sturn (2006); Maskus (2000); various contributions in Fink and Maskus (2005); and, critical with respect to pharmaceuticals, Lanoszka (2003).
38. The joint study on 'WTO Agreements & Public Health' (WHO/WTO 2002) indicates that there are a few fields where there has been some long-term institutionalized cooperation, as in the field of the SPS Agreement and the role of the Codex Alimentarius. In many other areas, however, the authors identify 'potential for complementing each other's work' (ibid.: 143) and 'increasing opportunities for taking of synergies' (ibid.: 144), which implicitly recognizes that there has been little concrete cooperation in the past (seen from 2002).
39. For the development of the campaign since 1996 see Mayne (2002); Helfer (2004); and Sell and Prakash (2004).
40. Following Burris (2004) and Burris et al. (2005), one could try to define the 'Geneva connection' in terms of their concept of 'nodal governance'.
41. These interviews covered different types of CSOs (ICTSD, MSF, and 3D, the Quaker UN Office), IFPMA and WHO.

3

From Conflict over Compromise to Cooperation? Big Pharma, the HIV/AIDS Crisis and the Rise of Countervailing Power in the South

Jan Peter Wogart

Introduction

During the last ten years, there have been a number of spectacular confrontations between government and private sector representatives of the North and the South[1] in the global health arena. The rapid spread of HIV/AIDS from a limited number of individuals in the industrialized nations to an ever-increasing number of people in the developing countries became the igniting spark for open conflict, pitting the national authorities of South Africa and Brazil against the transnational pharmaceutical companies (TNPCs, 'Big Pharma') and their governments. The results were remarkable, both with regard to the unexpected shifting power positions of the contestants as well as the implications for global health governance (GHG). The South succeeded in getting the prices of anti-retroviral drugs (ARVs) against AIDS significantly lowered so as to make 'treatment for all' an accepted norm in GHG. At the same time, the developing countries have also been able to strengthen the application of safeguards within the stringent patent right protection legislated under the Trade Related Intellectual Property Rights (TRIPS) agreement as part of the World Trade Organization (WTO) package that became international law in 1995.

This chapter will analyse the power and politics of the large research-oriented TNPCs, their accomplishments and current problems, and the increasing significance of the pharmaceutical industries in newly industrializing countries (NICs). It will focus on the two conflicts, their major causes as well as their resolution in the context of the multiple interactions of major actors in both rich and poor countries' health arena in general and its pharmaceutical markets in particular. It will address three issues proposed in the book's introduction concerning the role of 'Big Pharma', namely: (1) the major characteristics of TNPCs as actors in GHG and their changes over the last ten years; (2) the nature of their interfaces with the other actors in the context of the rapidly spreading HIV/AIDS crisis; and (3) the processes at these interfaces linked to the structure of and changes within national and global health governance.

After presenting a summary evaluation of the major characteristics of the TNPCs, a step-by-step analysis of the major interfaces the industry has had with public and private entities in the face of the HIV/AIDS crisis will form the heart of this chapter. The relationship between the interfaces and the emerging global health governance as well as the efforts of the business actors to come to terms with the new institutional structure are considered in the context of the latest developments of globalization and the TNPCs' particular efforts to move from a more defensive to an offensive strategy in tackling the access to medicines in developing countries.

The analysis will work with elements of strategy models, which have been used increasingly by economists, business analysts and legal experts. It will combine these approaches with a political science framework which examines the emergence of GHG in the context of multilevel governance outlined in Chapter 1. Particularly useful for analysing the TNPCs in the multiple public and private negotiations is a game theory-oriented approach and the notion of 'forum' or 'regime shifting' (Helfer 2004), used by the corporations and the governments of the North in internationalizing intellectual property rights (IPRs) in the context of TRIPS. Not surprisingly, the international civil society organizations (CSOs) and representatives of the South reacted by using the same strategy in fighting for a 'Development Agenda' in the World Intellectual Property Organization (WIPO) and an increased public responsibility for 'Essential Health Research' in the World Health Organization (WHO).

Both groups of actors perceived their goals within a socio-political structure and an institutional setting which has allowed them to pursue these different objectives. In doing so, they have changed the very economic and social structure of the global health architecture, and with it the new concerns, activities and rules of GHG have emerged. At the same time, the emerging GHG is now shaping the perceptions and strategies of the very actors which have been so crucial in building it. In brief, the social interaction analysed here has been co-determined by the property of actors and the existing socio-political structure (Sell 2000).

Major features of the pharmaceutical industry

The purchasing price of pharmaceuticals, sales of which make up about 15 per cent of total health expenditures in rich countries but are estimated to reach between 20 and 25 per cent in poor countries, can vary by hundreds of per cent, depending on which class of drugs they belong to and which country they are sold in. The 'innovator' drugs are protected by patents, granting the producer a monopoly rent in compensation for past and future research and development (R&D) efforts. While not officially disclosed, after passing a series of tests and approval from public regulatory authorities, the TNPCs base and rationalize their pricing decisions not on short- and long-term costs but on the degree of competition from similar drugs, the elasticity of demand, and the extent to which the new patented drug substitutes earlier treatments of the disease, many of which have been expensive, especially when it entailed medical treatment in hospitals (Neukirchen 2004: 93).[2]

Patents, prices and profits of the major pharmaceuticals

In the past the industry has reaped the benefits of that type of pricing and the protection rather extensively granted to them by law, even if governments intervened with price controls. In the US, the authorities have refrained from using price controls. Instead, the firms enjoy a great number of positive incentives, ranging from tapping results from superior public sector institutions to tax reductions for locating in special US territories.[3] The legal and policy framework has made it possible for the major companies to consistently remain among the top financial performers of all industrial branches, irrespective of whether profitability is measured by return on revenues or on assets. Despite recent legal and development problems, the pharmaceutical industry's net revenues averaged close to 30 per cent of shareholders' equity, remaining one of the leading industries in the annual ranking of *Forbes* magazine. Large legal departments ensure that nobody infringes on the patents. Furthermore they try to prolong them by applying for additional patents for innovations that can be added on to the make-up of the existing drug.

For an industry that is faced with high fixed costs for R&D, mergers and acquisitions to reach ever larger economies of scale are a must. As a consequence, the concentration of the industry has accelerated in the last two decades.[4] While there were still over thirty major pharmaceutical companies engaged in R&D in the 1980s, the number has shrunk to about half of that, all of them concentrating on the goal to invent, produce and sell a 'blockbuster', that is, a drug which reaches annual sales of over US$1 billion.[5]

Table 3.1 Vulnerable giants: sales, market value and R&D expenditures of the large pharmaceutical companies (in US$ billion)

Rank	*Name*	*Sales 2004 (a)*	*Market value*		*R&D spending*
			2000	**2004**	
1.	Pfizer	45.2 (51.1)	290	201	7.5
2.	GlaxoSmithKline	30.6 (32.8)	178	145	4.5
3.	Sanofi-Aventis	25.0 (27.4)	49	128	4.0
4.	Johnson&Johnson	21.8 (24.7)	146	200	4.7
5.	Merck	21.7 (23.9)	216	71	3.8
6.	AstraZeneca	21.4 (21.7)	89	69	3.4
7.	Novartis	20.9 (22.9)	128	131	3.8
8.	Roche/Genentech	15.7 (17.8)	91	112	4.0
9.	Bristo-Myers Squibb	14.9 (15.6)	146	50	2.5
10	Eli Lilly	13.1 (13.7)	105	66	2.6
11.	Wyeth	13.1 (14.3)	83	58	2.1
12.	Abbot Labs	11.2 (14.3)	75	75	1.6
13.	Amgen	10.4	n.a.	n.a.	1.9
14	Takeda	10.4	n.a.	n.a.	1.1
15.	Schering-Plough	6.3 (6.9)	83	29	1.6
16.	Bayer	5.6 (6.4)	39	25	1.1
Total		287.3 (314.3)	1718	1360	50.2

Sources: IMS Health; Thompson Data Stream, ECONOMIST, June 2005.
Note: (a) sales data are for prescription medicines and generics, numbers in brackets include OTC sales; if healthcare products and diagnostics are included, some companies such as Bayer and Roche easily doubled their total sales in 2004.

As Table 3.1 indicates, the sixteen largest research-oriented pharmaceutical companies had annual sales averaging US$18 billion in 2004, with some of their major products bringing in over US$1 billion per year. The statistics on the market value of those companies' stocks, however, reveal that the majority of them have faced significant buyers' sell-offs in the recent past, reflecting the growing competition from the generic industries, the problem of negative side-effects showing up only after their drugs had been pushed on to the market too soon, and the increasing wave of informal marketing channels at discount prices, of which the Canadian imports into the US are only the most prominent example.[6]

An increasing portion of pharmaceuticals are generics that enter the markets at significantly lower prices once the patents are terminated. Their production was fostered by the 1984 Hatch-Waxman Act, which allows the producers of generics access to the research results and the long series of tests of the R&D companies in order to be ready for their own production once the patent has been terminated.[7] Other countries followed with similar legislation, and recent examples of more intense competition can be found everywhere.

The rise of pharmaceutical production in the South

Production of generic pharmaceuticals in the South is mainly taking place in the larger industrializing economies and is undertaken in both private and public sector firms. In Brazil, for example, patented products are imported or receive only the final touches by the TNPCs' local plants. Legal generics are just beginning to establish themselves and have reached market shares of merely 10 per cent. An estimated 40 per cent of pharmaceutical consumption is still being produced in several small and some large local plants and are called 'similars', that is, unauthorized copies of patented drugs. It is this part of production which the TNPCs have been fighting against by arguing that they are not only violating patents but that they are also potentially dangerous to patients.[8] Indeed, both industry and independent sources estimate that counterfeit drugs make up 25 per cent of medicines sold in developing countries, with specific drug counterfeits reaching 40 per cent in some Latin American and Asian markets.[9]

Production, distribution and exports of generics have been more important in India and China than in the advanced Latin American countries. By declaring patents valid only for processes rather than products, India's major pharmaceutical companies have achieved specialized manufacturing capabilities through reverse engineering, by producing generic drugs from antibiotics to Viagra, including medication against AIDS. While the fourteen leading companies' sales only reached US$2.9 billion in 2003, or about 1 per cent of the above-mentioned TNPCs, the plants of India's leading firms have become significant suppliers of active ingredients for the European and US generic industries, receiving export revenues of over US$1.5 billion during the same year.[10]

Most of the drugs sold in other developing countries have also been copied from patented medication without the local producer holding a licence from the original producer of the drug. While the amount of sales was too small to really hurt the big TNPCs in the past, they have actively supported the introduction of new and tougher IPRs legislation in the developing world for years, and they were partly successful when, with the TRIPS agreement, IPRs became an important part of the Uruguay Round Agreements that led to the establishment of the WTO.

As a consequence of the vast number of different suppliers, international price comparisons of the very same drug are difficult to make, even before the multiple interventions of governments and/or insurance companies enter into the picture. Nevertheless, there is the 'WHO Model List of Essential Medicines', which not only provides specific classification of each drug but also information about its availability and price. Moreover, the CSO Médecins Sans Frontières (MSF) has been doing research on the prices of important drugs against major diseases in developing countries, the results of which are regularly posted on the internet (MSF 2004).

R&D efforts to cure new and traditional diseases

As Table 3.1 has indicated, the major TNPCs' annual outlays for R&D average over US$3 billion, making up 17 per cent of their sales. These expenditures are a significant amount both in absolute and relative terms, and are routinely used by the industry representatives in their defence of the high prices they cover for innovator drugs. While the industry's quoted cost of each new drug development amounting to US$800 million has been questioned,[11] there is no doubt that the R&D outlays have advanced rapidly in the last fifteen years, reaching close to US$106 billion in 2004 (Global Forum for Health Research 2004: xi), which was triple the size of fifteen years earlier. However, what has perplexed the industry and the public is that the results in terms of new products and licences have not caught up with the expenditures but in fact show a declining trend, falling from an average of forty in the mid-1990s to less than thirty in the earlier years of this decade, as illustrated in Figure 3.1. There seem to be several reasons to assume that, in spite of proceeding at an ever increasing pace of R&D, the industry has been losing ground in providing the public with innovative products. Among them, the more important problems appear to be:

- Essential drugs against killer diseases like diphtheria and tetanus with relatively simple cause-and-effect relationships have been developed and are on the market. Diseases like cancer and HIV/AIDS are more complicated and harder to fight, requiring substantially more R&D resources.
- The deciphering of the human gene promises great advances in the future, but the change from scientific research to practical application is requiring many more years than originally anticipated.
- Extensive marketing has put the R&D departments in a position to produce ever more effective medication, which has required larger inputs of human and financial resources per unit of output than used in the past.

Higher research outlays require more liquid funds, which the companies get from the capital markets. Investors in those markets follow closely the industry's development quarter by quarter, looking at the production and

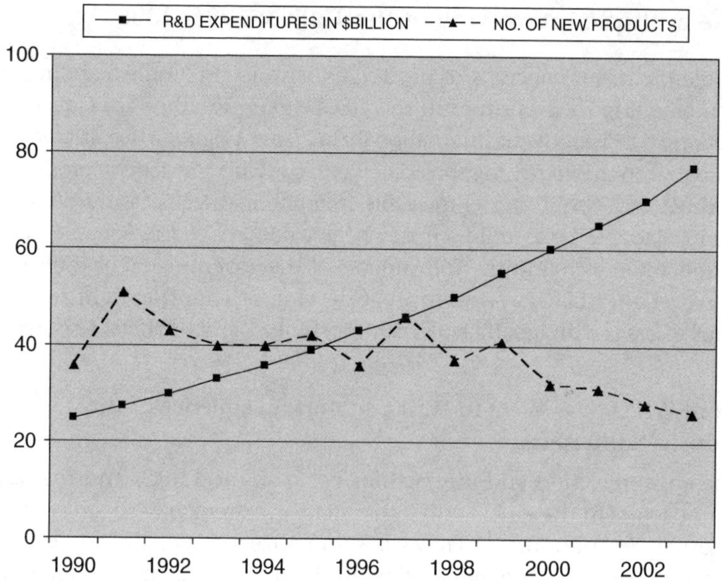

Figure 3.1 R&D outlays and new pharmaceutical products
Source: European Federation of Pharmaceutical Industries and Associations, Yearbook 2004.

pipeline of profitable products that sell in the rich countries. Under this institutional set-up there is little incentive for the industry to engage in large-scale research of medication required by the developing countries (DCs). As a consequence, only thirteen new medicines for tropical diseases entered the market between 1975 and 1999, at a time when the industry licensed nearly 1400 new chemical entities worldwide (Trouiller et al. 2002). Most of the major pharmaceutical companies had closed their research labs for tropical and other diseases affecting poor people in the 1980s and 1990s: the rate of return was too low (Neukirchen 2004: 215). At the same time there has been a rapid upturn in the transmission of infectious diseases, which were expected to be under control for some time. One example is tuberculosis. About one third of the world's population is currently infected with the mycobacterium tuberculosis, with two million people dying every year. Many strains of the bacterium have become resistant against one or more antibiotics, which were once hailed as an effective weapon to wipe the illness off the planet. Similar problems have occurred in the case of dengue fever and malaria, two well-known tropical diseases affecting over 360 million people each year, most of whom live in the developing countries (WHO 2001b).[12]

The multiple interfacing of the TNPCs: 1995–2006

While the major concerns of the TNPCs have focused on expanding and strengthening their position in the OECD countries, they have also been working consistently on internationalizing patent rights. Their strategy has been to stop the increasing spread of illegal copying and generic production of drugs by introducing enforceable international legislation around the world. Those efforts would seem to be a legitimate and reasonable undertaking and also found the full support of the governments of the North. However, they failed to convince the developing countries fighting infectious diseases with insufficient scientific, human and financial resources.

From WIPO over WTO to WHO: summary sequence of the industry's interfaces

The ensuing action and interactions between the TNPCs and the other major actors in the global and national health arena have been analysed in other contributions.[13] They are summarized below, and some of the 'deadly games' are then discussed in detail. In principle, there were numerous encounters, some memorable and others not. Most occurred at the time the HIV/AIDS virus spread around the globe and were part and parcel of the worldwide discussion to fight the disease, with governments in DCs trying to take on the responsibility and costs of prevention and treatment. Here are the major events and their perceived outcomes:

- Overture: The TNPCs and other hi-tech industries receive government support in OECD countries for strengthening international IPRs in international organizations such as the World Intellectual Property Organization (WIPO).
- *Act 1*: Initiated by the TNPCs, the North practises regime-shifting from WIPO to TRIPS promising more effective enforcement of IPR rules through potential trade sanctions (Game 1: TNPCs win without serious opposition).
- The South's response to TRIPS: they negotiate on the use of safeguard clauses resulting in the Doha Declaration of 2001. The North fights to keep the use of safeguard clauses as restricted as possible, prolonging and delaying discussions on the crucial paragraph 6 of the Declaration and Article 31 of the TRIPS agreement, which nevertheless led to amendment of TRIPS in 2005 (Game 2: while officially a draw, the compromise was considered a loss by TNPCs because of 'soft' evasion clauses).

- *Act 2*: TNPCs go to court in South Africa to fight against a law that allows domestic production of generics, but decide to withdraw under pressure of transnational public opinion and CSO action (Game 3: TNPCs lose decisively).
- Negotiation with Brazil on ARVs that lead to steep price reductions, despite calls for the USTR to threaten legal action at WTO (Game 4: another resounding loss for TNPCs).
- *Act 3*: The TNPCs support the formation of global public–private partnerships (GPPPs) and increase involvement in fighting neglected diseases (Game 5: outcome too early to tell; while possibly used and abused for public relations, it may become a win-win situation).
- A second regime shifting of the North and increased emphasis on bilateral trade agreements with legislation going beyond the TRIPS agreement (TRIPS+) (Game 6: won by the North and TNPCs against considerable but unsuccessful CSO opposition).
- *Act 4*: The South/CSOs respond with own 'regime shifting' of IPR issues from the WTO back to WIPO by introducing development agenda (Game 7: uncertain outcome, with little chance of adoption without major changes).
- Simultaneous introduction of medical R&D treaty (Global Framework on Essential Health Research) into the WHO, amplifying the worldwide discussion on the use and abuse of patents and access to knowledge (Game 8 is controversial, but could produce more than two winners and with it an increasing amount of lives that can be saved and/or improved).

These events took place between 1995 and 2006, many of which are also highlighted in the other chapters of this book.[14] What is unique in this case is that the TNPCs were both directly and indirectly not only the major actors in the fight over prices of the ARVs against AIDS, but were also responsible for the introduction and negotiations of TRIPS and TRIPS+ in the bilateral treaties, although those were officially purely governmental interfaces. Their involvements in turn were based on the fact that TNCs have not only vast financial resource-based power, but also have become increasingly involved in decision-making and formal norm-setting of GHG.[15]

As a consequence, the TNPCs found themselves in a number of interfaces, ranging from legal ones like the encounters with the South African government in the country's courts, to organizational ones, which entailed the drafting of the TRIPS legislation and its discussion with the US Trade Representative, to resource transfer-based interfaces occurring in the fight over drug pricing with Brazil and increased efforts to support R&D of neglected diseases. They were also involved in discoursive interfaces, both through their major associations on the national and international level (PhRMA and IFPMA) and also via top executives of the major companies taking part in key discussions with public and other private partners and opponents. With the TNPCs using their vast financial resources quite extensively on all fronts, most of the encounters were really a combination of at least two or three of those types of interfaces. By putting too much emphasis on the legal interfaces at the beginning of the discourse on access to medicine in poor countries, they did not get the expected results, as they admitted quite openly afterwards.[16]

Big Pharma's strategies for and beyond the market

Analysts of the pharmaceutical industry have long used game theory in their strategic advice to management. In deciding among alternative research projects, which not only face a significant risk of failure but also the possibility of strong competition even after many years of successful R&D, management was well advised to use this approach to help them choose which projects to sponsor and which to drop or delay.[17] In the case of internationalizing IPRs, the TNPCs chose the regime-shifting strategy, which they considered secure since it had the backing of the US government. That strategy did seem to work out well at the beginning, when the shift of a new legal and enforceable base for IPRs from WIPO to WTO was accomplished without major opposition, as highlighted in Figure 3.2.

By simultaneously pressing for the internationalization of IPRs at WIPO, into which the US government introduced the Sustained Patent Treaty, attaining a successful introduction and legislation of the TRIPS agreement at WTO, and insisting on even tougher IPR regulations (TRIPS+) in various bilateral treaties, Northern governments in general and the US Trade Representative in particular followed the script designed and proposed by the hi-tech TNCs, among which the TNPCs played a crucial role.[18]

Once accepted, the WTO's Secretariat was quick to point out that 'TRIPS attempts to strike a balance between the long term social objective of providing incentives for future inventions and creation, and the short term objective of allowing people to use existing inventions and creations' (WTO 2003: 1). Many of the developing countries saw it differently. Respected free-trade advocates like Jagdish Bhagwati described the WTO's intellectual property protection as a tax that most poor countries pay on their use of knowledge, 'constituting an unrequited transfer to the rich producing countries' (Sexton 2001: 10).

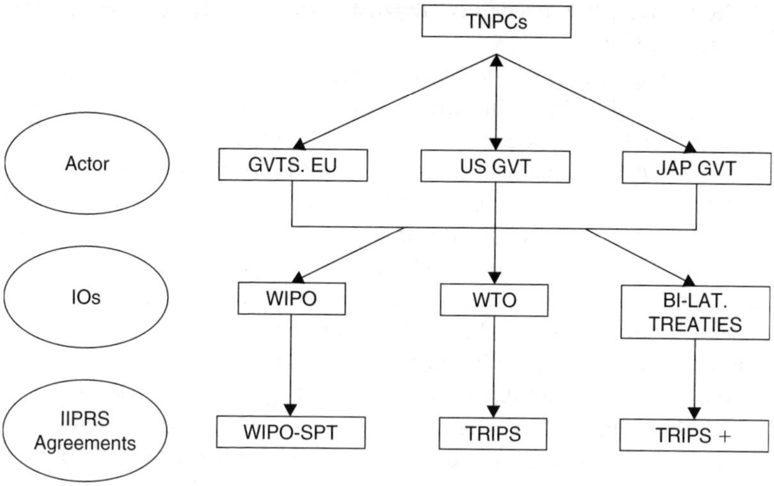

Figure 3.2 Internationalizing patent rights as proposed by the North
Source: Own graphic.

HIV/AIDS, Doha and the battle over drug prices

It was the rapid spread of the HIV/AIDS virus in developing countries that made officials in both the developed and developing countries realize that the stringent conditions of the IPRs in the TRIPS agreement made it nearly impossible to treat even a minority of patients in the developing economies. As a consequence, discussions of how to ensure that poor countries would have access to low-cost medicines in the case of serious diseases endangering the public health of those nations got underway in the late 1990s and led to the Doha Ministerial Declaration on the TRIPS Agreement and Public Health in November 2001.[19]

Game strategies of the TNPCs and Brazil over the pricing of ARVs

Before the negotiations over the TRIPS amendment in the halls of the WTO in Geneva became ever more entwined in the definition and interpretation of specific clauses and paragraphs, the real battles had already taken place in the marketplace for ARVs. As Latin America's leading industrializing country, Brazil had an ongoing discussion with the US government regarding the enactment and implementation of full-blown legislation covering patents. This issue became a major point of contention when the government-owned generic industry started producing two of the twelve ARVs needed by Brazil to effectively treat its HIV/AIDS-infected patients.

The federal and some local government authorities had become seriously involved in initiating the production of ARVs in the late 1990s. During that time period, Brazil had already managed to cut mortality rates of AIDS by half, lower the hospitalization of the victims by 80 per cent and reduce the mother-to-child transmission significantly (Bacon et al. 2004; Ministério de Saúde 2005b). Since the Brazilian government provided the treatments free of charge to every patient in need, the case for lowering the public sector costs of the patented ARV medicines became a priority for Brazilian policy-makers.

Encouraged by the willingness of the North to confirm Southern rights for issuing compulsory licences in the case of a national emergency, Brazil entered into negotiations with a number of TNPCs to ask them for significant price reductions or face the threat of the country issuing compulsory licences. That encounter itself led to a perfect game scenario with possible moves and countermoves, containing considerable downward risks on both sides should they lose the battle. For the Brazilian challenger, there were considerations beyond the payments of royalties for the licence, starting with a serious test of the production capability and cost containment of its government-owned laboratories, and ending with the availability and costs of the required ingredients. For the TNPCs, the adherence to their stipulated high prices meant facing the possibility of the firms being shut out from a large and growing market of a major emerging economy and the undesirability of setting a precedent for compulsory licences detested by most TNPCs. Cohen and Lybecker (2005) have developed a scenario borrowed from simple game theory, which reflects well the options one of the TNPCs faced by bargaining with the Brazilian government authorities. A slightly changed version of their diagrammatic presentation is depicted in Figure 3.3.

It is fairly easy for the TNPCs to realize that it would be foolish to immediately opt for a large discount, especially since the companies are believed to have the US government's support. On the other hand, while it might have been possible to bluff and hang tough, believing that the issue of compulsory licensing is even more distasteful to the Brazilians than it is to the industry, it might be the best strategy to start with a relatively small discount, which will not have the best outcome (after all, X is less favourable than W but better than Y and Z), but may find Brazil's willingness to agree, since that outcome is at least second best for the country (B is worse than A but better than C). In case Brazil rebuffs

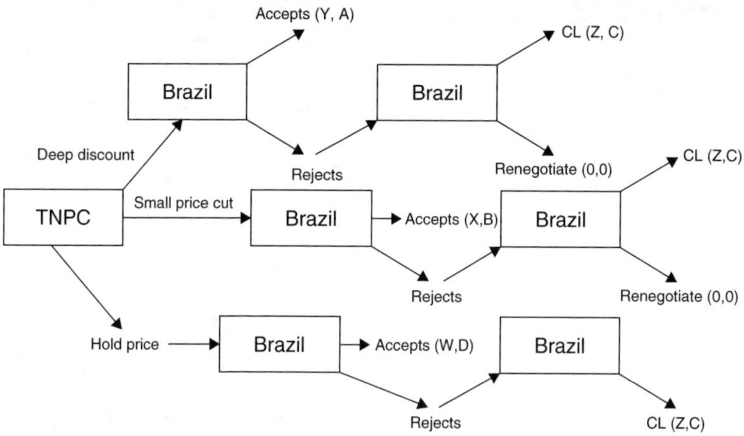

Figure 3.3 Price bargaining for prescriptions
Source: Graphic modified from Cohen and Lybecker (2005: 220).

the offer of a small discount, further negotiations would seem a probable outcome rather than an immediate issuing of a compulsory licence.

What is missing here are the probabilities attached to the expected reaction of the Brazilian policy-makers and with it the outcome of the game. Clearly, the large discount would have a fairly high probability of being accepted, but would leave no room for any further manoeuvres to improve the outcome for the TNPC. On the other hand, the probability of the government's willingness to return to the bargaining table with the TNPC remaining unwilling to give in an inch would also be high and lead directly to the issuing of a compulsory licence. So to start with a relatively small price reduction would seem not only to provide both parties with intermediate outcomes and room for further negotiations, but it would also appear to be the choice with the highest probability attached.

The actual negotiation between Brazil and Hoffmann-La Roche over the ARV Nefivanir did indeed take that route. The company started off with a 13 per cent price reduction, which the government of Brazil rejected. At the same time as the state-owned Far-Manguinhos prepared for the production of that medication, the health minister asked the company to cut prices by 40 per cent. Roche replied with a 30 per cent discount, but saw its situation further weakened by other TNPCs granting significantly larger price reductions, with Merck leading the pack by offering reductions of over 60 per cent for its patented ARV (Rich 2001; Cohen and Lybecker 2005).

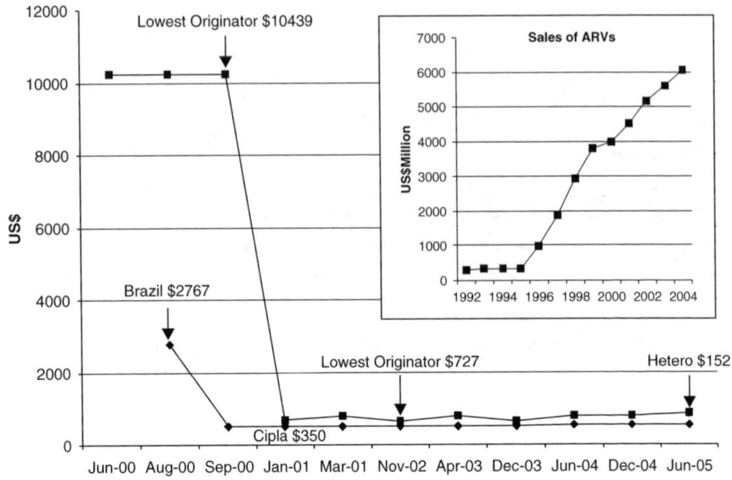

Figure 3.4 Patents, the rise of generics and their impact on prices and sales of ARVs
Source: Drafted from statistical sources of MSF, IMS Health (2005: 5 and 11).

The breakthrough on the domestic front of pharmaceutical production came in August 2000, when Brazilian firms were able to produce some crucial generics that cut treatment costs per person by 70 per cent, enabling the health service agencies to treat up to three times the patients they had been able to during the early and mid-1990s. As Figure 3.4 indicates, that breakthrough and the ensuing negotiations with the multinational companies, which the Brazilian health minister threatened with the issue of compulsory licences unless prices were cut sharply, occurred in 2001. The production of cheaper generics in India decreased the annual treatment costs to even lower levels, apparently without stopping the continuous rise in total sales revenues of ARVs.

Three additional factors contributed to Roche eventually giving more generous price reductions. First, the earlier unsuccessful attack by the TNPCs in the South African High Court against Medicine and Related Substances Control Amendment Act had led to the TNPCs' eventual withdrawal under the strong protest of the international health community, especially by CSOs such as Oxfam and MSF. Secondly, the continued public pressure of both the local and international civil society converged in Brazil to a powerful movement, encouraging health minister Serra to ride the wave of popular support by challenging the TNPCs, and with it increase his chances as a presidential candidate. Thirdly, the TNPCs' trump card to have the US government and/or the EU invoke trade sanctions to have Brazil punished for being in conflict with Article 27 of the TRIPS agreement (non-discrimination), and legislation of its own concerned about industrial rather than human life protection,[20] failed. The US Trade Representative withdrew its complaints against Brazil at the WTO in mid-2001 and agreed to a mutually acceptable compromise with the country.

The success on the national front encouraged Brazil and the CSOs also to play an increasingly more active and demanding role on the global health arena. The outcomes were realized in two initiatives at WIPO and WHO. After successfully renegotiating TRIPS, the developing countries, under the leadership of Argentina, Brazil and Kenya, introduced a 'Development Agenda' into WIPO's General Assembly, hoping to provoke further discussion of the value and the best timing of IPR legislation in developing countries. At the same time, those countries took up a plan from one of the CSOs concerning the change of patent rights in light of the need to increase not only the people's access to medicines at reasonable prices but also to liberalize the access to knowledge in general.

The TNPCs' counteroffensive: new initiatives and further regime-shifting

At the time of the conclusion of the TRIPS agreement, the US Trade Representative had also begun to introduce strict IPR legislation into bilateral trade treaties, starting with the NAFTA agreement and continuing with a number of trade negotiations, which resulted in very similar outcomes and strengthened IPRs beyond the compromises reached at the WTO. The TNPCs played an indirect though important role in the bilateral trade agreements. In addition, they reacted more forcefully on other fronts of developing countries' concerns after the public attacks and surprising losses against the major players of the South. Among others, more resources were committed and spent on research for vaccines and treatment of the 'neglected diseases'.

TNPCs support of the North's second round of regime-shifting

The strengthening of the original TRIPS to become TRIPS+ was the basis for almost all trade negotiations the US Trade Representative undertook either with individual countries or a group of countries in the South. In the case of Latin America, the pressure put on the small countries 'south of the border' became particularly severe and provides a good example of the continuous strength of the discoursive interfacing of TNPCs with the US government authorities. Negotiations between the

US Trade Representative and the five Central American economies plus the Dominican Republic lasted for well over three years. Although trade with those economies make up only a fraction of the overall US exports and imports, President George W. Bush made it a major policy issue and lobbied Congress for the passing of the bill. While the usual interest groups of the agricultural sector (sugar, cattle) and industry (textiles) were the major opponents and nearly had the bill toppled, the IPR issues in general and the patents legislation in particular became important points in the debate of the House of Representatives.

Supported by assessments from Oxfam and MSF, the Committee on Government Reform prepared a report for a number of Congress members who had been fighting the excessive influence of the pharmaceutical industry in government for some time (US House of Representatives, Committee on Government Reform 2005). That report stipulates the major concerns, which were found in most IPRs negotiated in other free trade agreements the US has recently undertaken.[21] These concerns are also taken up by the UNCTAD ICTSD Project on Intellectual Property and Sustainable Development.

The number one issue includes restrictions on compulsory licensing, which limit the circumstances under which the Central American Common Market (CACM) countries (and also most other nations negotiating free trade agreements with the US) can issue the compulsory licences authorizing generic manufacturers to produce low-cost versions of patented drugs. Closely related to it is the prohibition of parallel importation, preventing developing countries from importing patented drugs from the most favourable available source. The other two issues revolve around the extension of patent protection for new uses of already patented products and the requirements to have the drug regulatory authorities in the CACM countries adjudicate patents despite their lack of expertise in the area of patent enforcement.

On the other hand, there are no provisions that would promote greater access to affordable medicines, such as the 'Bolar-type' provision to ensure that countries permit testing and experimental work required for the registration of a generic medicine during the patent period of the original product so that generics can enter the market immediately after the expiration of the patent. Neither are there requirements for patent holders to disclose the 'best mode' for reproducing an invention so that society can benefit from it after the patent expires. Finally, there are no caps on patent extensions for delays in the issuance of a patent or the marketing approval process. The report concludes: 'Taken together, these trade provisions will significantly impede the ability of developing countries to obtain access to inexpensive, life-saving medications. Contrary to the Doha Declaration, these provisions in the trade agreements advance the financial interests of large multinational drug companies at the expense of the developing world's ability to address public health problems' (US House of Representatives, Committee on Government Reform 2005: 5).

Addressing R&D needs for drugs and vaccines against neglected diseases

Learning from the clashes with South Africa and Brazil and their impact on world opinion and civil society action, the pharmaceutical companies have been engaged in an increasing number of partnerships, both with public agencies and CSOs to fight infectious diseases. In the case of HIV/AIDS, eighteen of these networks were active in October 2004, and in the case of tuberculosis and malaria there were eight and eleven respectively (IFPMA 2004b). Table 3.2 provides an overview of some of the PPPs in which the companies are involved that concern medication for and vaccines against HIV/AIDS.[22]

The first results of R&D activities undertaken in the area of neglected diseases by large and small pharmaceutical companies as well as by PPPs have now been evaluated. In a 2005 report entitled *The New Landscape of Neglected Disease Drug Development*, researchers at the LSE Health and Social Care Unit report that the ongoing debate over the lack of R&D for those neglected diseases no longer holds true (Moran et al. 2005). Between 2000 and 2004 over sixty projects have tackled these neglected diseases. Two new drugs are now at the registration phase and eighteen new products in clinical trials, half of which are at the final stage.

The TNPCs are conducting about 50 per cent of those projects, half of which they are carrying out on their own and the other half within a PPP.[23] Even in the case of their own research, the idea is to finally test and market the product together with public partners because of the public sector characteristics of the markets for those medications. Moran et al. (2005) found that of the US$250 million funding spent without market incentives to support the PPPs, only 16 per cent came from governments, while the Gates Foundation alone has contributed nearly 60 per cent of the funds.

It is still premature to provide a comprehensive evaluation of those efforts, since most of them have only started recently. Some public sector involvement has led to high administrative costs and poor management of such programmes. The legal status, corporate governance and operational efficiency are issues which will have to be analysed in some detail before well-founded judgement can be made. However, for the pharmaceutical companies participating in the PPPs, one would expect an efficient

Table 3.2 Examples of pharmaceutical firms' involvement in public–private partnerships against HIV/AIDS

Programme	***Pharmaceutical firm***	***Partner***	***Public health objective***
ACADEMIC ALLIANCE for AIDS CARE and PREVENTION in AFRICA (AAACP)	Pfizer	Makarere University, Uganda	Training of medical personnel in HIV/AIDS
Accelerating Access Initiative (AAI)	Abbott, Boehringer-Ingelheim, Bristol-Myers Squibb, GSK, Gilead Sciences, Merck, F. Hoffmann–La Roche	UNAIDS, WHO, UNICEF, UN Population Fund, World Bank	Preferential pricing of retrovirals for prevention and treatment of AIDS
DIFLUCAN® PARTNERSHIP PROGRAMME	Pfizer	Governments and CSOs in Africa, Asia, the Caribbean and Latin America	Donation of its antifungal medicine, Diflucan®
GLAXOSMITHKLINE'S POSITIVE ACTION ON HIV/AIDS	GlaxoSmithKline	Community-based organizations around the world	Capacity building, strategic management, leadership, advocacy
SECURE THE FUTURE®	Bristol-Myers Squibb and the Bristol-Myers Squibb Foundation	Government leadership and local organizations in southern and western Africa	Food security and poverty alleviation; epidemiological and medical research in HIV/AIDS
International AIDS Vaccine Initiative (IAVI)	Merck, Phizer	Governments, foundations, World Bank, other corporations	Development of safe, effective, accessible, preventive HIV vaccine

Source: IFPMA (2004a: 13).

execution of the commitments undertaken combined with the necessary supply logistics, storage and documentation.

With respect to health outcomes, the PPP model showed better results than the medication developed by the industry alone. While it is still too early to tell, the rapidly increasing PPPs may under certain circumstances become a major provider for low-cost medicines against the formerly neglected diseases.[24] However, critical issues like the sustainability of these efforts, the consequences of the proliferation of PPPs, and their potential use for purely public relations purposes must be taken into account (Caines 2004; Ollilla 2003; Richter 2004).

Resulting impact of interfaces with national and global health governance

The South African and Brazilian fights against HIV/AIDS in general and the confrontations between the government authorities and the TNPCs in particular not only present a most interesting example of 'public vs. private' conflict and its resolution in the global health arena, they also highlight the incredible amount of actions and interactions that have taken place and are still occurring among official and unofficial representatives on the local, regional national, and – particularly in this case – on the global level.[25]

TNPCs and the global health architecture

A broader perspective of how the increasing responses of the South interacted with the initiatives of the North is provided in Figure 3.5, which brings together the multiple interfaces among the major actors in the health arena today. From earlier discussions regarding the TNPCs' interactions with and influences on the governments of the North in pressing for internationalizing IPRs in various fora and the response from the developing countries to fight for an amendment on TRIPS and introduce new initiatives at WIPO and the WHO, it has become clear that those major pillars of the global health architecture have changed substantially.

They will continue to do so in the near future. While neither the TNPCs nor the CSOs belong to those 'pillars', their actions and interactions have played a major role in bringing about the change of such venerable institutions as the WHO and World Bank, the WIPO and the WTO, the latter two of which would not have imagined becoming part of wide-ranging discussions and decisions concerning global health issues fifteen years ago.

The confrontation and dialogue between the Northern and Southern representatives have not been limited to exchanging legal opinions and

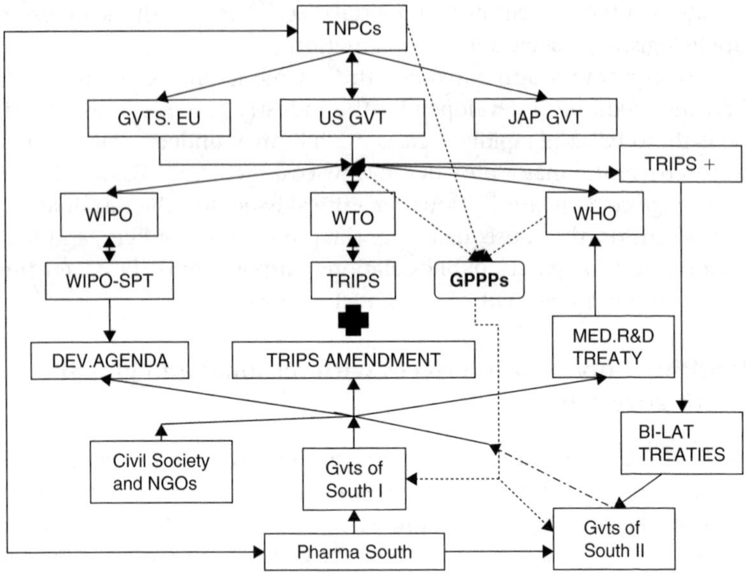

Figure 3.5 TNPCs and global health governance in the making 1995–2005
Source: own figure.

issuing threats, but have taken place on many other levels, both formally and informally. In addition to the discussion within the IGOs and in the government buildings in New York, Geneva, Washington, Brasilia and New Delhi, there were numerous meetings where senior representatives of the WTO, the respective governments, the TNPCs and the CSOs discussed the major issues.

One example was a 2001 conference sponsored by the Foreign Policy Centre in London, the report of which (Walters et al. 2001) stated that

> despite dissonance over many of the fundamentals, the seminar opened several doors for potential solutions among which were:
>
> - The introduction of a tiered patenting system
> - Increased flexibility of TRIPS for developing countries
> - The creation of an international fund to support the consolidation of health systems in those parts of the developing world hardest hit by the AIDS virus.

By 2004, two of these proposals were translated into reality. The Doha Declaration gave a wider and much more flexible interpretation of the

TRIPS agreements and the Global Fund to Fight AIDS, Tuberculosis and Malaria (GF) had been installed to grant financing for prevention and treatment programmes against those diseases in the affected developing countries. In the meantime, experts of intellectual property rights are rethinking some of the rules written into the legislation of both the developed and developing countries, and the multinationals are trying to figure out how to manage a multitiered pricing system, which benefits the poor in the developing countries but not traders who re-export the discounted drugs to the high priced markets of developed countries.

With all the heat created over the pricing of drugs, exemplified by the number of proponents fighting the TNCs over monopoly rights, participants of the debate tend to forget or to play down the fact that drug prices are but one part of the story, as many poor countries have discovered when they had to administer the ARV therapy. Similar to earlier statements of industry representatives and their associations, Adelman et al. (2004: 1) brought home the point that 'ARV therapy is only effective if there is a healthcare infrastructure – doctors, nurses, clinics, supplies, storage and distribution systems. This infrastructure is often lacking in developing countries, where the majority of the AIDS victims live.' Even in the narrower confinement concerning the supply of essential medicines, price is only one variable. Without strategic procurement, improved logistics and training of pharmacists, the reliable supply of drugs cannot be guaranteed. As a consequence, the OECD countries and the multilateral institutions have committed an increasing amount of resources to support programmes which provide the necessary framework.

In spite of these efforts there is a remaining gap between the demand for and supply of AIDS medication. The development of the national, state and local social infrastructure will take time. The fight against HIV/AIDS continues, but while proper treatment is increasing, recent information indicates just how far the vast majority of the countries are away from treating many of the current victims. With the exception of Latin America, where close to two thirds of the population infected by HIV receive treatment, the reach to victims in other regions of the world is considerably smaller, with estimates setting the treatment coverage to between 11 and 14 per cent of the infected adult population (see: www.avert.org/aidsdrugs.htm 2006).

Conclusion: back to the future

In the meantime, the major TNPCs have joined forces with the other major actors in developing countries as had been predicted thirty years ago by

Perlmutter. The latter visualized a gradual shift that TNCs would have to make from directing international trade solely in their own best interest to adjusting to and coordinating with the growing priorities of nation-states and civil society (Perlmutter 1972). Many of those predictions were indeed part and parcel of the TNPCs' strategies and have been evident in their behaviour during the last three decades of the 1900s. However, some have been hastened by the challenges the firms faced from other actors in the health arena and the rapid changes of GHG in the last ten years.

Because of their amazing accuracy, it may be interesting to summarize Perlmutter's ideas at this point. The first set of observations pertaining to the 1980s are still perceived as the area of worldwide dominance by the TNCs and follow from an analysis of the strategies and impact the multinational enterprises had on the world economy during the 1960s and 1970s.[26] In the context of further concentration of firms and increased global reach, the second set of observations foresaw an increasing, tougher environment for all TNCs, which would have to prove their mettle in a number of innovative moves, facing challenges not only from national governments, but also unions, consumer associations, and other new interest groups within civil society.

For the TNCs' international investments to continuously engage in profitable business, it meant not only an increase in the transfer of capital but also technology, as well as an improvement of efficiency and economic performance of local businesses taken over by the TNCs. At the same time, Perlmutter maintained that policy-makers in developing countries would be pressing the companies to increase the host country's competitiveness and provide further employment and training. While a lot has been researched and written on the TNCs' contribution towards the latter four goals in developing countries, the pharmaceutical firms have hardly been engaged in either taking over local business or transferring technology. Being a research-intensive sector, only some of them are sharing research on tropical diseases in the few centres described above (Table 3.2).

The first order of any business is to make profits, and the pharmaceuticals seem to have championed that cause by making sure first and foremost that the emerging competitors in the major markets play by the rules, that is, respect patent rights. As has been shown, they have been pressuring and are succeeding in introducing patent rights into major developing country markets. In the case of HIV/AIDS, the TNPCs went one step further and narrowly fought for their 'monopoly rents' in the face of a worldwide pandemic, a costly mistake as the top executives admitted afterwards. As a consequence, they have not only lowered the prices and recently doubled their efforts in providing free medication, but also entertained an increasing number of new business models, among which the public–private partnership is only one. More often, there have been business alliances in both developed and developing countries, which combine the relative advantages of each type of enterprise.

In this context it is interesting to follow up with the final set of Perlmutter's predictions concerning the behaviour of TNCs towards people, ideas and resources, which can be expected to be most intensive in those regions and countries in which the TNCs have a significant share of foreign current and future production, and where the share of foreign employees and/or foreign shareholders is significant. In brief, the 1972 prognosis maintains that (a) the TNCs will enter into coalition with public entities, (b) the TNCs will entertain and then participate in joint research and development units and laboratories, and (c) there will be an increasing number of consortia and TNCs from the emerging economies. All three predictions have become or are becoming true in the case of the pharmaceutical industries, as was shown above. In addition, worldwide generic competition is putting the TNPCs under increasing pressure to lower prices or to launch their own generic brands. Attempts to come to terms with those rivals in special agreements have been attacked by ambitious attorney generals in various states.[27]

In sum, joint action and dialogue between the private sector companies, their associations and agencies representing or favouring the market system and its existing legal framework, and those within or outside government pursuing the welfare function are ongoing and will have to be dealt with not only on the global, but also the national and the local level. While a study on a very particular illness can only highlight the potential for progress in pursuing a generally accepted framework within the rules and commitments of global health governance, it would seem that the TNPCs' confrontations and disagreements with the developing countries have led from open conflict to compromise and even to cooperation in some undertakings.

The extent to which the pressure of civil society and of some of the leading developing countries will induce pharmaceutical production to yield an ample supply of low-cost medication for the poor as well as for the better-off around the world is open to question. It would seem that increased competition from the rapidly growing generic producers in the North and the South will be a more important force in enlarging supply and lowering prices. Last but not least, innovative legal interpretation and negotiations that bring about changes of intellectual property rights in general and patent rights in particular should provide a further impetus to limit monopoly pricing and rent seeking.

Notes

1. The terms 'North' and 'South' are used to characterize the dominant positions; it does not mean that *all* Northern and *all* Southern countries supported the respective positions.
2. Increased competition has narrowed the considerable differences among various international markets. We are still far from achieving a convergence to one price, but the globalization of markets is working in that direction among OECD countries. 'The ten oldest drugs, launched before 1988, are up to four times more expensive in America than elsewhere, the ten newest drugs, launched after 1997, are only twice the price' (*The Economist* 2005a: 12).
3. For a critical discussion of multiple incentives for Big Pharma in the US see Young and Surrusco (2001); *The Economist* (2005b); Abramson (2004).
4. In the last two decades of the twentieth century, there were close to fifty mergers in the pharmaceutical industry, valued at over US$1 billion, seventeen of which crossed the US$5 billion mark (Zeller 2001).
5. The most successful 'blockbuster' drug is Lipitor, an anti-cholesterol medication which provided its producer Pfizer with annual sales of over US$3 billion in 2004. Its patent is currently being challenged by India's largest manufacturer Rambaxy in various courts around the world. For a discussion on the battle in British courts see *The Washington Post*, 13 October 2005.
6. For a good summary of the major issues facing Big Pharma, with special emphasis on the problems in the largest and most profitable US market, see *The Economist*, 18 June 2005.
7. At the same time, the Hatch-Waxman Act also granted a number of benefits to the research-oriented pharmaceutical companies: among others longer time periods for patents (Angell 2004).
8. Clearly stated in a letter by PhRMA to the Office of the US Trade Representative on 15 February 2002.
9. For a summary review of the counterfeit problem, see Seiter (2005a).
10. *Financial Times*, 22 January 2004. The leading companies are Ranbaxy, Dr. Reddy's, Aurobindo and Lupin, ringing up 70 per cent of total Indian sales.
11. The US$800 million R&D spending on each new drug was taken from a Tuft's University study funded by the industry, which also supplied selected data from ten of their major firms. DiMasi et al. (2003) analysed the R&D costs of sixty-eight randomly chosen drugs (on the basis of data provided by the pharmaceutical industry). A thorough examination by the Public Citizen Congress Watch came to the conclusion that average R&D costs for each new product came closer to US$100 million during the late 1990s (Young and Surrusco 2001), a figure which DiMasi et al. (2004) again vehemently criticized. It should also be noted that the latest cost estimates for R&D in public–private partnerships are relatively low. Drugs developed by the TB Alliance for example, have been estimated to be between US$115 and $240 million (CIPIH/WHO 2006: 93f.). For a good account of the issue of serious public sector involvement in early drug research, see Goozner (2004).
12. The most recent changes in tackling these neglected diseases both within the industry and in the new institutional set-up of public–private partnerships will be discussed below. For research on PPPs, see Bartsch (2003); Buse and Walt (2000a, 2000b).

13. For the conflict between Brazil and the TNPCs, see Wogart and Calcagnotto (2006). For the discussion on TRIPS see Wogart and Hein (2006). For a broader background see Wogart (2006).
14. Besides Chapters 2, 4, 7 and 8, see Von Soest and Calcagnotto (2006) for most of the interfaces between the TNPCs and the Brazilian and South African government. For the discussion of TRIPS developments, see Wogart and Hein (2006).
15. For a discussion of the direct involvement of the TNCs in national and global politics, see Sell (2000) and Jawara and Kwa (2003).
16. *The Economist* (2005b).
17. See for example Senn (1996); 'Game Theory and Business Decisions', URL: http://faculty.haas.berkeley.edu/xuanming/147/.
18. For an extensive discussion of the TNPCs' role in drafting the TRIPS agreement, see Sell (2000).
19. Declaration on the TRIPS Agreement and Public Health (14 November 2001), DOC WT/MIN(01)/DEC2.
20. The US complaint against Brazilian legislation authorizing compulsory licences and parallel imports in cases where international patents were not executed in the domestic market within a time period of three years (UNCTAD/ICTSD 2005: 372).
21. These are mainly smaller countries, including Singapore, Jordan and Morocco, and hemispheric nations like Chile, Peru, Colombia and the Central American countries. The larger economies of Asia, such as Thailand, South Korea and the Philippines, were still negotiating in 2005/6, particularly the IPR part of the agreement.
22. In addition, a growing number of them are becoming very active in supporting the fight against malaria and TB as well as such tropical diseases as dengue fever; some have joined the Global Alliance to Eliminate Leprosy, the Sleeping Sickness Program and the International Trachoma Initiative. They are also actively participating in important initiatives against vaccine preventable diseases such as the Global Alliance for Vaccines and Immunization (GAVI) and the Vaccine Fund (VF). A good overview on partnerships in health is given by the various studies conducted by the DFID Health Resource Center in 2004.
23. Most of the work is done by four companies: GSK, Novartis, Astra-Zenica and Sanofi-Aventis.
24. Four country studies on the impact of PPPs in addressing the access to low-cost medicine issue provided some other encouraging findings (Caines and Lush 2004). While the researchers admitted that the quantification of benefits for public health derived from donation programmes such as AIDS medication to prevent mother-to-child transmission of HIV was difficult to establish, several indicators showed that the programme had led to favourable short-term results. A similar positive evaluation was given to the Joint Novartis WHO discounted drug programme for tropical diseases.
25. A more complete narrative of this process in Brazil has been treated in an earlier essay (Wogart and Calcagnotto 2006).
26. They include, among others, global exploitation of technological innovations, worldwide gathering of information on consumer needs and demands, education, training and mobilization of business leaders around the world, realization of worldwide exporting patterns reflecting 'comparative cost advantages', and contributions to nation-states' balance of payments and tax revenues.
27. For a discussion of that issue in the special case of the world's second biggest selling drug Plavix, see *The Economist*, 19 August 2006: 48–9.

4
The Role of Civil Society Organizations in Global Health Governance

Sonja Bartsch and Lars Kohlmorgen

Introduction

Civil society organizations (CSOs) have been around much longer than the current debate suggests, with the Anti-Slavery Society (1839) and the International Committee of the Red Cross (1863) being among the first CSOs to be established in the nineteenth century. Particularly in the field of health, CSOs have always played an important role in the provision of medical services or the realization of humanitarian relief, especially in the developing world. However, it can be observed that both the quantity and the quality of their activities as actors of global health governance (GHG) have increased since the 1980s. According to different studies (for example Anheier et al. 2004; UIA 2004) there are now approximately 3000 international CSOs that belong directly to the health sector (of approximately 51 000–59 000 international CSOs altogether).

This great number is closely related to the general changes in the economic and political sphere that are often subsumed under the term globalization. As observed in the previous chapters, these developments have led to a larger influence of international and transnational actors and an increasing relevance of private forms of regulation through non-state actors and hybrid forms of regulation through the cooperation of public and private actors. CSOs interact with other CSOs, governments and bureaucracies of nation-states both in the North and the South, bilateral donors, international governmental organizations (IGOs) and transnational corporations in the newly emerging structures of global health governance.

While the greater importance of non-state actors is a general characteristic of politics in the era of globalization, in many regards, non-state actors and CSOs play a more important role in the health sector than in other sectors of global politics. One general reason for this is the historical tradition of non-state actors' involvement in health affairs (due to private physicians, insurances, pharmaceutical companies, church-related organizations, and charity and relief organizations like the Red Cross Federation). This involvement increased particularly in developing countries in the process of political globalization and due to problems of IGOs in fulfilling some of their functions. Moreover, the role of CSOs refers to the ethical obligations that derive from the fact that millions of poor people are suffering and dying from diseases, which are not always curable but treatable in industrialized countries and which *could* be treated also in the developing world since effective drugs and measures exist. This ethical pressure, which also influences the activities of other actors, such as pharmaceutical companies and governments of industrialized countries, gives CSOs insisting on human rights a position in global health politics that enables them to exert pressure on the other actors and to influence policies (Bartsch and Kohlmorgen 2005b; Hein 2005).

In this chapter, we will address the various activities of CSOs in the health sector and scrutinize their patterns of interaction at the different interfaces in global health governance. For this purpose we will first discuss the concept of global civil society, address the special case of faith-based organizations (FBOs), and give a short overview on definitions and types of CSOs. We will then deal with the different types of activities of CSOs and distinguish between political, operational and self-empowerment functions. In order to capture the relationship between these functions and the interactions of CSOs with other actors of GHG at the different types of interfaces in more detail we will then look at three exemplary issues that are crucial for the fight against HIV/AIDS: the political conflicts around the access to ARVs in developing countries; the operational activities of NGOs and FBOs at country level; and the processes of empowerment of affected populations through self-help and support groups at local, national and global level.

Global civil society, civil society organizations and faith-based organizations

Before we deal with the role of civil society in global health governance, in the following we will briefly outline our understanding of the terms 'civil society', 'civil society organization', 'non-governmental organization' and 'faith-based organization'.

Civil society

Our understanding of the term civil society is not normative – establishing the roles civil society should fulfil – but analytical – describing and interpreting the activities we can observe. From this perspective, civil society is, next to state and economy, one of the three parts of society as a whole and thus refers to the sphere of ideas, norms, activities, institutions and individuals between state and market (Kaldor 2003: 6f.). It must be added, however, that these three spheres cannot always be explicitly separated, so that civil society is partly connected with and influenced by the two other spheres. Additionally, civil society is always characterized by power relations. Referring to Antonio Gramsci (1971), it can be said that civil society is an important arena where conflicts over the balance of power and strength between the different societal actors take place and where the political and economic power relations are culturally shaped and legitimized (Gramsci: creation of hegemony).

One can distinguish between national civil societies and global civil society. The latter can be interpreted as the societal sphere between (national and international) state-run institutions and the global market, which functions beyond the limitations of the national society (Anheier et al. 2001b: 17). Global civil society is more than the sum of national civil societies, as it develops its own inter- and transnational forms and structures of society that differ from the national. It is obvious that the social and political interactions in the global realm are not as dense as in the national sphere. However, particularly with regard to the increasing transnationalization of political and social interactions beyond state and market, it has become more and more reasonable to treat global civil society as a category on its own (Scholte 2000; Kaldor 2003, Keane 2003; Anheier et al. 2004; Hein 2005)

Civil society organizations

The term 'civil society organization', according to our understanding, refers to all non-state, non-profit and mostly voluntary organizations and initiatives that act in the political and social sphere of civil society. According to our remarks on global civil society we have to take into account that CSOs operate at different levels: some just work on the local or national level, whereas others are active at all governance levels. Moreover, many CSOs explicitly operate in the transnational/global realm without focusing on one particular country. However, they are characterized by a number of common features:

- organizationally and financially not dependent on governments;
- non-profit orientation;
- resource inflows on a voluntary basis and/or voluntary membership.

This definition excludes business associations from civil society although their activities do not directly aim at making profits. However, as most of their work is targeted on improving the political and economic conditions for companies to increase profits, they are seen here as belonging to the realm of for-profit organizations. Moreover, in some cases they do not generate their resource inflows on a voluntary basis, but have mandatory memberships, so they do not meet the third criterion either.

Thus far, however, the definition of CSOs is still rather broad. In the following we will therefore further differentiate between different types of CSOs (Kaldor 2003):

(a) *Social movements*: In the strict sense, social movements are not collective actors. They are rather informal networks of different organizations, groups of people and individuals, 'who act together to bring about transformation in society' (Kaldor 2003: 12). In doing so, they can take up the same stance on specific issues and pursue the same goals so that they can be perceived as collective actors when their activities are – in spite of their informality – accompanied by some organizational constancy at least for a certain phase. Social movements mostly focus on one particular issue. Often – and particularly in the field of global health – social movements act via campaigns and try to educate the public and to exert pressure on decision-making bodies and policy-makers. Social movements can be distinguished with respect to scope (radical–reformist), method of work (peaceful–violent) and degree of institutionalization (spontaneous, situational, and loose–continuing and more formalized).

(b) *Non-governmental organizations* (NGOs): Whereas social movements are networks of different individual and collective actors, NGOs definitely have the status of actors (that can be involved in social movements). The scientific debate on the adequate definition of NGOs is still ongoing, and an agreement has not been found yet (and probably never will be). Combining the arguments of different authors,[1] we define NGOs as those CSOs that bear the following attributes:

  - they are characterized by professionalization and sustainability in terms of their organizational structure;

- they do not follow criminal or illegal goals;
- they act as agents for others and advocate for their interests; the interests of those groups can be broader or narrower in nature, but should not stem from exclusively individual or private motivations;[2]
- they work towards the public benefit and general charity; private resources (donations, membership fees) are transferred into public goods;
- they are self-determined and develop their own organizational structures;
- they focus on specific issues or policy fields.

This detailed definition excludes both social movements and certain local grassroots groups (which are not formalized enough to qualify as NGOs) and unions (which represent mainly the interests of their members).

(c) *Social membership organizations*: Most of the facets associated above with NGOs apply also for social membership organizations – as we call the third type of CSOs. The crucial difference to NGOs is that these social membership organizations mainly and by constitution work for their members' interests. This may, nonetheless, also include advocacy activities for non-members and often means that political questions are addressed that fall under general policies (as in the case of unions).

(d) *National and ethnic organizations and movements*: Whereas Mary Kaldor (2003: 18) subsumes religious and national movements into one category of civil society actors and characterizes them as 'based on particular sections of society, defined in terms of culture, kin or religion' and as 'neo-traditional', we think it is necessary to distinguish between national/ethnic organizations on the one hand and religious organizations on the other. The ideologies and worldviews of these two types of civil society actors clearly differ. Since religious or faith-based groups play an important role in global health activities, we deal with them as a special kind of civil society actor below. With respect to national and ethnic organizations and movements we can differentiate roughly between 'old' nationalist movements, which normally connect the aim of national self-determination with democratic, participatory and inclusive values, and 'new' nationalist and ethnic movements, which usually lack progressive and democratic values and are mainly based on identity politics and exclusion (Kaldor 2003: 19).

(e) *Foundations*: Finally, we also add foundations to the realm of civil society and thus to CSOs as far as they are clearly devoted to non-profit interests and goals. This, however, turns out to be a problem, as in many cases we cannot separate between the profit interests of companies and the philanthropic objectives of foundations that were established by these companies. For example, the foundation itself may be non-profit but it might function to sanitize the public image of the company, which could contribute to increasing profits. Considering foundations as part of civil society is associated with a changing view on CSOs in global health governance, as for example the Bill and Melinda Gates Foundation, which due to its large resource-based power is a very influential actor. After Warren Buffet's gift of more than US$30 billion and with an estimated annual spending of US$3 billion per year it is one of the greatest funders of global health promotion and the fight against infectious diseases. Following the logic that the Gates Foundation qualifies as a CSO, we could say that global civil society is not only an important actor of global health governance but is at the heart of it. For the moment we can maintain that non-profit foundations are part of civil society. However, they are in somewhat of a grey area between civil society and the private for-profit sector, as the interests behind most of them are not clear and may be induced or at least influenced by profit interests.

The special case of faith-based organizations

Faith-based organizations (FBOs) are a special case in the landscape of civil society activities. On the one hand, they take part in public life like other CSOs, but on the other hand, they are based in religious organizations mostly with a long history of shaping social life and orienting the identity of people. Catholic orders have continuously played an important role in health care since the early Middle Ages; religious values have for a long time mobilized people to take a stand on issues that have been secularized under the banner of 'human rights' – at least with respect to economic and social rights – while with their focus on 'religious truths' they have frequently polarized opinions related to civil and political rights.

We define FBOs as organizations that emanate from or are established by religious communities and take over certain social services (for example in community work, humanitarian relief, poverty reduction, health provision), advocative functions in political conflicts (mostly related to ethical, social and cultural issues) as well as missionary activities (education, preaching for certain patterns of behaviour). This understanding of FBOs includes both organizations in industrialized countries and developing countries where FBOs often have important roles at the local and national level and are deep-rooted in people's everyday lives. Although FBOs are religious organizations, they sometimes also take the form of a social membership organization or an NGO.

The role of FBOs in health politics has been reinforced by the specific attention US politics has paid to them during the last decade. The Charitable Choice legislation in 1996 was designed to improve access to federal funding for faith-based organizations with a particular view on strengthening the activities of these groups in welfare services. This has been enforced by George Bush's initiative called 'Rallying the Armies of Compassion' from August 2001 stressing that 'America is richly blessed by the diversity and vigor of neighborhood healers: civic, social, charitable, and religious groups . . . We must heed the growing consensus across America that successful government social programs work in fruitful partnership with community-serving and faith-based organizations – whether run by Methodists, Muslims, Mormons, or good people of no faith at all.'[3] In the context of fighting HIV/AIDS, this has gained significant importance as a background to the PEPFAR initiative (see case study II).

Functions of civil society organizations

It has already become apparent that the interactions between CSOs and other actors take different forms and follow different logics, and that CSOs thus fulfil different functions in global health governance. These can be separated analytically into three categories: political, operational and self-empowerment functions.

Political functions

The political function of CSOs refers to a number of activities, which take place mostly at the global level, but can also be found at other spatial levels of politics. CSOs thus make proactive use of the emerging system of multilevel governance in global health. Their activities often relate to more than one policy field (for example, trade and health, human rights and health; or, more generally, global welfare and market creation), which also gives them an important advantage in knowledge and communicative relations compared to other actors.

One of the most important activities in this context is the representation of interests from civil society which are not mirrored sufficiently in other types of organizations. CSOs act as agents for marginalized and weak groups and advocate for their belonging. Important means to do so are the development and realization of political campaigns (for example,

Access to Essential Medicines, Make Poverty History), the dissemination of information and knowledge on specific issues (for example, Guide to ARV prices, 10/90 gap in R&D for neglected diseases), and the lobbying of decision-making institutions both at national and international level.

While these activities relate especially to the discoursive interfaces in global health governance, a second group of activities targets more the organizational interfaces. In this context, the following fields of CSO engagement can be highlighted in particular: the participation in international conferences (for example, the series of large UN conferences in the 1990s), the establishment of consultative relationships with international governmental organizations (for example, consultative status in ECOSOC, official relations with the WHO), the participation in the decision-making bodies of IGOs (for example, the Programme Coordination Board at UNAIDS), and the participation in newly emerging global public–private partnerships (for example, the Global Fund).

A third important political function of CSOs is the observation and control of international, national and transnational activities of state and non-state actors. CSOs act as watchdogs to monitor, for example, the outcomes of UN conferences (for example, Social Watch, which focuses on poverty eradication and gender equality), the results of specific programmes carried out by IGOs (for example, participation of CSOs in M&E activities), the quality of national politics (for example, Global Health Watch, Transparency International), or the behaviour of transnational companies ('naming and shaming', monitoring of codes of conduct). These activities refer to a certain extent to legal interfaces, although judicial enforcement, of course, is not possible in this case. The activities of CSOs, however, can contribute to an improved voluntary compliance with existing rules and might in the long run also support a further legalization in global politics and a stricter enforcement through the respective institutions at the national and international level.

Operational functions

In terms of the operational functions of CSOs we can also observe a number of different activities which aim at supporting people suffering from ill-health and diseases at the local and national level. We can distinguish between operational functions CSOs fulfil on the basis of their own resources and those which are mainly financed by other actors.

The first group of activities includes the realization of own health projects in developing countries (for example Oxfam and MSF), technical and financial support to in-country intermediary organizations (for example International HIV/AIDS Alliance), and the provision of medical aid and humanitarian relief in emergency and crisis situations (for example MSF, Red Cross). The second group refers to those activities where CSOs take over responsibilities in the provision of health services from national or international public actors. The most prominent example is the so-called 'contracting' in health systems, where CSOs are given certain – formally public – tasks, for example in the areas of prevention, treatment and/or care, and are financially compensated for doing so (for example in the Brazilian HIV/AIDS programme).

For many CSOs, these operational functions combine with political ones, and especially in the past few years, an increase of advocacy and political activities can be observed, which is related to the social problems in the context of neo-liberal globalization (Gebauer 2001: 97; Lindenberg and Bryant 2001: 173f.). Operational functions are related to resource-transfer interfaces if the provision of services implies the allocation of resources by CSOs. If CSOs are involved in contracting without providing own resources they interact with other actors at organizational interfaces.

Self-empowerment function

Especially in the health sector, a third type of function can be identified, which we would like to call the self-empowerment function. CSOs in this field (for example GNP+, ICASO) consist of people who are affected by certain diseases and aim at improving their living situation and advocating for their rights. They are not acting as agents for the interests of other marginalized civil society groups but pursue first and foremost their own interests. These types of CSOs played a crucial role both in shaping the discourse on HIV/AIDS and in helping the affected individuals to take their lives into their own hands.

They thus combine political and operational functions as they represent the interests of the affected populations at the local, national and/or global level and aim at influencing political decisions on the one hand, while they engage in operational activities that directly support the affected people (for example, through projects for prevention, treatment and/or care at the local level) on the other. Thus we can find the self-empowerment function at discoursive, organizational and resource-transfer interfaces as well as at legal interfaces.

Civil society organizations in global health governance

In the following we will deal with the interactions and interfaces of CSOs with other actors of global health governance and give examples for the three different functions of CSOs introduced above: the conflicts around the access to ARVs in developing countries (political function), contracting in national health systems to CSOs in general and faith-based organizations in particular (operational functions), and the processes of self-organization and empowerment of affected communities (self-empowerment function).

Interfaces of CSOs with other actors of global health governance

In global health governance, CSOs interact with a multitude of different actors at various spatial levels, ranging from local self-help groups, national administration and IGOs to transnational corporations (TNCs). With respect to the actors involved and to the different modes of governance, we can differentiate between four forms of interactions: (a) between different CSOs, (b) with state actors, (c) with private sector actors and (d) between all three types of actors (for example in PPPs or in participatory bodies of IGOs). The forms of interactions at the interfaces vary between the poles of *conflict* and *cooperation* and depend on the interests and strategies of the actors involved and on the type of interface. CSOs can pressurize other actors politically or even fight against them. Yet they can also cooperate with other actors, either to strengthen and exert political influence or to take over concrete projects in the provision of health.

When we analyse the organizational interfaces *between different* CSOs in the health sector we can identify three trends. First, the challenges of transborder interdependence problems bring about the emergence of CSO families (Lindenberg and Bryant 2001: 139f.). Individual CSOs can join relatively weak coordination networks ('umbrella coordination'), affiliate themselves under a common roof, where they yield some autonomy with regard to decision-making, standard-setting and resource allocation ('confederation'), or they can join far-reaching forms of transnational cooperation such as 'federations', where the headquarters play a central role with regard to decision-making, resource allocation and so on. The latter model of a CSO family is often regarded as an organization in its own right. Second, we can observe an increased transnationalization of CSO activities. Local, national and transnational CSOs of different kinds of CSO families link their activities beyond national borders and work in issue-specific networks (for example, International Baby Food Action Network, IBFAN) or engage in multisectoral networks in broader transnational social movements (for example People's Health Movement, PHM) (Lindenberg and Bryant 2001; Keck and Sikkink 1998). The increasing virtualization of the CSO landscape is the third trend: this involves the onset of virtual networks that operate with a minimum of staff and administration efforts and whose activities primarily relate to the internet via websites, email lists, discussion forums, online publications and so on (for example Health and Development Networks, HDN).

Although forms of cooperation prevail with respect to the interactions among CSOs there are also areas of conflict. For instance, CSOs compete for members, attention, publicity and resources. According to an OECD report on European CSOs, the top quintile of CSOs received more than 90 per cent of all financial resources (Woods 2000: 17). The consequences of this competition are a professionalization and a kind of commercialization of CSO activities as well as an adjustment of CSOs. Furthermore, in the course of this competition, a certain 'oligopolization' of the CSO landscape occurs (Stubbs 2003:1), which causes great potentials of conflict among CSOs.

With respect to the interfaces *between CSOs and state actors*, it is reasonable to distinguish between interfaces at the national and at the global level. For health CSOs at the national level, the respective ministries of health and finance, local and national administrations as well as the state institutions of the health system are the most important partners of interaction. CSOs cooperate mainly in three different forms: as recipient of funds in order to conduct own programmes, as contracting partner in the fulfilment of public responsibilities, and via the participation in political bodies and forums. Thus, both organizational and resource-based interfaces play an important role in the relationship between CSOs and state actors at the national level.

At the global level, crucial state actors in public health are, of course, the WHO and UNAIDS. The WHO has cooperated with CSOs since its establishment in 1948. In the year 2002, 189 CSOs were in official relations with the WHO (including so-called non-commercial CSOs of the private sector). CSOs that are in official relations with the WHO have the right, for example, to attend the World Health Assembly and the meetings of the Executive Board – though without voting or decision-making rights – and they are entitled to be heard by WHO bodies. Another 284 transnational CSOs cooperate with the WHO mostly in the operational field without being part of the system of official relations. Finally, there are several hundred CSOs that cooperate with the WHO at national and local level (WHO/CSI 2002). Basically, the relationship between CSOs and the WHO is ambivalent: on the one hand, many CSOs try to strengthen the WHO and regard it as an ally in the pursuit of their goals. On the other hand, CSOs criticize the WHO for supposedly flawed policies or slow reactions, and frequently turn to other organizations and institutions because the opportunities to participate are greater there. UNAIDS offers – compared with other IGOs – a rather far-reaching participation of CSOs at the organizational interfaces, at least formally. Besides twenty-two governments of industrialized and developing countries and the ten co-sponsoring UN organizations, five CSOs are members of the highest body, the Programme Coordinating Board – without, however, the right to vote (Kohlmorgen 2004; Chapter 5).

The interfaces *between CSOs and private-for-profit actors* are traditionally characterized by mutual mistrust, different patterns of thought, and diverging logics of action. Health CSOs mostly define themselves as counterweight and corrective to the activities of TNCs and try to repel their influence as well as to mitigate the effects of their activities. In the focus of CSO activities and campaigns at the discoursive interfaces are pharmaceutical corporations, tobacco corporations and major food producers, which are accused of pursuing their interests at the expense of people particularly in developing countries. Since the mid-1990s, we can, however, observe a slightly increasing cooperation between CSOs and TNCs. The type of cooperation varies from singular or continuous financial assistance for CSOs and the exchange of information to common operational activities (for example in workplace programmes to fight HIV/AIDS). Whereas both types of actors hope to benefit from cooperation and partnerships – TNCs through improvements in their image, CSOs through increased funding for their activities – the risks involved – financial risks for the companies, the danger of cooptation, and a loss of reputation for CSOs – are obvious and quite substantial, so that the cooperation of CSOs and the private sector is regarded critically in most cases.

More frequent, in contrast, is the *cooperation of all three types of actors* – CSOs, TNCs and state actors – in global public–private partnerships (GPPPs). Currently there are about 80 GPPPs in the health sector (Buse and Walt 2000a, 2000b; Widdus 2001; Buse 2004). The DFID recently commissioned a number of studies on global health partnerships (for a synthesis see Caines et al. 2004) and introduced a typology based on the main areas of activity. Following that typology we can distinguish between partnerships active in R&D (product discovery, development of new diagnostics, drugs and vaccines), GPPPs in the area of technical assistance and service support (service access, provision of discounted or donated drugs), GPPPs that concentrate on advocacy activities at the global and national level (including resource mobilization), and partnerships in the area of financing (provision of funds for specific disease programmes). Among the most prominent of these GPPPs is the Global

Fund to Fight HIV/AIDS, Tuberculosis and Malaria (see Chapter 6), which covers the three most important poverty-related diseases and disposes of a large influence at the resource-based interfaces. To what extent GPPPs are characterized by cooperation or conflict depends on the particular internal governance structure, the forms of decision-making, on the interests and the logics of action of the participating actors as well as on the degree of trust and transparency within the partnership (Bartsch 2003). Since partnerships are normally weakly formalized and institutionalized, they tend to dissolve in case of too severe conflicts, so that functioning PPPs show mostly cooperative patterns of interaction.

Case study I: the conflict on access to medicines

In recent years, the question of universal access to treatment of AIDS patients became one of the most important and conflictive issues of HIV/AIDS politics and global health politics in general. At the discoursive interfaces of global health governance in the last few years, the conflict regarding drug prices came to the fore, which includes the issue of patented drugs and intellectual property rights and which has, of course, important implications for the amount of finance required.

As already explained in Chapter 2, the negotiations concerning the TRIPS agreement within the World Trade Organization (WTO), in particular, became the centre of the CSO campaigns. From 1996 onwards, Health Action International successfully developed a campaign against the effect of TRIPS on limiting the access of poor people to patented medicines, scandalizing the coincidence between high prices of drugs and large profits for pharmaceutical companies on the one hand and the suffering and dying of millions of AIDS victims on the other. They argued that intellectual property rights were not only a trade but also a public health issue and thus managed to link these two aspects. Since the late 1990s, a large network of CSOs, led by Médecins Sans Frontières (MSF)[4] have been advocating and campaigning for access of poor AIDS victims to ARVs in the 'Essential Drugs Campaign', which included advocacy and lobbying against efforts of industrialized countries within the WTO to establish international patent protection for drugs that are needed in developing countries (Sell 2002; 't Hoen 2002; Schultz and Walker 2005; Chapters 2 and 3). The campaign for low-cost medicine was not only carried out at the global level – by means of activities and lobbying within the WTO and other IGOs – but also in particular countries.[5]

The Doha Declaration that supplemented the TRIPS agreement and the agreement on §6 of that declaration on 30 August 2003, can be interpreted as a result of these activities. CSOs not only lobbied representatives of IGOs and Northern governments, but also became increasingly important as advisers to developing country members of the WTO and helped them coordinate their positions in the subsequent renegotiations of the TRIPS agreement. Governments of developing countries cooperated with CSOs during the negotiations and CSOs brought in their political, legal and technical knowledge and their contacts with governments of industrialized countries (UNDP 2002: 104ff.). Hence, during this process, CSOs were changing their character from basically mobilizing and advocatory actors towards cooperating experts and actors with a negotiating role in the global political process. CSO networks were highly efficient in four domains: creating media attention and public interest, mobilizing support both from the public and the private sector, lobbying representatives of IGOs and governments of industrialized countries, and empowering poor Southern countries to take a strong position in the negotiations. They managed to establish a functioning private governance scheme in which the relevant discourses were framed. Both through the strategic use of the media and through personal networking, CSOs then managed to disseminate information and transfer ideas to another governance scheme: the state-based WTO.

The institutional setting thus enabled CSOs to exert considerable influence in one of the most important discourses in global health. Norm- and agenda-setting processes through private governance modes played a crucial role in that context. The discoursive power of the CSO networks, combined with the decision-making power of the developing countries in a conventional forum of state regulation, and supported by the exercise of legal power by the national governments in South Africa and Brazil in the conflict on parallel imports and compulsory licensing, accounts for the relatively strong position of both state and non-state actors from the South at the discoursive interfaces.

Meanwhile, the prices for AIDS treatments in developing countries dropped noticeably, on the one hand because of generic competition, and on the other hand because of CSO activities – which, aside from TRIPS-focused activities, include campaigns against transnational pharmaceutical corporations (TNPCs) with the objective of reaching low prices – and the increased global consciousness concerning the need for AIDS treatment. This influence of CSOs also becomes apparent if we look at the initiative for a 'Global Framework on Essential Health Research', which is currently under discussion in the WHO. This initiative was influenced and kicked off by a proposal for a 'Medical Research and Development Treaty' made by the US NGO Cp-Tech and supported by many CSOs in 2005. It was brought into the Executive Board in January 2006 by Kenya and Brazil and thereafter debated in the Word Health Assembly in May 2006, which then decided to establish an intergovernmental working group on this issue (see Chapter 5).

The political conflicts on drug prices point to the fact that CSOs in global health governance often work together with governments and IGOs to strengthen and realize poor people's interests in developing countries. Often, the activities of CSOs are focused on strengthening state actors (such as governments of developing countries or the WHO), so that these can improve the health situation in poor countries. Depending on the represented positions and pursued strategies in health policy, governments of nation-states and IGOs are in many cases partners of cooperation and at the same time targets of political campaigns. The activities of CSOs are not only limited to conducting campaigns and political actions, but also imply the collaboration in partnerships and other forms of cooperation with IGOs and states. Forms of hybrid regulation in the health sector have become more important not only regarding operational but also in terms of political functions.

Conflict and cooperation are also characteristics of the relationship between CSOs and TNPCs as well as other private companies, but conflict obviously prevails. For example, MSF indeed searches for cooperative forms of interactions with TNPCs – both with the producers of patent-protected drugs, with whom issues such as prices and the development of new drugs are negotiated, and also with the producers of generics, who produce low-cost drugs that are distributed by MSF in African countries. However, at the same time, MSF and other CSOs exert pressure on TNPCs to obtain price reductions. Concerning the concrete conflict of intellectual property rights and access to medicines, CSOs represented the interests of the affected groups, whereas TNPCs primarily pursued their interest in gaining profits. Thus, CSOs acted as a counterweight to the activities of TNPCs and the governments of some industrialized countries that clearly supported the position of the TNPCs. This function of CSOs contributed to the establishment of the aforementioned political compromises at global level.

In sum, the political function of CSOs is characterized by both conflicts and forms of cooperation with public actors and private for-profit actors. However, the conflicts prevail, especially regarding the interactions with the latter. From the analysis of the political interaction of CSOs with other actors of global health governance we can conclude that CSOs influence governance processes mainly through the discoursive interfaces of global governance – even though other actors are more powerful in terms of decision-making and resources. This relatively strong position might lead to a greater inclusion of CSOs in organizational interfaces such as decision-making bodies, which could further increase their power in global health governance.

Case study II: NGOs and FBOs as contractual partners

National and international CSOs not only deal with the question of access to medicines for AIDS patients from a political point of view, but also consider this issue in operational terms. They are active in the acquisition and distribution of drugs, conduct programmes to enhance prevention, treatment and care for AIDS patients, and support national health systems in developing countries.

The increasing role of CSOs in the health systems of developing countries is influenced by several processes. First of all, the integration of private actors and CSOs into the health systems of developing countries has – because of the colonial past and the historical engagement of FBOs – a long-lasting tradition. This tradition was interrupted by the aspirations of many countries during the post-colonial phase to strengthen the influence of the nation-state and to dispose of the remnants of colonialism. Due to a lack of resources and capacities, however, the construction of public health systems proved to be difficult, especially in the poorest countries, so that after a while private (international) actors were increasingly being brought in again. This development is enforced by an accelerating integration of CSOs in development cooperation in the context of the promotion of 'good governance' through bilateral and multilateral donors since the 1990s. CSOs are often seen as alternatives to bureaucracies and administrations affected by corruption (Clayton et al. 2000: 2). Moreover, in the 1990s, neo-liberal reforms in the health sector led to a transfer of certain public tasks to non-state actors such as international and national CSOs (Clayton et al. 2000: 3; Robinson 1997: 61). Finally, the HIV/AIDS epidemic confronted many countries with weak governing capacities and limited financial means with nearly unsolvable problems which required support through external actors both from the state and the non-state sector (Green and Matthias 1997: 12f.).

CSOs support health systems of developing countries by cooperating with governments and public authorities in the realization of projects, by being authorized through national governments or international organizations to conduct certain activities (*contracting*, which leads to a stronger orientation of CSOs towards market principles), or by being active – with toleration of the state – in spheres where the government is on the retreat (Clayton et al. 2000: 12; England 2004; Harding 2003; Mills and Broomberg 1998: 18f.; Robinson 1997; Slack and Savedoff 2001; especially for HIV/AIDS: Barnett et al. 2001).

The integration of CSOs into the Brazilian HIV/AIDS programme between 1993 and 2002 is a sound example of successful contracting. More than 200 mainly national CSOs managed altogether 794 projects with a total volume of US$25.6 million in the fields of prevention, treatment and care. The projects were assigned by the Ministry of Health and financed by the government of Brazil and the World Bank (Connor 2000). The World Bank declares that in 1997, 60 per cent of all its projects concerning health were carried out with the participation of CSOs (World Bank 1998: 4). Meanwhile, in sub-Saharan Africa, CSOs are among the largest service providers in health. For example, hospitals managed by CSOs are responsible for 43 per cent of all medical services in Tanzania, for 40 per cent in Malawi and for 34 per cent in Ghana. In Asia the role of CSOs is not as prominent. Their share in the provision of health services is, for example, 13 per cent for Bangladesh and 12 per cent for Indonesia. In India as well as in most of the Latin American countries, where the state is the primary service provider in health, CSOs play an even less important role (Loewenson 2003: 5; Medicus Mundi 1999; Clayton et al. 2000: 2; England 2004: 18f.). The degree of CSO integration in national health systems thus differs, depending on the power of the state: whereas in middle-income countries such as Brazil, CSOs are primarily assigned and contracted by the national government, in many low-income countries with a lack of capacity and resources, IGOs and development banks often play the most important role in this context.

In the academic discussions on the role of CSOs in national health systems, both advantages and positive effects as well as disadvantages and dangers are pointed out (for the following see: Clayton et al. 2000: 7; Green and Matthias 1997: 44f.; Loewenson 2003: 6f.; Mills and Broomberg 1998: 23f.; Robinson 1997: 62f.; World Bank 2004a: 151). On the one hand it is emphasized that CSOs bring in additional resources, are more flexible in their work than public authorities, offer services of high quality at low costs, and are better able to take into account the needs of local and indigenous populations. Some researchers, on the other hand, argue that there is no proof that CSOs are more effective in providing health services to the poor, and that public authorities are better suited to care for local communities. They also contradict the common assumption that CSOs are always more flexible than public institutions and refer to the need to evaluate CSO performance in concrete cases. A comprehensive integration of CSOs into national health systems is often considered problematic, as this could prevent the development of sustainable structures and lead to a dependency on private, often foreign, institutional and financial capacities. In addition, large CSOs could enter into competition with the government and even replace it in parts. It is generally argued that – in order to reach positive results – more synergies are necessary between CSOs and public institutions, too. If these cannot be created, it will result in a duplication of structures and competing activities, which leads to inefficiency and a limited effectiveness of the health system.

In many cases, however, despite – or maybe because of – the divergence of CSOs from public concepts, one can observe positive effects on the provision of health services and the integration of the poor, as the interests of the national elites frequently do not focus on social aspects and therefore tend to ignore the situation of poor people. In that case, international and national CSOs represent a counterbalance to national politics and represent the interests of the poor and marginalized. For this reason there are several tensions between CSOs and the state, especially if CSOs conduct not only operational functions but develop political activities. This tends to happen frequently, as CSOs in developing countries are generally confronted with an inadequate health system and widespread poverty, which they are unable to reduce on their own and therefore push towards an intensification and/or a reorientation of public activities. This demonstrates that the mixture of diverse functions of CSOs in global health governance also often concerns those CSOs who primarily want to be active as service providers in the health systems of developing countries.

This mix of operational and political functions can also be stated for faith-based organizations, which play an important role in the global fight against HIV/AIDS. In this context we have to distinguish between FBOs in developing countries and those based in industrialized countries, which operate in developing countries and pursue humanitarian and/or missionary objectives. Although apparently their main field of activity is operational, as they are involved in service provision and the support and care of ill people, their engagement also has political and discoursive effects (for example, if a certain prevention method is favoured or if Christian values are dispersed implicitly).

In most developing countries, local and national FBOs (that are mainly associated with Christian belief, but also relate to other religions), play an important role in the fight against HIV/AIDS because they are an integral part of life and society and are rooted in local structures. Thus, FBOs in many countries build a large network covering most of the local communities. This presence and involvement in local communities is often accompanied by having the trust of the people in general and also of the people living with HIV/AIDS. Of course the activities of FBOs differ from country to country and also within the country from region to region. Thus, the function and the activities of FBOs in the area of HIV/AIDS range from low-level responses such as publishing messages on prevention on World AIDS Day in some regions and communities, to an intense and continuous commitment in prevention, care and treatment, and a major contribution to the national reaction to HIV/AIDS in other communities (Parry 2003). The important role of FBOs in the national HIV/AIDS response in some countries also has to do with their general engagement in the health sector. For example, in many developing countries, FBOs provide 40–50 per cent of health care (Mathai and Galbraith 2004).

Due to FBO involvement in the fight against HIV/AIDS, they are also part of governance structures in the sense that they participate in organizational interfaces such as National HIV/AIDS Councils (NACs) or Country Coordinating Mechanisms (CCMs) that are a precondition for receiving money from the Global Fund and should include all important stakeholders (Chapter 6). In fact, international and local FBOs act as principal recipients for some Global Fund grants and are sub-recipients in many countries. In the first five rounds of Global Fund grants, FBOs, on average, made up 5 per cent of members of the CCMs.[6] However, some FBOs themselves complain that they receive too little information on the Global Fund and claim that their degree of participation in the CCMs is unsatisfactory (Lee et al. 2003). Furthermore, some FBOs give accounts of a level of reluctance of donors to support FBOs in developing countries: 'International donors fund governments, not usually FBOs. Donors withhold funds from FBOs because of a perception that they are funding "a denomination" ' (Parry 2003: 14).

At least for the area of HIV/AIDS, this changed with the President's Emergency Plan for AIDS Relief (PEPFAR).[7] As it is a general priority of development cooperation of the Bush administration to increase funding for FBOs both from the US and in developing countries, PEPFAR channels a considerable share of its funds through FBOs (about 25 per cent of all PEPFAR money). In the fiscal year 2004, PEPFAR had 248 FBOs as partners comprising over 20 per cent of all partner organizations (GAC 2005). In 2006, the Office of the US Global AIDS Coordinator specially launched the New Partners Initiative with the objective of finding new partners among FBOs and community CSOs. Analysing these efforts, we can state that with this initiative, which accounts for US$200 million of the PEPFAR funds, and by encouraging new actors to enter the field of HIV/AIDS, the US government tries to change the landscape of HIV/AIDS and development-related CSOs according to its own interests.

This strengthening of FBOs, together with the general policy of PEPFAR to strengthen abstinence as the main prevention method,[8] yields considerable influence on the HIV/AIDS policies at country level. Many FBOs reject the use of condoms, whereas most of the other CSOs favour condoms as the main prevention method and claim that this is based on scientific approaches. This indicates that there are conflicts between FBOs and other CSOs due to their different worldviews and policies. However, there are not only conflicts in the interaction of FBOs and other CSOs, but also in the global HIV/AIDS policy of the US government, as Holly Burkhalter (2004: 8) observes: 'The future of U.S. global AIDS policy will be complicated . . . because the conservative groups interested in the issue have different tactical priorities than their liberal counterparts and the broader medical establishment.'

The increasing involvement of some conservative FBOs in service provision in developing countries and in the overarching global fight against HIV/AIDS shows that the realm of (global) civil society is not only a domain of progressive NGOs, social movements and grassroots organizations, but also of organizations that are more conservative in nature and favour corresponding approaches and policies. This, however, is also a characteristic of global health governance.

Case study III: self-empowerment in the field of HIV/AIDS

One example for self-empowerment functions are the activities of organizations of HIV-positive people and AIDS patients (People Living with HIV/AIDS, PLWHA). They advocate for the rights of affected populations because the group of PLWHA is not sufficiently represented in political campaigns of the CSOs, in the process of supplying health services, and in health politics in general. The reasons for the low level of inclusion of their interests and needs in health and HIV/AIDS policies are the stigmatization and discrimination in many countries, the low sensibility towards the HIV/AIDS epidemic in some countries, as well as the fact that PLWHA are often seen only as passive recipients of medical care instead of as active participants in the making of (global) health policy. Against this background, CSOs of PLWHA fulfil political and operational functions by working (through advocacy and disseminating information) towards a changing political perception regarding the role of PLWHA on the one hand, and by conducting operational activities to improve the health provision of affected persons on the other. The starting point of their activities is the conviction that PLWHA should be more integrated into strategies for fighting HIV/AIDS, in order to overcome political and social exclusion, pursue their interests, and make available their potential for the fight against the AIDS epidemic (Hetzel 2002).

After the establishment of local self-empowerment organizations during the 1980s at first in industrialized countries and then also in developing countries, regional and global networks[9] developed during the 1990s, which are not only active in local capacity-building but also in advocacy at the global level. Meanwhile, there are at least 350 PLWHA organizations outside Western Europe and North America (228 in Africa, 63 in Asia, 10 in Eastern Europe, 59 in Latin America; USAID 2004b).

In the following, we mainly examine the activities of PLWHA in the discoursive field of the global fight against HIV/AIDS. At the global level, repercussions of the activities and demands of numerous PLWHA organizations can be found in three central documents: the Denver Principles (1983), the Declaration of the Paris AIDS Summit (1994) and the UNGASS Declaration of Commitment on HIV/AIDS (2001). The Denver Principles denote the first international declaration of PLWHA, demanding an end to stigmatization and discrimination, the participation in all political processes and the acceptance of their rights. The principles were adopted in the US by activists at the second National Forum on AIDS. The Declaration of the Paris AIDS Summit, signed by forty-two states, for the first time formalized the principle of a 'Greater Involvement of PLWHA' (called 'GIPA'). Based on the objective to promote the participation of PLWHA at the national, regional and global level, states committed themselves to protecting and promoting the rights of PLWHA and to include respective CSOs in HIV/AIDS politics. The GIPA Principles have been confirmed in the 'UNGASS Declaration of Commitment on HIV/AIDS', signed by nearly all UN member states. In addition, this declaration asks governments to develop national strategies for strengthening health systems and improving the treatment for HIV/AIDS patients.

The means of interaction between PLWHA-CSOs and actors of the public and the private sector varies according to the function CSOs fulfil (operational/political) and also according to the degree of participation of such organizations in political and economic processes. If PLWHA organizations are active in the political field of advocacy and lobbying – as could be observed, for example, in the preparation of the UNGASS Declaration – they often come into conflict with state actors particularly from developing countries, who sometimes do not assess the HIV/AIDS epidemic as a great danger and are often reluctant to relinquish sovereignty and public responsibilities to other (non-state) actors. With respect to the involvement in public bodies, the degree of conflict rises with the increasing scale of participation (for a discussion of the steps of participation, see UNAIDS 1999: 3): when PLWHA are not seen merely as addressees of activities or as providers of health services, but their participation in political processes and decision-making structures is concerned, the relationship with state actors becomes more and more conflictive. PLWHA organizations only have the right to vote in the Executive Board of the Global Fund; at UNAIDS they are a member of the Programme Coordinating Board, but do not have the right to vote. The interfaces with private actors – at the level of political debates – play only a moderate role, although many CSOs appeal to the companies to take responsibility in supporting PLWHA. When PLWHA-CSOs are mainly operationally active in the country and communities by being involved in the care and treatment of PLWHA or by conducting education and information campaigns, the relationship with state actors is normally cooperative, although CSOs in such cases often receive stronger support from bilateral and multilateral donors than from national authorities.

Conclusion

Our analysis shows that CSOs play an important role in the health sector both in terms of their political, operational and empowerment functions and as actors at the various interfaces of global health governance.

One general reason for this is the governance structure in global health and, in particular, in the fight against HIV/AIDS. The field of HIV/AIDS policies and access to medicines was first introduced by Northern and Southern CSOs and by some governments of developing countries – both types of actors with mainly human rights and social policy interests in this case. Governments from the North and, accordingly, most of the IGOs that are shaped by them reacted hesitantly to the increasing HIV/AIDS epidemic in developing countries and particularly in sub-Saharan Africa during the 1990s. There was thus a window of opportunity for the self-empowerment of weak actors due to the lack of coherent regulations at the global level and the low-level activities of more powerful actors.

CSOs influenced policy-making processes through their campaigning activities, which pointed to the deficits in the health systems of many developing countries, the insufficient international activities to improve public health, and the failures in the fight against specific diseases. The negotiations around the Doha Declaration can be seen as an illustrative example for this case, as CSOs, through their cooperation with certain developing countries' governments and their lobbying and campaigning activities, were able to shape the resulting compromise considerably.

This shows their discoursive power in global health governance. Also, the integration of CSOs in the governing bodies of the Global Fund opened an important channel of influence by increasing their decision-making power at the global level. In operational terms, CSOs are indispensable for the most basic health services in quite a few developing countries, and play a considerable role in the health systems of most Southern countries. Moreover, CSOs with a primarily self-empowerment function are important parts of the global health architecture and contribute to putting those groups at the centre of attention who should be the final addressees of all health-related policies: the people affected by ill-health, diseases, poverty and lack of health services especially in the developing world. If we take a closer look at the interaction of CSOs with other (state and non-state) actors of global health governance and scrutinize the patterns of conflict and/or cooperation in these interactions, we can observe the following.

The *political function* of CSOs is characterized by a dualism of cooperation and conflict. First of all, we can observe an increasing integration of CSOs in consultations (ECOSOC, WHO) or decision-making structures (UNAIDS, Global Fund). In certain conflicts with public or private actors they enter into coalitions with IGOs or certain nation-states. These coalitions, however, are mostly temporary and issue-specific in nature, and in other contexts or on other occasions the former partners in these coalitions can become political opponents and targets of political campaigns. The WHO and UNAIDS, for example, are partly seen as allies in the fight for an improvement of health systems in the developing countries and the conditions of the poor, and at the same time are criticized for their general strategies or for taking or not taking certain measures. With regard to the interaction with actors from the private sector, scepticism and opposition prevail, despite some political cooperation or partnerships. Transnational corporations as representatives of a globalized world economy, in particular, are often regarded as a creator of health-related problems (for example unfavourable working conditions, rigid patents and high drug prices, lack of R&D for diseases of the poor) so that, in most cases, conflictive patterns dominate interactions between them and CSOs. In these conflicts, CSOs define and position themselves as welfare-oriented correctives to processes of neo-liberal globalization and the growing influence of private, market-oriented actors and their respective strategies.

The *operational function* of CSOs is mostly characterized by non-conflictive forms of interaction. The cooperation of CSOs with state actors and the taking over of formerly public activities has increased considerably. Also, at the global level CSOs are increasingly integrated in the operational activities of IGOs and global public–private partnerships. At the same time, however, many operational CSOs start to react politically to problematic situations, criticizing, for example, the retreat of the state and advocating for a stronger engagement of public actors in global health. The relationship to the private sector in terms of operational activities in the last few years is increasingly characterized by cooperation and partnerships, although different interests, logics of action, and political positions tend to lead to conflicts which have a negative impact on the performance of these endeavours.

The *self-empowerment function* includes political and operational elements, as it aims both at the representation of the interests of affected communities and at their direct support through specific projects and activities. PLWHA organizations are often supported by governments in the industrialized countries, which aim at promoting the GIPA principles and at the same time influencing the HIV/AIDS policies of countries in the South. The lines of conflict in the field of self-empowerment thus quite often run between alliances of CSOs, industrialized countries and IGOs on the one hand, and governments of developing countries on the other hand. The interaction of PLWHA-CSOs with private actors is relatively limited, although especially those TNCs active in Southern countries could contribute to a greater participation of affected communities through workplace programmes or employment patterns. That these possibilities are not more utilized can be attributed to the fact that most PLWHA organizations take a critical position with regard to the private sector and thus focus more on national governments (legislative competencies) and on IGOs (agenda-setting power) in order to enforce their interests and rights.

It has been shown that, in the health sector, private and hybrid forms of regulation have gained an increasing importance, supplementing or complementing traditional forms of state regulation. This opens up new channels of influence for non-state actors at the various interfaces in global health governance.

This influence is most visible at the *discoursive interfaces*, where CSOs were able to make use of their large discoursive power and their perceived legitimacy as advocates for the human right to health, since norm- and agenda-setting processes through private governance modes played a crucial role in this context. Other actors, such as TNPCs, which are normally considered much more powerful than CSOs and dispose of a large resource-based power, did not manage to accomplish an optimum of their goals in the conflict on patents and drug prices, as their type of power did not converge with the specific type of interface where that conflict was carried out.

Also at the *organizational interfaces*, the influence of CSOs increased, as traditional forms of state regulation were supplemented by new hybrid forms like the Global Fund, where CSOs are provided with actual decision-making power. Hence the influence of non-state actors at the organizational interfaces is closely related to the prevailing governance modes, as they have an impact both on the degree of inclusion/exclusion of certain actors and the power relations at the different organizational interfaces.

At the *resource-based interfaces* – except for the large foundations – their influence is more limited because their financial power is comparatively small (although they do, of course, pursue activities in developing countries which contribute to an improvement of the health situation of poor or marginalized groups). If we add non-monetary resources (like information, knowledge, people), the picture changes slightly, but it can still be said that CSOs are among the weaker actors of global health governance at the resource-based interfaces.

Legal interfaces mostly play a role in the context of national legal disputes, as in South Africa (Chapter 8), where CSOs supported the position of the South African government in its lawsuit with the Pharmaceutical Manufacturers' Association of South Africa, or they initiated court procedures against violators of legal provisions. At the global level, processes of legalization are still in their infancy, so that at the current stage evidence on the role of CSOs cannot be provided. It can be assumed, however, that CSOs, through their activities, can contribute to a larger voluntary compliance with existing norms and rules and also – in the long run – support processes of further legalization and judicial enforcement.

Considering the current architecture of global health governance, it can be said that the increasing importance of private and hybrid forms of regulation on the one hand entails the inclusion and participation of CSOs, groups of affected people, and local organizations, which contributes to political processes that are closer to the needs of affected populations and which might eventually increase the legitimacy of global health politics. Weak actors and affected communities are empowered at the global and national level, which exerts some pressure on the governments (both of industrialized and developing countries) and also on private for-profit actors to intensify their efforts in improving the health situation of those groups. Moreover, this global governance structure with forms of hybrid regulation presents the opportunity to pool available resources and knowledge and allows different actors to bring in their particular skills.

In general, it has turned out to be more flexible than state-based regulation. The effectiveness of governance and thus the output-legitimacy may increase.

On the other hand, it should be considered that state actors (such as governments of industrialized countries) can functionalize hybrid and private regulation to pursue their own interests and instrumentalize CSOs. Furthermore, as a result of the greater number and variety of actors, we face a fragmentation of activities that can lead to a certain governance ineffectiveness both at the global and national level. Due to the involvement of non-state actors, questions of legitimization and accountability also arise, as private and hybrid governance modes can undermine the formal and – more or less – democratically legitimized IGOs and the coordinating capacity of governments in developing countries.

Global health governance as 'the totality of collective regulations to deal with international and transnational interdependence problems' in the health sector (as defined in Chapter 1) is thus characterized by numerous and changing patterns of conflict and cooperation. Politics at the interfaces is influenced both by the different modes of governance involved and the constellation of actors defined by their interests and power resources. CSOs as actors of global health governance have to weigh up the chances of realizing their own, welfare-oriented goals and the danger of being coopted by state or private actors in the pursuit of their political strategies and market-based interests.

Notes

1. See Heins (2002: 44); Hirsch (2001: 15); Kaldor (2003: 78f.); Martens (2002); Take (2002: 38f.); Willetts (2002: 5).
2. Following that criterion, certain self-help groups – as in the case of people living with HIV/AIDS (PLWHA) – could not be considered as NGOs, as they pursue first and foremost the interests of their members. On the other hand, they also advocate for broader goals like participation of PLWHA and non-discrimination, so that their classification as NGOs is once again justified.
3. See: http://www.whitehouse.gov/news/reports/faithbased.html.
4. MSF invested the money they received for winning the Nobel Prize in 1999 for a greater part in this campaign.
5. Prominent examples are the conflicts concerning patents and drug prices in South Africa and Brazil; see Chapters 7 and 8.
6. For a comparison: PLWHA-CSOs: 4 per cent; local and national NGOs: 15 per cent; international NGOs: 3 per cent; governments: 37 per cent (Global Fund 2004).
7. The bilateral programme PEPFAR was launched in 2004 to fight HIV/AIDS in developing countries with US$15 billion up to 2009 (cf. Chapter 5).

8. For example, in 2005, the US Congress mandated that one third of HIV prevention funds go to programmes that promote abstinence and fidelity in marriages and partnerships.
9. Regional networks: for example, Asia Pacific Network of People Living with HIV/AIDS, Network of African People Living with HIV/AIDS; global networks: for example, Global Network of People Living with HIV/AIDS (GNP+), International Council of AIDS Service Organizations (ICASO), International Community of Women living with HIV/AIDS (ICW).

5
International Governmental Organizations and Global Health Governance: the Role of the World Health Organization, World Bank and UNAIDS

Lars Kohlmorgen

Introduction

This chapter focuses on the World Health Organization (WHO), the World Bank and the Joint United Nations Programme on HIV/AIDS (UNAIDS) in global health governance, particularly in the fight against HIV/AIDS, and analyses the interactions and interfaces between each of them as well as with other relevant global health actors.

In the previous chapters we outlined the institutional change in global health governance and thus the impact of the changing conditions and contexts for international governmental organizations (IGOs) on their interfaces with other actors and in fulfilling their modified functions in a globalizing world. One should assume that in the process of political globalization, IGOs would play an increasingly significant role due to the greater relevance of political processes at the global level. However, due to the inflexibility of the organizational settings of many IGOs in general and due to the lack of leadership of more powerful actors and their hesitant reaction to the increasing HIV/AIDS epidemic in developing countries in particular, there was a window of opportunity for actors, who normally do not dispose of much resource-based, decision-making and legal power, for setting the agenda and influencing global policies in this field. Civil society organizations (CSOs) operated in the discoursive field of global health governance as well as at the respective interfaces and strengthened their discoursive power with the focus on access to medicines. One can safely claim that this particular field of global governance was to some extent already 'occupied' by normally weak actors in the global power structure when more powerful Northern governments and IGOs (re-)entered this field.

Furthermore, the altered context of global health problems, such as increasing transborder spread of infectious diseases and the increasing interconnection between poverty and certain diseases in developing countries, challenged IGOs and to some extent overstrained their capability to react to these problems. Additionally, the general process of the transnationalization of governance and the greater importance of hybrid and private forms of governance affected the basically international and intergovernmental structures of policy-making and governance.

This is the complex political and institutional setting of the current global health governance system in which the WHO, the World Bank and UNAIDS play important roles. If we acknowledge that current processes and structures of global health governance are strongly influenced by nation-states and keep in mind the important role of non-state actors, we have to question the role of IGOs as the classical organizations of cooperation between nation-states. What is the role – at least formally – of the 'anchor' organization (Murray 2005; Shakow 2005; Ivanova 2005: 8) of global health, the WHO?

This analysis is based on institutionalist approaches of International Relations (Rosenau 2002; Keohane 2002), governance theories (Scharpf 1997; Kooiman 2003; Mayntz 2005) and on the concept of interfaces (as outlined in Chapter 1). Furthermore, I refer to the approach of forum-shifting (Braithwaite and Drahos 2000), which can help to analyse how actors use different institutions and fora to pursue their goals in global health governance – a question that is extremely important if we want to understand the role of IGOs. Forum-shifting in global governance can be defined as the attempt to influence and change politics and pursue goals by using the forum that seems most appropriate to achieve one's objectives. According to Braithwaite and Drahos (2000: 564), forum-shifting comprises three different strategies: 'moving an agenda from one organization to another, abandoning an organization, and pursuing the same agenda in more than one organization'. This concept of forum-shifting is a promising attempt at analysing the relationship between the discourses, the strategies of different actors, and the institutions in which they act; and it can contribute to a better understanding of global governance. However, the concept is still in its infancy and further conceptualization and empirical research are necessary.

Furthermore, if we analyse IGOs in global governance, one must distinguish between two different functions of these organizations that imply different perspectives of analysis. First, IGOs are *fora* and organizational *interfaces*. They are a forum for nation-states and for other actors like other IGOs or non-state actors, inasmuch as these are involved in formal structures. The interactions of these actors constitute these organizations. Furthermore, there are internal interfaces between different departments and single staff members. If we analyse IGOs from this perspective we have to examine the single actors that are part of the organization, and we have to deal with the interactions between these single actors. Second, IGOs are *actors* of global governance. This means that they – albeit influenced by their stakeholders – have some level of autonomy, and that, although there are often different interests and preferred strategies within one organization due to conflicts at the internal interfaces, they have their own organizational interests. Looking at IGOs as actors implies examining their interactions and interfaces with other actors of global governance both horizontally (at the global level) and vertically (global–national). Whereas in reality both functions are closely interrelated and do in fact mix, I attempt to separate them analytically in a first step and then combine them afterwards. This enables an analysis of the internal and external interfaces of IGOs as well as the interrelation of both, so that we can understand the functions and roles of IGOs in global governance.

The following are the main propositions of this chapter:

- Set against the background of a complex and fragmented system of global health governance, social policy-oriented IGOs such as the WHO are weakened due to new modes of governance and as a result of the interests of powerful nation-states. Public–private partnerships (PPPs) and private actors take over some of the responsibilities and functions of the WHO, or deal with newly emerging problems. Governments of industrialized countries shift the forum of action, at least in some important fields of global health, away from the WHO and try to bypass the latter.
- At the same time, the current institutional structure of global governance with its relatively strong influence of CSOs and its impact on national governance strengthens policies to fight poverty-related diseases and to enhance access to medicines. In this context, there are several challenges and opportunities for IGOs to reaffirm or regain their central positions in global health governance, for example, as interface managers.

This chapter begins with a brief analysis of the WHO as a forum and organizational interface by looking at its internal organizational structure. It then discusses the WHO as an actor first in global health governance in general and second in the fight against HIV/AIDS. The role and power of the WHO will be addressed by scrutinizing the WHO's interfaces with the World Bank and UNAIDS and also with the Global Fund to Fight HIV/AIDS, Tuberculosis and Malaria, as well as the President's Emergency Plan for AIDS Relief (PEPFAR). Continuing, the chapter makes some brief remarks on the role of the World Bank in global health governance. Finally, it focuses on UNAIDS as new form of IGO by analysing again the two forms of its interactions.

The World Health Organization in global health governance

The WHO was founded by the members of the international community 'for the purpose of co-operation among themselves and with others to promote and protect the health of all peoples' (WHO Constitution). Therefore, it is *the* organization of nation-states to promote global health. The WHO is an IGO that comprises 192 governments, with the World Health Assembly (WHA, all member states) and the Executive Board (32 member states) as their main decision-making bodies.

Among others, the main objectives and functions of the WHO are:

- to develop internationally common solutions and goals for crucial challenges in the health sector;
- to set internationally accepted norms and standards and to give technical guidance and advice for member countries in promoting health (this includes the classification of diseases and causes of death, standards for medical provision, treatment, and drugs);
- to help countries develop political strategies and public health concepts to reach these goals and to implement norms and standards;
- to fight communicable and non-communicable diseases (for example, smallpox eradication, the fight against HIV/AIDS, tuberculosis and malaria, vaccination programmes).

Thus, the WHO has both normative and technical functions and it does not – by definition in its constitution – have a political function, although, of course, in reality it is not as clear-cut. Also, in comparison to UNICEF or UNDP, the WHO does not have a strong function of programme implementation in developing countries. With respect to interfaces we can state that, on the one hand, the WHO is a forum with organizational interfaces where governments (and also other actors) negotiate and make health policy. Thus, political processes within the organization are important if we want to understand the WHO. On the other hand, the WHO is also an actor with its own interests and strategies, as it is a specialized agency of the United Nations, and the Secretariat has a semi-autonomous status. Although it is accountable to the WHA and remains a 'servant' to the member states, the Secretariat has some autonomy and has an impact on designing the WHO's strategy and policies.

Organizational interfaces are not only crucial within the WHO, but also when it operates as an actor and interacts with others in global health governance and engages for example in hybrid institutions such as PPPs. Moreover, one of the WHO's foremost functions is to coordinate international health-related activities and policies of its member states and other actors. This, however, relates also to discoursive interfaces. As the WHO's mission is to set norms and guidelines for the health sector, it interacts intensely with other actors at discoursive interfaces of global health governance and enjoys an important discoursive power – also due to its accumulated expertise. With respect to its function in setting norms and guidelines and providing technical assistance for the countries, the WHO is also involved in resource-transfer interfaces. The WHO is not a funding organization and thus its power in terms of financial resources is not strong; however, it does have some power and influence due to its ability to provide knowledge. Finally, legal interfaces are also of some importance for the WHO as it offers an institutional basis on which to propose and negotiate rules, conventions, and thus forms of international law (for example the WHO Framework Convention on Tobacco Control, International Health Regulations). Though the WHO is involved in all four types of interfaces of global health governance, the following analysis will concentrate on organizational and discoursive interfaces, which are of foremost importance for the WHO in the fight against HIV/AIDS.

The World Health Organization as a forum: internal interfaces

The WHA is the highest decision making body of the WHO with some legislative functions. Thus, relating to our concept of interfaces, it is the most important organizational interface within the WHO where governments of member states interact. The WHA makes all important decisions regarding the WHO's internal and external activities, like the approval of its strategies and policies regarding institutional reforms, the work programme, approval of the biennial budget, election of the Director General, decisions on conventions and legal issues, and publication of recommendations for nearly all issues in the health sector. The WHA comprises delegations of all member states, each of whom has one vote.

The WHA has to interact closely with the Executive Board, which includes thirty-two health experts of member states chosen by the WHA for a period of three years. At least three member states per WHO region have to be represented on the Executive Board. The Executive Board prepares the meetings of the WHA, gives advice to the WHA and develops the programme and the budget that is then discussed and approved by the WHA. On the other hand, it functions as a kind of executive organ of the WHO as it has to translate the decisions of the WHA into policies. Due to these functions the Executive Board can be considered powerful and influential within the WHO. Although the Executive Board members are formally independent, single member states can exert substantial influence on the technical and political direction taken by the WHO via the Executive Board.

The technical work as well as the realization and implementation of measures and programmes – the day-to-day work – is done by the Secretariat, the staff of the WHO. If one looks at the WHO as an actor, it is mainly the work of the Secretariat that counts. The Secretariat is organized into the headquarters, six regional offices and close to 150 country offices and has at present about 8000 employees. The headquarters in Geneva has about 2000–3000 staff – depending on the strategic decisions of the respective administration, the work programme, and on the basis of extra-budgetary funding. According to the WHO constitution, the Secretariat should act as a kind of 'servant' to the member states. Hence it should not act on behalf of the WHO's organizational self-interests, but instead to the advantage of the member states. However, at the same time the WHO constitution stipulates that the Secretariat should not act at the member states' disposition and should have some autonomy (WHO 1946; interviews[1]).

The division of the WHO into headquarters, regional offices and country offices gives rise to some problems for the organization. If we look at this division of the WHO in a different way – and in keeping with Ruger and Yach (2005) – we can distinguish between global and operational functions at the regional and country level. Global functions include activities such as norm-setting and defining goals at the global level, whereas operational functions include all those efforts to give advice to governments and authorities, to strengthen capacity, and to develop infrastructure at the national level. Without going into the details of this complex and contested discussion it can be maintained here that there is tension between the headquarters and the six regional offices as well as between the global functions and the operational functions in the countries. Some argue that the relative power of the regional offices weakens the WHO as an effective and influential actor at the global level (Ruger and Yach 2005; Murray 2005). Then again, some of the WHO's power derives precisely from this decentralized structure, because the governments have great influence on the WHO and therefore consider it an accountable and legitimate actor. They regard the WHO as 'their' organization and thus might follow its guidelines and recommendations. However, many experts claim that there is no proper management of relations between the different offices and that regional offices to some extent are poorly led, hence effectiveness is reduced (Murray 2005; interviews). Thus it seems that one of the sources of power (the regional structure and the strong influence of member states due to the WHA and the Executive Board) at the same time hampers and weakens the ability of the WHO to fulfil its function as a global actor.

Analysing the interfaces of governments inside WHO generally, we can state that governments of developing countries – compared to the World Bank for example – have a relatively strong position within the WHO (as, for instance, the WHA functions according to the principle 'one country, one vote'). In particular, newly-industrializing countries (NICs) such as Brazil and South Africa have a certain influence and power within the organization. This relative great weight of developing countries also becomes apparent when we acknowledge that since 1966 more than half of the biennial budget was spent on programmes and operational activities in developing countries (Koivusalo and Ollila 1997: 8). This shows that the WHO works, for the most part, for developing countries and that development issues and the relationship between poverty and health are of great relevance. However, the WHO's great efforts in assisting poorer countries has led to a divide in donors and recipients and thus to unequal positions.

We see that organizational and resource-transfer interfaces mix in reality. This is particularly so with internal interfaces within IGOs as they are mostly financed by member states. In fact, the shape and constitution of organizational interfaces within the WHO is based mostly on resource-transfer interfaces, since providing funds for the WHO means having more informal power and influence. It is therefore worthwhile to take a look at the WHO's budget: its total budget for 2004/2005 was US$2.8 billion, but the approved biennial regular budget (based on assessed contributions from member states according to the UN scale) for 2004/2005 was only US$880 million (see Table 5.1). Two thirds of the total budget

Table 5.1 Programme budget WHO 2003–2007 (in US$ 1000)

	2002/2003	2004/2005	2006/2007
Regular budget	855 654	880 111	915 315
Voluntary contributions	1 380 500	1 944 000	2 398 126
Total budget	2 236 154	2 824 111	3 313 441

Source: WHO (2005).

come from voluntary contributions from member states and also from CSOs, foundations and the private sector. Northern governments (or government-run bilateral ODA agencies) account for most of the extra-budgetary funds. The high and ever-growing share of extra-budgetary funds means that donor countries and also increasingly private actors have huge potential to influence the WHO's strategies as well as its political and technical decision-making and policies. In addition – returning to the North–South relations – as many of the WHO's activities in developing countries are financed with additional budgetary contributions, industrialized countries' governments exert indirect influence on health policy in developing countries via these funds.

Due to their resource-based power, governments of industrialized countries influence – often informally – decisions and policies of the WHO both via the WHA and the Executive Board and also by exerting influence on the Secretariat and its staff in particular. There is some informal influence and pressure by relevant donor countries (mainly the US) on decisions concerning top level staff (such as the Director General (DG) and also Assistant DGs) and concerning key policies and programmes. This does not mean that the WHO Secretariat always follows the instructions of Northern governments, but it does mean that serious conflicts arise in cases where interests and strategies differ: 'WHO has great difficulties in criticizing or acting against the interests of the government of an influential Member State' (Murray 2005: 14).

WHO as an actor of global health governance

Before analysing the role of the WHO as actor in the current structure of global health governance one needs to take a brief look at its history. In the first three decades of its existence, the WHO was predominately a technical organization dominated by medical professionals and focusing on the eradication and containment of specific diseases. Whereas political conflicts were not of great importance during that time, the WHO experienced a politicization in the context of the so-called North–South conflict in international politics and UN organizations in the 1970s. Discussions on development and health were on the agenda and the awareness of linkages between both was prevalent in the WHO and other organizations of international health. At the same time, problems in the efforts towards the eradication of malaria and the evaluation of related programmes led to a questioning of the focus on the technical-medical solutions to tackle specific diseases as the dominant practice within the WHO (Koivusalo and Ollila 1997: 11f.).

Thus, in the late 1970s a more horizontal and comprehensive approach came to the fore. The International Conference on Primary Health Care in Alma Ata in 1978 proposed a Primary Health Care strategy, endorsed by the World Health Assembly in 1979, to achieve the objective of 'Health for All by the Year 2000' not just by giving the poor a minimum of health services (in a more neo-liberal sense), but by providing health services for all as the foundation of a comprehensive health system (in a universalistic sense). However, ideologically charged conflicts within the context of the North–South confrontation and a certain aloofness on the part of industrialized countries hampered the implementation of the Primary Health Care concept. In keeping with the hegemony of neo-liberal concepts in the global economy, the assumption that the Alma Ata concept of Primary Health Care was too idealistic and not feasible gained increasing acceptance among IGOs, and in the 1980s the concept of Selective Primary Health Care became dominant in discourses and in health activities. This strategy focused on specific diseases in developing countries and on the lack of immunization and also defined so-called attainable goals. Some donors, IGOs and scholars favoured this concept, its influence extending even to the current focus on fighting specific (mainly infectious) diseases.

However, not only the hegemony of neo-liberal concepts – highlighting targeted, selective help and private provision instead of comprehensive health care – but also failures in some developing countries in implementing this strategy have reduced the acceptance of the Primary Health Care approach in current global health policies (Cueto 2004; Sanders 2003; Thomas and Weber 2004: 192 ff.; Lee 2004; Brown et al. 2006).

After the period of internal political debates and the WHO's more political role in international health in the 1970s and 1980s under Director General Halfdan Mahler, the term of Hiroshi Nakajima was characterized again by a more technical, medical and managerial approach. There were some debates on the WHO's strategy and policy under Nakajima. For example, it was assumed that the influence of some powerful nation-states and the pharmaceutical industry had increased; moreover, internal governance issues were criticized. Looking back, this period saw a decline of the WHO's political role and is often interpreted as one reason for the weakening of the organization in the 1990s (Koivusalo and Ollila 1997: 6f.; Horton 2002; Brown et al. 2006). The political weakness of the WHO occurred at a time of institutional change in global health governance, characterized by a greater political influence of private actors and a greater weight of the World Bank. From 1998 to 2003, under the aegis of Gro Harlem Brundtland, the WHO once again stressed its political functions as a global health actor. One important element of the WHO's work as a global actor was the creation of the Commission on Macroeconomics and Health that tried to strengthen the promotion of health for economic reasons. It was in this period that the WHO began to react to the changed institutional setting and tried to regain power and political influence.

If we analyse the WHO's current role in global health governance we can identify some strategies that should strengthen it as a central actor in this arena. One of these strategies has been to engage more intensely in PPPs or even to create them (for example, Stop TB, Roll Back Malaria). Relating to this, Brundtland tried to improve the relations to the private sector and pharmaceutical companies, which was criticized by many experts as they feared a loss of the organization's independence (Horton 2002; Lee 2004: 15; Brown et al. 2006). Another initiative that strengthened the WHO as a global health actor was the negotiation of the WHO Framework Convention on Tobacco Control (FCTC). This process led to some conflicts with tobacco companies. However, the WHO and the member states finally withstood the massive lobbying attacks from these companies. With the FCTC, the WHO for the first time made use of Article 19 of the WHO constitution, which provides it with treaty-making power (Fidler 2002; Taylor et al. 2003; Collin et al. 2002; Aginam 2005).

Finally, the flexible and fast reaction of the WHO to SARS in 2003 and the successful conclusion of the renegotiation of the International Health Regulations (IHRs) reveal the potentially strong role the WHO can play in disease surveillance and response. The new IHRs are applicable to a much wider range of international and transnational public health problems and risks (not only infectious but also non-communicable diseases, not only naturally occurring but also intentionally caused). Moreover, the new IHRs include non-governmental sources of information into the surveillance system, which can be interpreted as an adaptation to the emerging governance structures that differ from the state-centred governance structures in the phase of the onset of the old IHRs. All in all, the revised IHRs give the WHO more authority and capacity to act in health and diseases control (Fidler 2005; Sell 2006: 33).

Although these processes and functions of the WHO indicate some strengths and power, research shows that there are also attributes and aspects of this organization and the entire system of global health governance that cause an enervation of the WHO in some fields of global health governance.

(1) We can generally observe that the neo-liberal hegemony has put social policy-oriented IGOs such as the WHO in a somewhat defensive position, while market-oriented organizations and regimes (like, for example, the WTO) have gained influence in global politics.
(2) Like other UN organizations, the WHO acts relatively slowly because its activities depend on a decision-making process that has to aggregate the interests and commitments of member states. One consequence of this is that some donors prefer to cooperate with other organizations or – in certain cases – to conduct bilateral programmes.
(3) The WHO is not only disregarded by the governments of some industrialized countries because of its assumed ineffectiveness, but in some cases also due to reasons of political power. As governments of developing countries have a relatively strong position within the WHO, it is sometimes difficult for governments of industrialized countries to pursue their interests. If they perceive their own interests to be different from the majority of other countries they try to circumvent the WHO and focus their activities and resources on other organizations.
(4) In the context of the institutional change of global governance, so-called new actors and governance modes at the global level (like CSOs and PPPs) challenge the WHO and take over some of its functions and are used increasingly by governments of industrialized countries instead of the WHO.
(5) Finally, since the WHO is not a funding organization it has no resource-based power in terms of financial resources (Horton 2002; Lee 2004: 15; Global Health Watch 2005; Brown et al. 2006; WHO 2006b: 61f.; interviews).

The WHO in the global fight against HIV/AIDS: interfaces and forum-shifting

The UN's first comprehensive reaction to HIV/AIDS came with the setting up of the Global Programme on AIDS (GPA) under the auspices of the WHO in 1987. The GPA's objective was to enhance international discourses on HIV/AIDS with an emphasis on empowerment and emancipation, provide technical assistance for developing countries, and mobilize the donor countries for a multilateral reaction to HIV/AIDS. Due to an increasing engagement of other UN organizations and the often criticized limited capacity of the GPA to reduce the inter-organizational rivalries within the UN system, the GPA was dissolved in 1995 and transformed into UNAIDS (Altman 1999: 20; UNAIDS 2002: 3; Söderholm 1997: 125f.).

After the establishment of UNAIDS in 1996 the WHO transferred its competencies, personnel and resources in handling HIV/AIDS to this new joint venture of UN organizations. In spite of several problems in coordinating the UN member organizations, UNAIDS was seen as the leading UN organization in the fight against HIV/AIDS as far as normative and strategic aspects were concerned, until the WHO started to develop its own HIV/AIDS policy again in 2000/1 (for a detailed analysis of UNAIDS see below). If we look at the interfaces between the WHO and UNAIDS we can identify conflicts. Both actors compete for the leading role in the global fight against HIV/AIDS, though according to official statements they complement each other. Experts criticize the duplication of structures as a result of the existence of UNAIDS and a relatively large HIV/AIDS department in the WHO. However, this parallel structure can also contribute to more effective activities if the HIV/AIDS department and UNAIDS cooperate closely. Particularly in the day-to-day work, this cooperation often depends on the relationship between the individual staff members in both organizations.

Besides the WHO and UNAIDS, UNICEF and the World Bank also play an important role in the fight against HIV/AIDS and in the health sector in general. At country level UNICEF became the most important health implementation agency of the UN family in the 1980s (Koivusalo and Ollila 1997: 46f.). Since 2000, the World Bank has run the Multi-Country HIV/AIDS Programme (MAP), which so far has distributed more than US$1 billion to twenty-six African countries. The important role of the Bank in particular in the fight against HIV/AIDS and in global health in general raises the question of cooperation or competition between the WHO and the Bank. Although there is, of course, cooperation between both organizations (as, for example, in the case of the health-related MDGs) and both are connected in UNAIDS, and although official statements maintain that the World Bank and WHO complement each other in their work, organizational self-interests engender some competition for the leading role in global public health (interviews). Furthermore, although the WHO and the World Bank take similar positions with regard to the organization of health systems (Kaasch 2006), they have different concepts and strategies in some areas. One example is depicted in the series of conflicts in the 1980s and 1990s, when the

Bank began to add health loans to its portfolio: 'Particularly for areas such as health finance, this advice often ran counter to WHO advice and led to a decrease in the influence of WHO' (Murray 2005: 15).

In 2002, the Global Fund was launched by the G8 and Kofi Annan, which caused another change in the global health architecture (see Chapter 6). It was established as a finance mechanism in the form of a public–private partnership, separate from the UN and WHO, because the US, especially, but also Japan and Italy did not want to have it under the auspices of the UN. The official rationale given by the donor countries for its separate structure was the lack of flexibility within the UN system. However, we can safely assume some political interests in bypassing the UN. This, of course, led to controversial discussions because UN organizations and especially the WHO feared a further loss of influence on global health issues, and some health experts and CSOs were afraid of a privatization of governance. The fact that the WHO, UNAIDS and the World Bank are members of the Executive Board of the Global Fund but have no voting power shows that, at least formally, these actors function merely in an advisory capacity within the Board.

This separate construction of the Global Fund is a typical example of forum-shifting since certain powerful actors decided that an essential function of global health governance (the allocation of money to fight infectious diseases) can be better addressed in a PPP-like forum than in IGOs. Moreover, it is interesting if we look at the interests and strategies of powerful nation-states: nation-states use a hybrid network structure to circumvent IGOs. This means that hybrid regulation, which leads to a sharing of the states' power and influence with other actors, can be a result of specific nation-state interests in solving global problems.

If we analyse the interaction between the Global Fund and the WHO from an actor-centred perspective we can ascertain a power shift. The donor countries created a new player in the field of global health – though not officially a political organization – that is provided with substantial power as it disburses financial resources. This changes the structure of power relations of global health governance. The establishment of the Global Fund can also be seen as a challenge to the WHO in terms of direct cooperation and coordination. Besides coordination problems in the countries (Bartsch and Kohlmorgen 2005c: 270f., and the section of this chapter on UNAIDS), there are conflicts at the interfaces between the Global Fund and the WHO (and also UNAIDS and the World Bank) regarding the operational work in the process of application for Global Fund grants.

Many Country Coordinating Mechanisms (CCMs) – that are the required institutions to apply for funding through the Global Fund – only dispose of limited resources and capacities and consequently have problems in developing and writing the ambitious proposals for the Global Fund. Consequently, UNAIDS and the WHO assist the CCMs. Although staff members of UNAIDS and WHO see this assistance as a natural part of their work, it causes problems as it increases the workload for UNAIDS and the WHO without granting any financial compensation. This is not only an interface problem at the national level but also causes conflicts at the global level between the Global Fund Secretariat and UNAIDS/WHO. Meanwhile, after negotiations between the WHO and the Global Fund Secretariat, the Global Fund appeals to donor countries to give extra funds to the WHO and UNAIDS to strengthen their support for the CCMs. Moreover, the Fund advises the CCMs to dedicate 10 per cent of the requested funds to capacity building and technical assistance with respect to developing proposals. This, however, may lead to a situation in which the WHO and UNAIDS are seen as consultants that possibly compete with other consultants on contracts for assisting CCMs, something which may contravene the WHO's function as an organization of the countries and the WHO Secretariat's self-conception as 'servant' to the governments.

Continuing the analysis of forum-shifting in HIV/AIDS politics, we see that, meanwhile, the Global Fund itself is sidestepped and has problems attracting enough funds. While it is quite normal for donor countries to disburse most of their funds via bilateral programmes – as this is the best guarantee for them to pursue their interests – it is striking that the US government, for example, established the mainly bilateral programme PEPFAR[2] after playing a crucial role in creating the Global Fund. The general reason for this may be that forms of hybrid regulation such as the Global Fund have led to a stronger role of CSOs than the US government had anticipated.

If we take a look at the policies in fighting HIV/AIDS of the WHO, the World Bank and UNAIDS on the one hand and PEPFAR on the other, we see some differences in the policies as well as conflictive interactions. For example, PEPFAR comprises a hierarchy of prevention methods and accepts condoms only as a method of prevention for groups at risk. The WHO, UNAIDS and the World Bank advise the use of condoms as a normal prevention method and utilize them in most anti-HIV/AIDS programmes. Besides prevention, PEPFAR also focuses on treatment. Only when CSOs and also WHO and UNAIDS staff members heavily criticized the Office of the US Global AIDS Coordinator for only financing branded drugs, did PEPFAR slowly begin utilizing generic drugs. These conflicts reveal that the US government acts on behalf of perceived national interests. Due to a general scepticism towards multilateralism and due to vital interests of social groups in the US (Burkhalter 2004), which are reflected in government policies, the activities of the WHO, UNAIDS and increasingly also the Global Fund are partly circumvented.

Whereas there are some different approaches and conflicts between the actors particularly in the implementation and day-to-day work in the countries, official statements stress that different approaches do not cause any problems but in fact complement each other. Indeed, we see that, for example, the WHO's 3 by 5 initiative cooperated with PEPFAR to reach the proclaimed objectives. '3 by 5' was launched by the WHO (together with UNAIDS) in 2003 and aimed at providing three million people suffering from AIDS with ARV drugs until the end of 2005. This is an interesting turn in the WHO's policies, which is accompanied by a general turn in global HIV/AIDS policies: whereas, during the 1990s, the WHO and other IGOs focused on prevention, the treatment of AIDS patients has come into the foreground of the fight against HIV/AIDS since 2001. The main reason for this policy change is the decline in drug prices which made it possible to provide more AIDS victims with ARVs even in resource-poor countries (see Chapters 2 and 3). Additionally, this change in direction was influenced by some pressure from the Brazilian government to concentrate not only on prevention but also on treatment (interviews). Thus national policies of a Southern government (in this case, of a middle-income country) influenced the WHO's and UNAIDS' as well as general global policies in the field of HIV/AIDS. Moreover, the campaigning of CSOs for the realization of human rights and access to treatment showed some influence (Bartsch and Kohlmorgen 2005b; Hein 2005; Sell 2002; 't Hoen 2002; Chapters 2 and 4).

As the WHO is not a funding organization it had to rely on other actors such as the World Bank, the Global Fund and donor countries to achieve the goal of 3 by 5, which was defined as a movement that is only initiated and coordinated by the WHO. This initiative can be seen both as an organizational and discoursive interface at the horizontal level and also as a resource-based interface vertically. The WHO's main role and contribution was to advise national governments and IGOs to scale up national facilities in the provision of ARVs. The WHO needed extra funding for the increase in these activities. However, the WHO obviously had problems in scaling up its activities the way it originally had planned: in January 2004, the plan of raising US$350 million was reduced to US$174 million. Instead of 400 staff members as planned, only 112 worked for 3 by 5 (WHO 2006b: 67). Finally, the objective of providing 3 million AIDS victims in developing countries with ARVs by the end of 2005 was not attained. The number of people treated with ARVs increased from 400 000 in December 2003 to 1 million in August 2006 (WHO 2006b).

The effectiveness of 3 by 5 of course also depended on the governments of developing countries that had to make the decisions on the HIV/AIDS strategy and were responsible for implementing multilateral and bilateral programmes. Although the WHO certainly has considerable influence on health policies in most of the poorer countries, these governments maintain their autonomy and sovereignty. For example, some of the countries that were crucial for reaching the 3 by 5 goal, like South Africa, Nigeria and India, complained that they were not consulted sufficiently in the process of initiating the programme and thus only supported the goals to a certain degree.[3]

Summing up, we can say that with the 3 by 5 initiative and its focus on HIV/AIDS, the WHO tried to gain influence in global HIV/AIDS politics dominated by UNAIDS, the Global Fund and bilateral programmes like PEPFAR. The WHO tried to play a more prominent role in this central field of global health governance in order to defend its claim to be the legitimately responsible institution for global public health. However, at the same time, the dependence on other actors in implementing the initiative, for example, illustrates the WHO's weakness (similar to other UN special agencies). Moreover, some experts lament that 3 by 5, with its narrow approach to support treatment (and not health promotion) and with its focus on implementation and operational work, weakens the global functions of the WHO (Ruger and Yach 2005: 1100; WHO 2006b; interviews).

Since the objectives of 3 by 5 could not be reached, the WHO has now developed a framework for universal access to HIV/AIDS prevention, care, treatment and support in the health sector by 2010 ('Universal Access by 2010'). Moreover, the establishment of the Commission on Intellectual Property Rights, Innovation and Public Health (CIPIH) and the discussions on a 'Global Framework on Essential Health Research' can be interpreted as efforts to position the WHO in the field of intellectual property rights and trade-related fields of global health and thus more firmly in the complex architecture of global health governance in general.

In the conflicts on intellectual property rights and TRIPS the WHO – according to our differentiation between IGOs as fora and actors – had two functions. First, the WHO was used by governments and CSOs as a forum to promote their goals of low level IPRs and improve access to medicines in the debates on IPR. Also, the negotiation process of the TRIPS agreement as the cornerstone of the WTO has been dominated by governments of industrialized countries with an interest in strengthening IPRs. Second – and this of course links with its function as a forum – the

WHO as actor was to some extent part of the coalition of developing countries and CSOs fighting for the objective that TRIPS should not impede access to medicines in poor countries (Sell and Prakash 2004; Sell 2006; 't Hoen 2002).

These two functions of the WHO as forum and actor of global health governance are also obvious in the debates on the initiative for a 'Global Framework on Essential Health Research'. This initiative was influenced and initiated by a proposal for a 'Medical Research and Development Treaty' made by the US-CSO Cp-Tech some years ago and was supported by many CSOs and scientists in 2005. It was brought before the Executive Board in January 2006 by Kenya and Brazil and thereafter became a topic for controversy. Finally, a resolution was accepted by the Executive Board, which was discussed at the WHA meeting in May 2006. In both meetings, conflicts arose between most of the developing countries and the US, EU and Japan, because the richer countries, for example, did not accept the references to global public goods and expressed doubts concerning public and open research projects. The WHA decided to establish an intergovernmental working group to draw up a global strategy and plan of action in order to develop a medium-term framework based on CIPIH's recommendations (WHO 2006a). Even though it remains to be seen whether this decision will yield practical results with effects on health research and the development of drugs, it can be considered as an important step in the WHO's efforts to engage more intensely in the field of research and development and to strengthen its role in global health. Moreover, the processes leading to this decision show that the WHO is used as a forum to pursue goals in political conflicts.

The World Bank

The World Bank is basically a development bank (formally, a UN Specialized Agency) that aims at enhancing economic development in poor countries and – at least in recent times – emphasizing the fight against poverty. As an intergovernmental organization it is also a forum of global governance. However, it is one with organizational interfaces mainly between governments of member states which represent the Bretton Woods organizations. According to their capital shares, economically strong countries have greater voting power within the organization. As an actor, the World Bank has power due to its ability to provide resources, which it is able to obtain both from private capital markets and member states; it may also be due to the greater coherence between the economic power of member states and the decision-making power within the organization.

The Bank's activities in the health sector began in the early 1970s, but the first loans were not awarded until the 1980s. The 1993 World Development Report *Investing in Health* (which recommended a public–private mix for financing and organizing health systems) had a great conceptual influence on health system reforms in the 1990s. Furthermore, the Bank had (and still has) a great impact on health policies due to structural adjustment strategies that have now turned into poverty reduction policies (cf. Ruger 2005; Wogart 2003).

As already mentioned, the Multi-country AIDS Programme (MAP) has provided twenty-six African countries with more than US$1 billion since 2001. Participation of non-state actors at the country level and good governance are prerequisites for recipient countries to receive money in the MAP. Thus, although the MAP is a programme run by an IGO it empowers non-state actors at the national level and relies on networking.

The Bank is the greatest single donor in health and one of the greatest single donors in the fight against HIV/AIDS. But it is not only powerful because of its lending and granting activities but also – as a result of this resource-based power – because of its discoursive power in influencing political and operational strategies in the health sector. Both the substantial resource-based and discoursive power provide the World Bank with much influence at resource-based and discoursive interfaces with developing countries as well as at the discoursive interfaces with other actors of global health governance such as the WHO. The Bank's important role certainly traces back to the fact that the rich countries dominate World Bank policies due to their majority in shares whilst developing countries play only a minor role. It is broadly accepted that, since the 1990s, the World Bank has remained one of the leading actors of global health governance (Abasi 1999; Buse and Gwin 1998: 666; Lee et al. 1996; Thomas and Weber 2004: 194; Ruger 2005; interviews).[4]

UNAIDS

UNAIDS was created in 1996 as the successor of WHO's GPA and can be seen as a new kind of entity in the UN system uniting ten UN organzations,[5] which is intended to align their efforts in the fight against HIV/AIDS by focusing on their particular strengths and comparative advantages, and also including non-state actors to some extent. UNAIDS is a multisectoral programme dealing with a broad range of issues and problems that are associated with HIV/AIDS and can be interpreted as an attempt by the UN to react to the institutional developments in global health and to improve the effectiveness of the global fight against HIV/AIDS. Its main objective is to coordinate the UN system's response towards the HIV/AIDS challenge. Besides the ten UN organizations, delegates of twenty-two governments from the North and the South and from five CSOs (including groups of people living with HIV/AIDS) are members of the Programme Coordinating Board, the highest body of UNAIDS. Although the CSOs are only non-voting members, the participation of non-state actors in a formal decision-making body is a novelty for the UN system (apart from the tripartite International Labour Organization). This, in addition to UNAIDS' encouragement of CSO involvement at the national level, illustrates the importance of hybrid forms of regulation and networks between public and private actors in global health governance. The day-to-day work of UNAIDS is conducted by the Secretariat, which disposes of approximately 150 staff members in Geneva and more staff posted in over seventy-five countries. Moreover, UNAIDS' work in the countries relies on the staff members of the co-sponsoring organizations, which make up so-called UN Theme Groups on HIV/AIDS (Kohlmorgen 2004).

Besides the coordination of the UN activities, UNAIDS' objective is to advocate a global reaction to the HIV/AIDS pandemic (which means the involvement in discoursive interfaces of global governance) and to contribute to the coordination and harmonization of the related efforts of different actors (which affects organizational and discoursive interfaces). UNAIDS assists countries in developing national responses to HIV/AIDS and provides information and data on the HIV/AIDS epidemic. Looking at all these functions concerned with enhancing cooperation between different actors and looking at the institutional structure of UNAIDS, the definition that best describes UNAIDS as an actor is 'interface manager' (Benner et al. 2002: 18; Altman 1999: 20; Söderholm 1997: 125f.; Kohlmorgen 2004).[6]

UNAIDS as a forum: internal interfaces

Due to the integration of CSOs as well as its coordinating function, UNAIDS is often seen as an example for UN reform and for minimizing ineffectiveness and duplication of structures. So how can one evaluate the performance of UNAIDS as an interface manager among UN organizations? According to Benner et al. (2002: 18), UNAIDS was not successful in establishing itself as an effective interface manager; yet they do not substantiate this statement.

Indeed, evaluation and research show that the attempts to improve harmonization and coordination amongst organizations within the UN are fraught with many problems (GAO 2001; UNAIDS 2002; interviews). Most of the coordination problems result from overlapping mandates, different interests and objectives of co-sponsors both in the fight against HIV/AIDS and beyond in other policy fields such as development, poverty reduction and economic policies, as well as from organizational self-interests. The co-sponsors – at different degrees and in various fields – continue to conduct their own HIV/AIDS policies and they do not surrender much of their autonomy. For example, the World Bank with its substantial resource-based power insists on keeping control of the resources they offer, even if it works closely with other partners. And, although officially UNAIDS and WHO complement each other without any problems, at times there is in fact a duplication of structures and conflicts arise that relate to the mandates and the influence of each organization. The self-interests of the participating actors are for the most part related to the competition for scarce resources (interviews). Thus, the existence of UNAIDS has not abolished rivalries between UN organizations and has not solved the coordination and cooperation problems.

However, in considering these problems one has to bear in mind that UNAIDS is a relatively small organization with massive funding problems and hence limited capacities to act effectively. Against this background it is obvious that UNAIDS has problems coordinating and aligning the activities and policies of powerful and diverse actors such as the World Bank and the WHO. At the same time, there is some progress in improving cooperation between the co-sponsors as is shown by the fact that all co-sponsors align their budget for HIV/AIDS activities in the UNAIDS Unified Budget and Work Plan. Staff members of the WHO and World Bank underline that UNAIDS – under the prevailing circumstances – has managed the relationship of the co-sponsors skilfully.

The inclusion of CSOs in the Programme Coordinating Board and in other bodies of UNAIDS constitutes another crucial aspect of UNAIDS' internal interfaces. The empirical data, however, indicate that CSO involvement prevails mainly at the global level and is encouraged mainly by the UNAIDS Secretariat, whereas the involvement (and sometimes also the cooperation) at the country level differs from country to country and is often not very far-reaching. This can be interpreted as a consequence of vertical interfaces with national actors complicating the field of cooperation (interviews; UNAIDS 2002: 29).

UNAIDS as an actor of global health governance: managing the interfaces

If we look at UNAIDS as an actor we mainly speak of the small Secretariat with its headquarters in Geneva and its country officers in the field.[7] In the following, we would like to analyse briefly UNAIDS' work as an interface manager by looking at the coordination of HIV/AIDS-related activities in the countries and at the efforts of donor harmonization in the contexts of 'The Three Ones' and the Global Task Team, which both relate to organizational and discoursive interfaces.

The World Bank as well as UNAIDS favour the concept of creating National HIV/AIDS Councils (NAC) at the national level. The establishment of such an NAC is a precondition to receiving loans and grants through the MAP. The NAC should be headed by a government member, preferably by the prime minister, and should include not only all relevant ministries and authorities, but also other actors such as CSOs. The NAC's responsibilities include the guidance of the national efforts to fight HIV/AIDS, the definition of policies, and the coordination of activities (World Bank 2004b: 21f.). However, studies examining national HIV/AIDS governance in sub-Saharan Africa conclude that in some countries the results and effects are poor and that duplication of structures is a problem. James Putzel (2004: 1136) cites Uganda and Senegal as examples of countries where the governments had already built up relatively successful HIV/AIDS programmes and where the foundation of NACs has led to some disorder. In its evaluation of the first year of MAP, the World Bank itself points to this problem of the duplication of structures in the recipient countries (World Bank 2002: 11). These problems were addressed again three years later, when the Interim Review of the MAP assessed the 'governance aspect of the national response' as 'troubling' and concludes that NACs 'are not providing consistent leadership and oversight' (World Bank 2004b: iii).

We see that the establishment of NACs has already caused governance problems. These problems have further increased in many countries with the requirement to set up Country Coordinating Mechanisms (CCMs) for applying for money and receiving it through the Global Fund. According to the rules of the Global Fund, each CCM has to work like a public–private partnership and has to include non-state actors, which is somewhat different from the constitution of the more government-based NAC (Dickinson 2005).

As countries differ, we also find different forms of relationship between NACs and CCMs. In some countries both complement each other and no or only few conflicts can be detected, while in many other countries there appears to be a lack of coordination and an uncertainty about which should be the leading body in the national response to HIV/AIDS. Obviously, there are conflicts between the multilateral organizations favouring either the CCM (Global Fund) or the NAC (World Bank, UNAIDS) (interviews).

In addition to the main funding initiatives PEPFAR, MAP and the Global Fund, other funding and donor activities are, of course, being carried out in each country. Moreover, as HIV/AIDS is a multisectoral problem, many other actors have an impact on the efforts to fight HIV/AIDS. While this institutional setting might support the empowerment of originally weak actors, such as CSOs or self-help and support groups, and provide new flexible mechanisms to distribute resources, drugs and aid, it frequently causes a fragmentation of efforts. Some actors lack the willingness to cooperate, and many governments and authorities of developing countries are overstrained with this multiplicity of external actors and different governance modes. That, obviously, is a central problem of global governance: the programmes and concepts of the multitude of actors at the global level as well as the interactions between them are reproduced at the national level and additionally complicated by the interfaces with national actors.

Meanwhile, these problems are well known to IGOs and governments of industrialized countries. The efforts towards donor harmonization have increased in recent years.[8] In this context, UNAIDS in 2003/4 undertook necessary measures to enhance harmonization through the so-called principle of 'The Three Ones'. The following three aspects were identified as necessary conditions to improve effectiveness in the efforts to fight HIV/AIDS:

- one agreed HIV and AIDS Action Framework that provides the basis for coordinating the work of all partners;
- one National AIDS Coordinating Authority, with a broad-based multisectoral mandate;
- one agreed country-level Monitoring and Evaluation System.

The Three Ones were agreed at a high-level meeting attended by the most important donor countries (and also a few developing countries), the WHO, World Bank, Global Fund and UNAIDS in April 2004, which means that most of the relevant actors have committed themselves to following these principles. In March 2005, in the context of The Three Ones, another high-level meeting labelled 'Making the Money Work' was convened which decided to establish the 'Global Task Team on Improving Coordination Among Multilateral Institutions and International Donors'.

This Global Task Team can be described as a global governance process in a nutshell: it was a multi-stakeholder initiative established to deal with a global problem. The Global Task Team was facilitated by the UNAIDS

Secretariat; its objective was to make recommendations on the current status of coordination and harmonization and on options to prevent duplication in the global response to HIV/AIDS and to develop measures to improve the effectiveness of country-led activities. For this purpose, from April to June 2005, delegates from the relevant multilateral organizations, donor and recipient countries, and also from CSOs met to perform a stock-taking of cooperation and duplication efforts thus far and to make further recommendations. The final report of the Global Task Team first concludes that – despite the work of UNAIDS – the UN system's response to HIV/AIDS at country level is unevenly coordinated. For instance, it states that the UN Theme Groups on HIV/AIDS, which aim at coordinating UN activities in the countries, have not succeeded in establishing joint programmes that include the HIV/AIDS-related activities of UN organizations in most countries (Global Task Team 2005).

Undoubtedly, UNAIDS has increasingly taken over coordinating functions in the global efforts to fight HIV/AIDS both at the global and national level. However, some experts hold UNAIDS itself responsible for the cooperation and coordination problems in the countries and criticize UNAIDS for creating a duplication of structures and for being ineffective particularly at the country level. Other interview partners explained UNAIDS' somewhat poor performance at the country level with its dependence on the governments in the countries: the effectiveness and implementation of the various UNAIDS activities could only be as good as the member states allow them be in operationalizing their mandate. Despite these negative assessments many experts and also the evaluation reports highlight the successful activities that have been undertaken by UNAIDS at the national level in the efforts to assist governments in developing strategies and programmes against HIV/AIDS, emphasizing the potential that UNAIDS has for coordinating activities (GAO 2001; UNAIDS 2002; interviews).

We can conclude that there are indeed substantial problems and conflicts regarding cooperation between the various actors at the resource-transfer interfaces and at the organizational interfaces of global governance in combating HIV/AIDS. UNAIDS tries to improve the coordination and cooperation, but the organization is faced with problems in its function as interface manager. In spite of this rather mixed picture of UNAIDS' role as interface manager, we can maintain that its efforts in advocating for a global response to HIV/AIDS have been partly successful. It is of course difficult to measure the real impact of UNAIDS on the increase in global HIV/AIDS activities. However, we can assume that UNAIDS has contributed to the greater awareness of HIV/AIDS as a global problem, to the consensus that the activities have to be scaled up and finally to the increased activities at the global level (GAO 2001; UNAIDS 2002). Therefore UNAIDS is an important actor at the discoursive interfaces of global health governance in the field of HIV/AIDS.

Conclusion

We have shown that IGOs are faced with many challenges due to the current institutional structure of global health governance, which is expressed primarily in the dominant role of Northern governments and the importance of non-state actors and hybrid governance forms. Whereas IGOs reacted only hesitantly to the growing HIV/AIDS epidemic in the 1990s, CSOs and some governments of the South at the same time increased their activities early and began urging IGOs to support the fight against HIV/AIDS. Since the end of the 1990s, Northern governments have intensified their operations in global health and above all in the fight against poverty-related infectious diseases not only due to self-interests, but also as a reaction to the pressure from CSOs. The governance activities of most governments of industrialized countries in the field of global health are mainly located in bilateral politics and programmes. However, they increasingly include hybrid regulation as a means of reaching their goals – which can be best exemplified with the Global Fund. We have seen that governments can use networks and hybrid regulation and even CSOs as fora to achieve their goals (for example, to weaken IGOs like the WHO or to circumvent disliked governments in the South). Thus, the strong role of Northern governments and the relevance of hybrid regulation and private regulation are intertwined.

This constellation weakens social policy-oriented IGOs at least in certain fields of global health. If we look at the role of IGOs we see a mixed picture, depending on the type of organization and its particular functions.

The World Bank is one of the most influential actors and the most powerful IGO in global health governance, as it disposes of much resource-based and discoursive power. It has considerable influence on health policies through its impact on macroeconomics and fiscal policies in developing countries, but also through its lending and granting activities in the health arena. The Bank is dominated by industrialized countries and, consequently, these governments see it as an adequate forum to influence health policies at the global level and in developing countries.

Whereas eventually the WHO is also dominated by governments of industrialized countries, developing countries play a more important role within the WHO than in the World Bank. These power relations within the WHO and its functions as an organizational interface relate directly to the WHO's work as an actor of global health governance: the WHO acts to a large extent on behalf of the interests of developing countries. The WHO can also be characterized as a social policy-oriented organization aiming at the realization of human and social rights. Both can be interpreted as sources of power, since governments of developing countries see the WHO as an accountable actor and legitimized institution. However, at the same time, this is one reason for the WHO's weakness in some fields of global health. It is sidestepped by some Northern governments in certain cases where interests of Northern governments other than human rights dominate the agenda or they perceive the WHO as lacking in efficiency. In these cases, the powerful governments tend to use other fora such as the World Bank or the Global Fund. However, the WHO is not only challenged by 'new' modes of governance that can be used by powerful actors to bypass it. In addition, CSOs and PPPs take over functions of the WHO in general, and they increase the fragmentation of global health governance, which is a problem generally but a particular problem for the WHO as the formally central and responsible organization.

We can summarize that the strength of the WHO depends on the concrete policy field and the interests of powerful actors that influence it: whereas in the fight against HIV/AIDS the WHO is a relatively enervated actor, it is quite powerful in other fields such as norm-setting or infectious diseases control. When the WHO acts according to the interests of the major funding countries, it can be a strong actor. When it does not, the agenda in some cases is shifted to another forum and the WHO is bypassed. However, the WHO tried to react to the challenges and problems by engaging in public–private partnerships and by focusing on HIV/AIDS policies with the 3 by 5 initiative. Since the WHO is involved in all types of global governance interfaces it can be considered the central organization (or the anchor organization) of global health governance. However, as the WHO has little financial resources – and thus only some resource-based power due to its knowledge and expertise – it is not as powerful as the formal central position on the map of global health governance may suggest.

Some of the challenges described for the WHO exist also for UNAIDS; however, with some differences, because UNAIDS is not a typical IGO. UNAIDS can be seen as an attempt to react to the health-related challenges of globalization and to adapt to new forms of governance (by engaging in networks and including non-state actors) and to coordinate fragmented activities (interface manager). Against the background of the current architecture this is an important function of global health governance; however,

UNAIDS still faces rivalries between the different actors and strong organizational self-interests of the co-sponsoring organizations as well as other actors, which sometimes hamper cooperation and alignment of anti-HIV/AIDS programmes and activities. Thus, UNAIDS is faced with many difficulties in fulfilling its function as interface manager in the global fight against HIV/AIDS. However, UNAIDS showed some positive results in working at discoursive interfaces as it played an important role in enhancing the fight against HIV/AIDS by advocating and providing information. As an actor pursuing social rights and social policy objectives UNAIDS is sidestepped in some cases by donor countries, too.

Concluding, one can say that a complex variety of governance modes in global health governance causes problems for IGOs but can also be treated as an opportunity for improving governance structures globally and the health situation in developing countries, for instance by strengthening their role as interface manager in global health governance.

Notes

1. Source: more than 60 interviews with experts and with staff members of the WHO, World Bank, UNAIDS and CSOs.
2. PEPFAR was launched in 2004 providing US$15 billion until 2009 to fight HIV/AIDS (US$9 billion for new bilateral programmes in 14 African and Caribbean countries, US$5 billion for existing programmes in 75 countries and US$1 billion for the Global Fund to Fight HIV/AIDS, Tuberculosis and Malaria). PEPFAR is directed by the US Global AIDS Coordinator. The first Coordinator was Randall L. Tobias, a former CEO from the pharmaceutical company Eli Lilly & Co. In January 2006, he was nominated to lead USAID. PEPFAR is implemented mainly by USAID, but with the considerable involvement of US-based CSOs as well as CSOs from the recipient countries (see also Chapter 4).
3. Cf. interviews. The South African Health Minister Manto Tshabalala-Msimang said in May 2005: 'I don't want to be pushed or pressurized by a target of three million people on antiretrovirals by 2005. WHO set that target themselves. They didn't consult us. I don't see why South Africa today must be the scapegoat for not reaching the target' (source: http://www.kaisernetwork.org/-daily_reports/rep_index.cfm?DR_ID=29874).
4. It is, however, necessary to stress that different departments, programmes and staff members within the World Bank have different interests and views on which strategy is best. This means that, to be precise, in many cases we cannot speak of 'the Bank' as one monolithic actor.
5. The so-called co-sponsors of UNAIDS are: United Nation Children's Fund (UNICEF), the WHO, the World Bank, Office of the United Nations High Commissioner for Refugees (UNHCR), World Food Programme (WFP), United Nations Development Programme (UNDP), United Nations Population Fund

(UNFPA), United Nations Office on Drugs and Crime (UNODC), United Nations Educational, Scientific and Cultural Organization (UNESCO), and International Labour Organization (ILO).

6. UNAIDS staff members see themselves and UNAIDS as a 'broker of different ideas and interests and between different actors' (interviews with staff members of UNAIDS).
7. One interviewed staff member – referring to this small size and the chronic problem of lacking funds – characterizes UNAIDS as follows: 'We work like an NGO.'
8. See Rome Declaration on Harmonization and Paris Declaration on Aid Effectiveness.

6
The Global Fund to Fight AIDS, Tuberculosis and Malaria

Sonja Bartsch

Introduction

Hybrid forms of regulation between state and non-state actors became an essential part of global health governance in the beginning of the 1990s. In a phase where the UN system was increasingly criticized for being bureaucratic and ineffective, and where nation-states were losing regulating authority due to globalization processes, cooperation with non-state actors in the form of global public–private partnerships (GPPPs) seemed a promising way forward and was promoted by a variety of actors. Today we can find about eighty GPPPs in the health sector, differing in terms of legal status, disease focus and area of activity, and ranging from small initiatives for single issues to large institutions for multiple diseases.

Among the most prominent of these partnerships is the Global Fund to Fight AIDS, Tuberculosis and Malaria (GF) that has become one of the biggest players in global health since its establishment in 2002. It was designed as a financing mechanism in order to 'attract, manage and disburse additional resources' for the fight against the three major poverty-related diseases. By September 2006, it had approved US$5.6 billion to support programmes in 132 countries and received pledges of more than US$9.5 billion until 2008. The GF is the leading financing mechanism in the case of tuberculosis and malaria, where it contributes to 67 per cent and 64 per cent of all international funding, respectively. In the case of HIV/AIDS the GF strongly interacts with other financing institutions like the World Bank or the bilateral donors and makes up approximately 21 per cent of all international funding.

But the GF is not only an important financing mechanism in global health, it is also a major organizational interface, linking different kinds of stakeholder groups in its governing and administrative bodies. By choosing the approach of a public–private partnership, the GF represents a new way of doing business in the field of development cooperation and health that goes beyond the state-centred intergovernmental approach of other actors in global health governance. While its partnership approach on the one hand enables non-state actors – that have no or only a limited voice in established state-centred institutions – to participate in decision-making processes at global and national level, and also facilitates communication and learning processes between different constituencies, it is on the other hand associated with considerable transaction costs for the participating actors and raises questions of the legitimacy of the political processes and the accountability of the GF both to its stakeholders and towards the broader structures of global health governance.

As an actor of global health governance, the GF, of course, interacts with a variety of other institutions at the discoursive interfaces. Although the GF defines itself as a pure financing mechanism and basically acknowledges the leadership of the WHO and UNAIDS, through its activities it influences both general discourses on the poverty-oriented fight against diseases and more specific discourses between actors of global health on the respective programmes and strategies.

In the following, the establishment of this new actor of global health will be explained and the role of the GF in all three of the above-mentioned interfaces (organizational, resource-transfer and discoursive)[1] will be analysed. The first section deals with the creation of the GF and describes the factors on the demand and the supply side that explain why the GF was established at all, why it was structured in that particular way and what kind of difficulties were associated with the initial phase. The next section then examines the GF with regard to its internal structure and its functioning as an organizational interface of different types of stakeholder groups. It will take a closer look at the partnership approach, examine its strengths and weaknesses at global and national level, and discuss the issues of accountability and legitimacy. In the following section, the activities of the GF at the resource-based interfaces and its interactions with other actors of global health are scrutinized. As the GF is designed as a performance-based financing mechanism, its main activities can be summarized by the triad 'raise it, spend it, prove it' (as formulated by Richard Feachem), which will be analysed separately. The next section will then explore the activities of the GF at the discoursive interfaces. This entails a differentiation between the role of the GF in general discourses (e.g. prevention versus treatment, affordable medicines for the poor) and its role in programmatic discourses (e.g. the 3 by 5 initiative, The Three Ones). Finally, in the concluding remarks, the most important challenges at the three interface types will be summarized and an outlook on the future perspectives of the GF will be given.

Establishment of the Global Fund

Demand and supply

In order to explain the establishment of a new organization like the GF it seems suitable to distinguish between a demand and a supply side. The global governance discourse tends to focus on the former and highlights aspects such as interdependencies between different types of actors and difficulties of state regulation in an era of globalization to account for an increasing demand for new forms of regulation (Kaul et al. 1999; Reinicke et al. 2000). In the case of the GF, the inability of the existing (bilateral and multilateral) structures to mobilize enough resources to effectively fight HIV/AIDS, tuberculosis and malaria – the numbers differ, but at the time the GF was established the most cited number was approximately US$15 billion annually (CMH 2001) – was the most important argument on the demand side.

But the existence of a demand for additional financing to fight the three diseases can only be considered a necessary but not a sufficient condition to explain why the GF was established at all and why it was structured in that particular way. In the process of establishing the GF in 2000/1, a number of factors played a crucial role on the supply side. The first was the existence of *political commitment* among the donor community to tackle the most important poverty-related diseases. International attention towards health issues in developing countries was propelled by the renewed focus on poverty reduction that came with the Post-Washington Consensus (WDR 2000/2001; HDR 1997, 2003), studies on the relationship between health and macroeconomic development (CMH 2001) and an increasing perception of health as a global public good (Kaul et al. 1999) as well as the need to produce 'global public goods for health' (Smith et al. 2003). These three approaches deal with health at different societal and political levels, but all contributed to a stronger commitment of political leaders towards the fight against poverty-related diseases and inequalities. Without these developments, the July 2000 G8 meeting in Okinawa, where the idea of establishing a new financing mechanism was discussed for the first time, and the subsequent processes that occurred until the start of the GF in January 2002, probably would not have created such a momentum among the donor countries as they eventually did.

This high prominence of health, however, can only be partly explained by these three perspectives. A second important factor on the supply side was the perception that ill-health in developing countries and the global spread of infectious diseases represent a *threat to security* at national and international level (Ostergard 2002; Peterson 2002; Youde 2005). This is related to a broadening of the security concept that can be observed since the end of the Cold War. While security was traditionally perceived as military protection against external threats to one's own territory and population, the concept was expanded in the 1990s towards non-military threats, emanating from economic risks, illegal activities, environmental changes and social problems. Especially in the case of the US, the perception of health-related insecurities was decisive for the stronger orientation towards health issues (Youde 2005; NIC 2000, 2002) and its leadership role in establishing the GF as a new financing mechanism.

The third important factor that supported the establishment of the GF was the desire of some G8 countries – especially the US and Japan – to *circumvent the UN system* that had experienced serious difficulties and was considered inefficient and bureaucratic. The idea of installing a new institution outside that system – and thus more directly under the control of the donor countries – seemed appealing to these actors as it converged with their own interests in bypassing to some extent the established UN organizations in the field of health like WHO or UNAIDS and shifting their activities to a new forum. It was not until April 2001 that the UN agencies finally agreed to the creation of a single fund (previously the option of funds within and beyond the UN system had been discussed) and that UN Secretary General Kofi Annan called for additional resources to support that fund. Without the strong pressure from the G8 countries and the leadership of Japan and the US to form an entirely new financing mechanism – independent from the UN system – the GF probably would not have been installed the way it was. At least one needs to question, however, whether actors like the US government or the Bill and Melinda Gates Foundation, who were among the first to pledge substantial amounts to the GF (at the time US$200 million and US$100 million, respectively) would have considered a similar support for a fund within the UN system.

The legacy of the founding phase

Once the decision for the establishment of the GF was taken, issues of design and structure gained importance. These processes started in June 2001 with the first informal meeting in Geneva and gained momentum with the establishment of a Transitional Working Group (TWG) in

July 2001. The TWG consisted of nearly forty representatives from developing countries, donor countries, civil society organizations (CSOs), the private sector and the UN system. During the second half of 2001, it developed the GF's governance structure and guidelines for the Fund's operational activities. The TWG met three times and held regional consultations in Africa, Asia, Latin America and Eastern Europe, as well as thematic consultations with CSOs, the private sector and academia in autumn 2001. Both the civil society and the private sector constituency had a number of consultative meetings before the GF was established, where they discussed the suggestions of the TWG and decided on their representatives for the Board. In order to structure the selection process for Southern governments, WHO regions were taken as a basis and slightly adapted to allow for a stronger representation of African governments.

That the GF was established as a public–private partnership with considerable representation of non-state actors can to a large degree be attributed to the activities of a strong coalition of CSOs, mainly from the field of HIV/AIDS. While many developing countries preferred a fund with a strong representation of recipient and donor countries (largely modelled after the WHO) and an only marginal influence of non-state actors, the CSOs successfully claimed that they represent and advocate the interests of those people who would be at the centre of the GF's activities: the people affected by diseases, ill-health and poverty in the developing countries. It certainly helped in that process that, since the beginning of the 1990s, GPPPs represented a popular and 'fashionable' form of regulation that was supported by the UN system and many state and non-state actors alike.

It is interesting to observe that the GF was established in a relatively short time. It became operational just half a year after the initial meeting of the Transitional Working Group and the establishment of a Technical Support Secretariat. This was only possible because most of the participating actors were highly committed to the idea of the GF and dedicated a considerable amount of time and energy to the rapid development of structures and procedures. From the onset, the GF was designed as a learning organization with a large degree of flexibility and transparency. While these factors helped the GF to start its activities very quickly – the Executive Board conducted its first meeting in January 2002 and the first call for proposals was issued in February 2002 – they are also responsible for some difficulties that the GF has encountered over the years.

As there was not enough time to discuss divergent expectations and interests of the participating actors, conflicts on certain issues like the adequate resource mobilization strategy or the question of in-kind donations tended to come up frequently and are not entirely solved even today. Also, the division of labour between the GF and its partners was not defined accurately enough. The GF was structured as a public–private partnership but it was not at all clear what role the different types of partners would play. The GF assumed a win-win situation for all participating actors in the pursuit of the common goal to fight HIV/AIDS, tuberculosis and malaria and thus expected its partners to fully support all GF activities. It did not consider sufficiently, however, that competing interests, different organizational cultures, a lack of mutual trust, or resource constraints could hamper an effective cooperation. The discrepancy between the claim of having a partnership and the reality of in fact operating as one, is in parts still visible today, although the GF recently launched a couple of initiatives to improve the cooperation and division of labour with its partners.

Due to the GF's rapid establishment, processes and structures could not be developed in advance. The GF started with only a few basic documents (mainly the framework document and the By-Laws) and had to establish procedures for example for the proposal process, the CCM composition or phase 2 renewal as things evolved. Thus the first years of the GF can be described as a process of 'learning by doing', which on the one hand was positive, as it enabled the GF to correct imbalances and solve difficulties quite quickly, but on the other hand was associated with additional work, especially for recipient governments and supporting agencies providing technical assistance at country level.

The Global Fund as organizational interface

As organizational interface the GF manages the interactions between the different stakeholders of the partnership. At the global level, the bodies of the GF are the Executive Board (responsible for the GF's strategies, policies, operational guidelines, and funding decisions), the Secretariat (day-to-day operations), the Technical Review Panel (review of applications through independent experts) and the Partnership Forum (biennial gathering of stakeholder groups). At the national level, the central institution is the Country Coordinating Mechanism (CCM), which is responsible for the proposals process. The management of the grants is the task of the Principal Recipient (PR; in most cases the Ministry of Health). The Local Fund Agent (LFA; in most cases a private accounting firm) has a monitoring function and reports to the GF Secretariat.

In the following, the two central decision-making bodies of the GF – the Executive Board at global level and the Country Coordinating

Mechanism at national level – will be analysed in more detail and questions of legitimacy and accountability of the GF will be addressed.

The Executive Board

The Executive Board today consists of five types of constituencies[2] which are grouped into two voting groups of the same size and one non-voting group.[3] The donor group is composed of eight representatives from industrialized countries and two representatives from the private sector (one company, one foundation); the recipient group consists of seven representatives from developing countries and three representatives from the CSO sector (one north, one south, one affected communities). In the non-voting group are three representatives of international governmental organizations (one WHO, one UNAIDS, one World Bank) and a Swiss member (as the headquarters of the GF is in Geneva). While seats for governments in the donor group depend on the willingness to fund the GF and were allocated on the basis of initial pledges to the GF (minimum: US$100 million), the selection of the other Board members is up to the respective constituencies.

The Board composition as it is today, however, is not the same as in 2002, when the GF became operational. CSOs representing the people living with the diseases (the so-called 'affected communities') were initially part of the non-voting group. They, however, continued advocating for a third voting seat and received strong support at the first Partnership Forum of the GF in 2004. They finally managed to convince the Board – which for a long time was reluctant to touch the balanced governing structure – that it would be beneficial for the GF's reputation to change their status, as this would demonstrate that the interests of the people living with HIV/AIDS, tuberculosis and malaria in the developing world are really taken into account by the GF.

This shows that the role of *CSOs* in the governance structure of the GF increased over time, which can be explained by the important function CSOs have for the GF in terms of advocacy, mobilization of support, and implementation of programmes, as well as with regard to the legitimacy of the GF as a whole. The CSO constituency in itself, however, shows a considerable bias – not in terms of North–South relation, as in many other partnerships, but in terms of disease focus. All three Board members represent CSOs from the area of HIV/AIDS, and organizations from the areas of tuberculosis and malaria are also mostly absent from the wider CSO Board delegations. This can be considered critical, since the GF, as mentioned above, is the major international funder for these two diseases (67 per cent and 64 per cent, respectively), without having civil society interests from these areas represented at Board level.

The relative weight of governments from the *developing countries* decreased with the changes in the Board composition, as their number of Board seats remained the same, while the seat for the 'affected communities' was compensated with an additional seat for the donor countries in order to restore the balance between the two voting groups. This led to considerable tensions between them and the CSO constituency. Quite a few Southern governments take a critical position regarding extensive CSO participation as they are afraid of losing influence and policy options if they share decision-making responsibility with non-state actors. As already mentioned in the context of the establishment of the GF, many Southern countries favoured an institution basically modelled after the WHO – with a strong representation of governments from developing countries – in order to better advocate for their interests at the Board level of the GF. This was not considered necessary, however, since the principle of country ownership at national level together with a balanced representation at global level seemed to be appropriate to accommodate Southern interests. Thus recipient countries can be considered among the weaker constituencies in the Executive Board.

The strongest constituency is probably the group of the *donor countries*. This can be attributed to the fact that most of the GF funds are raised by the US, Japan and the European countries, which gives the donors considerable influence at Board level. Although decisions are mostly taken by consensus, the resource-based power of the donor group cannot be neglected. This can also be seen with regard to the Board Committees, which serve as working units of Board delegations to prepare the Board meetings. Both the Policy and Strategy Committee (responsible for core policies of the GF and strategic planning) and the Finance and Audit Committee (responsible for the GF's budget and resource mobilization) are currently chaired by representatives from the donor group, while only the Portfolio Committee (which gives advice on issues relating to the portfolio of grants) and the Ethics Committee (which oversees the Conflict of Interest Policy) are chaired by a member of the recipient group and the CSO constituency, respectively.

The pharmaceutical industry is represented only as part of the *private sector* delegation and was not given the possibility to act as a Board member for that constituency. It did not manage to gain significant influence on the strategies of the GF. In-kind contributions (of drugs and services) were discussed at various Board meetings, as they could contribute to an improvement of the resource situation of the GF, but the private sector until today has not been able to convince the GF members that this would be a suitable strategy at the global level. But it is not only the pharmaceutical industry that is relatively weak in the GF; this applies nearly to the entire private sector – with the exception of the Bill and Melinda Gates Foundation, which actively supports the GF. While the GF would like to see a stronger engagement of that constituency – especially in financial terms – the private sector favours other forms of cooperation, for example co-investment schemes for workplace programmes at country level, pro-bono services or marketing campaigns.

Summarizing the Board composition it can be said that – albeit being formally equal – the represented constituencies dispose of different types of power and influence. While the donor group – due to its large resource-based power – is probably the most influential constituency, CSOs follow second, as they dispose of substantive discoursive power both in the Executive Board and beyond. The recipient countries, of course, play a crucial role in the governance structure of the GF, but their main area of influence is the country level. At global level their relative weight decreased with the change of the Board composition. The private sector does not play a major role at the global level (except the Bill and Melinda Gates Foundation), as it does not contribute substantial financial resources, and the GF itself limits the private sector influence both through its governance structure and its decisions on in-kind contributions.

The balanced composition of the Board and the careful selection process of Board members must be seen in the context of the establishment of the GF. As it was positioned outside the UN and not hosted by any other organization, it was necessary to strengthen its legitimacy as an actor of GHG. By including state and non-state actors from the South, the GF strives at gaining legitimacy both in terms of input and output legitimacy (for the concept see Scharpf 1999). On the input-side the participation of those groups of actors that would be the ultimate addressees of GF decisions can help to establish some kind of congruence between 'the rulers and the ruled' – a basic feature of legitimate governance processes in a normative sense. On the output-side it can be argued that the ability to participate in the decision-making processes will positively influence the 'belief in legitimacy' in an empirical sense and thus contribute to a better compliance of the respective actors and – via the voluntary pooling of resources – enhance the effectiveness of the GF.

It must be seen, however, that the legitimacy of the GF as a whole also depends on the legitimacy of those who represent the different constituencies. While governments are elected by the people in their respective countries and thus can claim to be legitimized by democratic voting processes (although, in reality, in some countries this is at least doubtful), the case is different for civil society and private actors for two reasons: they are not democratically mandated through elections, and they do not represent larger groups of people, but advocate for special interests or pursue individual aims. While this is not seen as too problematic in the case of most CSOs, as it is assumed that they advocate for the right things (which should at least be questioned sometimes), the representation of private companies or foundations is often criticized as it is feared that their private agendas gain too much influence in the decision-making process (Ollila 2003; Richter 2003, 2004).

By limiting the influence of private actors and strengthening civil society organizations, the GF tried to enhance its legitimacy as an institution of global health governance. Additionally it introduced various mechanisms to ensure both internal and external accountability[4] of its own activities at the global level. Among them are clear rules for the composition and operation of its governing and administrative bodies, policies on conflicts of interest, an early-warning system, focal points for communication purposes, and a very high degree of transparency. Critical issues in this context are the relationship with its multilateral partners and the governance processes at national level. What has proven helpful for the GF operations in the Executive Board over the years is the fact that the GF defines itself as a pure financing mechanism and leaves politically delicate decisions like the use of generics, prevention strategies, or in-kind donations to the recipient countries instead of stipulating the respective policies at global level.

The Country Coordinating Mechanisms

While the GF functions relatively well as organizational interface at the global level and accountability mechanisms are in place, considerable governance difficulties are reported at the national level, especially with regard to the Country Coordinating Mechanisms (CCMs).[5] Although CCM structures vary from country to country, a number of typical problems can be identified.

One of the most problematic issues is the fact that many CCMs are *dominated by the respective governments*. Many governments in the recipient countries were either not prepared or not willing to work with non-state actors, hence CSOs were not represented sufficiently in the CCMs or were handpicked by the governments. CCMs were created because the GF required them in the proposals process but not because cooperation with civil society was a goal in itself. Especially people living with the diseases – due to the related stigmatization – as well as women's organizations were often not represented sufficiently in the CCMs. Thus the input legitimacy of the CCMs in many cases is limited.

A second problem can be identified in terms of *participation*. Even where formal representation of non-state actors is given, practical constraints often inhibit the respective actors from truly participating in the CCM processes. Travel costs, language barriers, lack of organization, scarce resources, information deficits, limited transparency, or short-term planning in many cases are obstacles for an effective participation of non-state actors especially from beyond the national capitals and also contribute to a low degree of accountability of CCMs towards their members and stakeholders.

The third important issue is the ambiguous *role of CCMs after the proposal* has been submitted. Although the CCMs are expected to oversee implementation, little support was given to CCMs to enable them to fulfil this role during the first funding rounds. The CCMs had to rely on the GF's bilateral and multilateral partners to receive support in the process of proposal development and the overview of implementation and were in a relatively weak position compared to the Principal Recipient, the Local Fund Agent and the GF Secretariat and Board. Since round five, technical assistance and capacity-building for CCMs can now be included in the grant proposal up to a certain degree in order to better equip CCMs for their oversight function and strengthen their position in the overall governance structure of the GF.

The GF also reacted to the critical points of representation and participation by changing its respective guidelines. CSOs for a long time had pushed, at Board level, for stricter CCM guidelines that would include requirements on CCM composition instead of mere recommendations. The idea was rejected at the eighth Board meeting as it was considered contradictory to the principle of country ownership. It was argued – especially by many developing countries – that if the GF wanted the countries to be responsible for strategies and policies it must not interfere with internal governance processes at national level. This position was harshly criticized at the Partnership Forum in July 2004. Country ownership, so the position there, should not be misunderstood as synonymous with government ownership. If the GF wanted to live up to its partnership approach, a more prescriptive model for CCMs seemed indispensable. The Board considered this critique and finally approved some CCM requirements (although not all) at the ninth Board meeting. A recent study by the Technical Evaluation and Reference Group – an advisory body providing independent assessment and advice to the GF

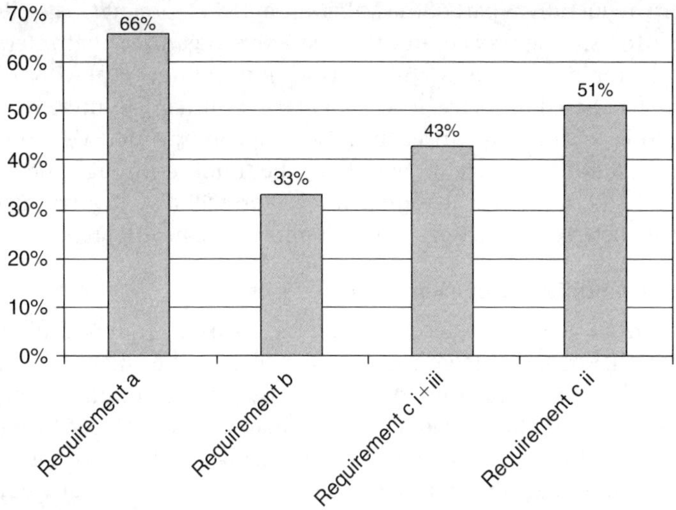

a: membership of people living with and/or affected by the diseases
b: members representing the non-government sectors must be selected by their own sector(s) based on a documented, transparent process
c i+iii: maintain a transparent and documented process for soliciting and reviewing submissions for possible integration into the overall grant proposal to the Global Fund and to ensure the input of a broad range of stakeholders in proposal development and grant oversight
c ii: maintain a transparent, documented process to nominate the Principal Recipient(s) and oversee programme implementation

Figure 6.1 Percentage of CCM requirements met
Own graph; *source*: http://www.theglobalfund.org/pdf/ccms/TERG_Report_CCM _Assessment.doc

Board – shows, however, that only a limited number of these requirements is met in practice (see Figure 6.1).

The Global Fund as resource-transfer interface

The goals of the GF are best summarized in an often cited statement, formulated in the central 'framework document' and the By-Laws: 'The purpose of the Fund is to attract, manage and disburse additional resources through a new public–private partnership that will make a sustainable and significant contribution to the reduction of infections, illness and death, thereby mitigating the impact caused by HIV/AIDS, Tuberculosis and Malaria in countries in need, and contributing to poverty reduction as part of the Millennium Development Goals.' While the partnership approach and the respective organizational interfaces were the topic of the last section, this section will now deal with the GF as resource-based interface. It will cover what former Executive Director Richard Feachem summarized as 'raise it, spend it, prove it', and focus on the issues of resource mobilization, the funding through the GF, as well as its performance at various levels, and will also discuss the relationship between the GF and other donors in the health arena.

Resource mobilization ('Raise it')

Since the GF was created as a funding mechanism to support the fight against HIV/AIDS, tuberculosis and malaria, the mobilization of resources was of crucial importance from the very beginning. Although it was clear that the GF would not be able to raise the US$15 billion identified as the annual international financing gap, it strived for a high level of additional contributions. Richard Feachem, in the early days of the GF, considered a 'cruising altitude' of US$7 billion desirable, and the latest calculations estimate that the resource needs of the GF will be US$3 billion in 2007 and between US$4 billion and US$8 billion in 2010 (GF 2007: 8). The first five proposal rounds cost an average of US$772 million for the first two years,[6] with a new round being established approximately every eight months. The figures are rising sharply for the years to come, as many grants enter their second funding phase, while at the same time new proposal rounds will be called for.

Resource mobilization – although critical for the GF operations – has become more difficult over time. While the US pledges initially made up for nearly half of all pledges, the government changed its policy in 2003 and declared that the US contribution would not be more than 33 per cent of the amount that is pledged to the GF until July of each year (the end of the US fiscal year). This led to the general formula for GF financing, as expressed by Jacques Chirac, that one third of the funds should come from the US, the EU countries and the rest of the world, respectively. The pledges from EU countries are clearly over-exceeding this target, while the US pledges – with only US$600 million pledged to the GF for the next two years – currently do not even amount to that percentage. The contributions of other actors also fall below the initial expectations. The private sector – with the exception of the Bill and Melinda Gates Foundation that thus far contributed US$150 million and just pledged another US$500 million – does not play an important role in funding the GF. Only 3.6 per cent of all contributions come from non-state actors, while the G8 countries alone finance two thirds of the GF (see Table 6.1).

Table 6.1 Funding sources of the GF

	Contributions 2001–2005		Pledges 2001–2008	
Source	**Million US$**	**Percentage**	**Million US$**	**Percentage**
United States	1,910	25.7	2,540	26.7
Europe	4,252	57.2	4,877	51.3
Japan + others	1,007	13.5	1,431	15.1
Non-state actors	268	3.6	654	6.9
Total	*7,437*	*100*	*9,503*	*100*

Own table; *source*: GF progress update 15 September 2006.

So in that sense the GF can be considered more a multilateral financing institution than a true public–private partnership (although contributions from the private sector and CSOs should not be limited to the funding issue alone).[7]

The current funding shortage of the GF can be attributed to a number of reasons. Many donor countries face *difficult economic situations*, with high budgetary deficits, unfavourable balances of payment, or low economic growth rates. Resources are therefore limited and contributions to the GF lower than expected. A second reason is the *decreasing attention to health issues* at the global level, while other issues – particularly after 11 September 2001 – moved into the centre of attention. Especially the US directed many resources to the promotion of homeland security and the wars in Afghanistan and Iraq. And also within the policy field of health, competition increased due to the *establishment of new initiatives* like PEPFAR. Of the US$15 billion that were approved by Congress to fight HIV/AIDS for five years, only US$1 billion were committed to the GF (US$200 million per year). A fourth risk for resource mobilization is what many CSOs call *donor fatigue* – an expression already used in former contexts of development politics. They are afraid that development issues in general will not receive enough attention in the future, as many donors tend to become pessimistic about the sense of aid.

In order to confront these risks and create a more solid resource base, the GF recently changed its resource mobilization strategy, rediscovering conventional mechanisms in international funding. While, since the creation of the GF, contributions had been on an ad hoc basis (which made medium- or long-term calculations difficult), a regular replenishment mechanism was introduced in 2005. The idea behind this mechanism is that donors declare their pledges for the next two to three years at fixed replenishment meetings and thus give the GF some planning reliability. The results of the replenishment process so far, however, have not met the expectations, and it remains to be seen how well that instrument will work to secure the future resource needs of the GF.

Many CSOs argue that the situation will not change as long as the contributions to the GF are on a voluntary basis and donor countries are free to determine the amount they wish to commit. Therefore, since 2002, they have been advocating for an 'equitable contributions framework' that links the contribution of the donor countries to their share in world GNP (France et al. 2003; Oxfam 2002a, 2002b, 2002c; Aidspan 2004). The idea behind the framework is that the GF should be demand-driven, in other words donors should be obliged to at least contribute the amount that is needed to fund all approved proposals of each round. It thus rejects the idea of a supply-driven GF that needs to prioritize the proposals with regard to the available funding. Although this CSO framework is not supported officially by the GF (and probably never will be due to political constraints), it can be considered an important advocacy tool, as it shows the GF members and the general public what is expected from each of the donor countries and helps in lobbying for a sustainable funding of the GF.

In order to improve the resource situation of the GF, the private sector delegation embarks on a different course and advocates for a less restricted position towards in-kind donations. Instead of expecting the private sector to contribute considerably in the form of financial resources, potentials of in-kind donations should be evaluated. A study commissioned by the private sector delegation in 2004 suggested that up to one fifth of all GF cash commitments could be replaced by in-kind donations, with drug donations even amounting to 30–35 per cent of all expenditures (Accenture 2004: 18). This idea was, however, rejected by the GF Board, since they feared undue influence of commercial interests and negative implications in terms of market impact, conflicts of interest and limited sustainability.[8] Moreover the majority of the GF partners would prefer more financial support from the private sector in the form of cash contributions instead of increased in-kind contributions.

While the main donor countries (especially the US and Japan) reject the 'equitable contributions framework' because of its mandatory character which would constrain them in their funding decisions, the CSOs and many developing countries oppose in-kind donations as they fear a predominance of commercial interests and a loss of country ownership. Hence, in order to mobilize enough resources in the future, the GF will continue to depend to a large extent on the G8 countries. Thus it must convince them that their money is spent effectively and prove the value of the GF principles of country ownership and performance-based funding.

Funding through the Global Fund ('Spend it')

The GF approved, in five funding rounds, US$5.6 billion for nearly 400 grants in 132 countries, of which US$2.7 billion are being disbursed until today. Table 6.2 depicts a breakdown of the GF portfolio by region, by disease, and by purpose for all five rounds.

The basic principle of the GF in terms of funding is 'country ownership'. This means that the GF does not have its own programmes or projects, but finances proposals that are developed by the countries themselves. The aim of this principle is to encourage bottom-up processes and Southern participation, and it represents a shift away from conventional development approaches as followed by other financing institutions in health like the World Bank or PEPFAR, where countries have to apply within much narrower strategic frameworks than in the case of the GF. It also allows the GF to leave politically delicate decisions such as the use of generics or the question of adequate prevention strategies to the recipient countries instead of defining the respective policies at the global level.[9]

The question, however, is how thoroughly this principle is applied in practice. As the GF itself has no country presence, it is not able to assist countries in the proposals process apart from providing them with information and guidelines. So in order to successfully apply to the GF (only an average of 36 per cent of the proposals are approved), the vast majority of countries require technical assistance from bilateral and multilateral institutions. This is an important channel of influence, as priorities,

Table 6.2 GF portfolio by region, disease and purpose

Region	Disease	Purpose
Sub-Saharan Africa: 56%	HIV/AIDS: 58%	Drugs & commodities: 48%
East Asia, Pacific: 14%	Malaria: 24%	Human resources, training: 22%
Latin America: 10%	Tuberculosis: 17%	Physical infrastructure: 11%
Eastern Europe, Central Asia: 8%	Health system strengthening: 1%	Administration: 11%
South Asia, Middle East, North Africa: 11%		Monitoring & evaluation: 2%
		Other: 6%

Own table; *source*: GF progress update, 15 September 2006.

norms or strategies of the respective actors are likely to find their way into the national proposal. In some cases a relabelling of the existing programmes of other donors was reported, so that national priorities may not be represented as clearly as the principle of country ownership suggests.

This construction also led to considerable tensions, especially between the GF on the one side, and the WHO and UNAIDS on the other side, which had to invest additional resources to provide technical assistance in proposal development without receiving any compensation. At the outset, the GF was not very sensitive towards these issues and took it for granted that the WHO and UNAIDS, as partners of the GF, would carry out these task in the context of their overall mandates in support of the countries. Resource constraints initially were considered just as little as possible objections against this new organization, which was established outside the UN system and has been competing with the traditional organizations for influence and resources in global health governance.

Over time, however, a learning process has taken place. The GF now seems to be more aware of the fact that it cannot expect its partners to support the GF for altruistic reasons, but has to offer them something in exchange in order to function efficiently as a partnership. The ruling opinion is still that no GF money should go to the headquarters of the WHO or UNAIDS, but that instead countries should be enabled to pay for technical assistance in the context of their grants. So at the tenth Board meeting it was decided that resources for technical assistance could be included in the grant proposal, which was not the case before. The support of The Three Ones and the 3 by 5 initiative as well as the engagement of the GF in global initiatives like the Global Task Team, the High-Level Meetings on the HMDGs, or the Global Joint M&E Facility also show that the GF is trying to improve its cooperation with other actors in global health.

At the national level, however, substantial challenges remain (some of which not only refer to resource-based, but also to organizational interfaces). Most important in this context is the issue of harmonization. Especially in the field of HIV/AIDS (where the GF is only one funder among others), a stronger coordination of activities is necessary to avoid duplication of activities and fragmentation of policies. Although donors committed themselves to better practices with the Rome Declaration on Harmonization in 2003 and the Paris Declaration on Aid Effectiveness in 2005, rhetoric and practice tend to differ considerably. The relationship between the CCMs and other coordinating institutions at national level (such as National Aids Councils, UN Theme groups) is often not clearly defined, although the GF states that – wherever possible – it strives towards an integration into existing structures instead of competing with them. In many cases, however, we can observe a duplication of structures and an unclear division of labour, which leads to substantial bureaucratic burdens for the recipient countries and stresses scarce country capacities (Dickinson 2005; UNAIDS 2003). While an increasing number of donors are channelling their assistance through larger frameworks of agreement with recipient countries like Sector Wide Approaches (SWAPs), Poverty Reduction Strategy Papers (PRSPs), basket funding or budget support, the GF to a large extent remains outside these structures. It mainly supports vertical, disease-focused initiatives and programmes that often do not align with broader horizontal approaches of public health and contribute to a further fragmentation of health policies at the national level.

Performance of the Global Fund ('Prove it')

Although it is one of the core principles of the GF to be 'performance-based', systematic monitoring and evaluation only played a minor role in the beginning. This can be explained by the development of the GF itself, where structures and processes were elaborated as issues evolved over time. So in the first years, the focus of the GF was on becoming operational, signing grant agreements and disbursing funds. As the first grants reached the end of their initial two-year funding in 2005, a 'Monitoring & Evaluation Framework' as well as procedures for the so-called 'Phase 2 Renewal Process' had to be elaborated.

The GF developed a ranking system for its grants that served as a basis for the further funding decision. Of the 74 grants reviewed in a GF progress report in September 2005 (GF 2005b: 59ff.) 28 per cent were rated category A ('met or exceeded targets'), 51 per cent achieved B1 ('adequate performance'), 18 per cent were considered B2 ('inadequate performance but demonstrated potential') and 3 per cent were in category C ('unacceptable performance'). Based on this ranking the GF Secretariat made recommendations to the Board that fell in four categories: go / conditional go / revised go / no go. Until 2006 the Secretariat had categorized four grants as 'no go'; two of these recommendations were rejected by the Board (Senegal: HIV/AIDS, Honduras), two were followed (Senegal: malaria, South Africa: HIV+TB).

A recent study (Gootnick 2005) summarizes a number of factors both at the global and national level that affected grant performance negatively. Among them are a lack of guidance for grant recipients from the national government or the GF Secretariat, poor coordination or rivalries between recipients and partners at the national level, and planning difficulties or incorrect time calculations that occurred in the GF proposal.

No significant association was found between grant performance on the one hand, and factors such as the type of PR, grant size, disease targeted, or percentage of funds disbursed on the other. This deviates from an analysis of the GF (2005b), which found that, in average, the grants that had a CSO as PR were performing better than those with government PRs.

Grant performance, however, is just one aspect of the GF overall performance. In order to systematically measure these issues, the GF developed a four-level model that distinguishes between operational performance (resource mobilization, proposal management, grant negotiation, disbursement and grant management, business services), grant performance, system effects (additionality, partnerships, sustainability), and impact (level of disease, contribution to MDGs). This model serves as a basis for the evaluation of the GF in 2006 that is currently underway. For future resource mobilization it will be crucial for the GF to show that it is indeed performance-based, that its funds are used in a cost-effective way and that its grants – together with the activities of other donors – have a positive impact on the level of disease in the recipient countries.

Relationship between the GF and other donors in global health

In order to effectively fight the three most important poverty-related diseases it is estimated that in 2007 international funding of approximately US$19.5 billion (and domestic spending of US$5.0 billion) would be necessary (GF 2006: 13). The largest amount (US$15.1 billion of international funding) is required for prevention, treatment and care in the field of HIV/AIDS, while interventions for malaria and TB would need international funding of US$2.6 and 1.8 billion, respectively. The current levels of financing, however, are much lower than the expressed needs. In the case of HIV/AIDS, the GF makes up approximately 21 per cent of all international funding (supplemented by the following international funding sources: bilateral donors: 28 per cent World Bank plus UNAIDS: 22 per cent, PEPFAR: 21 per cent, private funding: 8 per cent).

These figures show that the GF managed to become one of the most important actors at the resource-based interfaces in global health. However, as the G8 countries are the major funders of the GF, the question of additionality has to be addressed: is the money for the GF really additional or is it crowding out other donor activities? Positions on this issue vary, as it is difficult to define and measure additionality. In 2004, the GF commissioned work on the system-wide effects of its activities and subsequently created guidelines to measure, inter alia, the additionality both at the global and national level. In these guidelines, additionality at the national level is considered given if 'financing from the

Global Fund is a true net addition to aggregate support for effective interventions against the three diseases'. Also, global additionality is framed relatively broadly in the sense that additionality 'is assured if the GF and other donors together succeed in closing the financing gap' and 'fails if GF assistance displaces other donor commitments' (GF 2005c: 14, 17). Potential indicators for additionality at global level are recommended (although not investigated in detail): levels and trends in donor assistance, shares for health-related programmes, and progress in reducing 'unmet need' for HIV/AIDS, TB and malaria spending.

A study by Pearson (2004) used these and other indicators to assess the economic and financial impacts of the GF and other financing GPPPs and made a number of observations in terms of additionality: (1) The share of health in ODA has been increasing over the past decade. While overall ODA declined in the 1990s, health-related spending rose continuously. (2) It is still too early to definitely assess whether financing GPPPs occur at the expense of other types of ODA or whether they supplement existing spending; there are indications for both developments.[10] (3) There is concern, however, that the increased spending on communicable diseases is crowding out other health areas, such as reproductive health or family planning, and that the high levels of spending for health in general are at the expense of investments in other policy fields like agriculture, water, sanitation, transport or energy. (4) There is little evidence that donors have been able to leverage additional funds from a wide range of new sources.

The GF is sensitive towards these issues, but points to the responsibility both of donor and recipient countries in ensuring additionality. So the same pattern that was found in terms of conflict-handling at Board level can be observed here: a tendency to shift problematic issues away from the GF itself towards other actors or political levels. The organizational model of a public–private partnership supports this pattern, as responsibility in such a model is to be shared among the different stakeholders and is not carried by a single actor alone.

The Global Fund as an actor at discoursive interfaces

As the GF defines itself as a pure financing mechanism, it does not try to play a major role at the discoursive interfaces and basically acknowledges the leadership of UNAIDS and WHO. Through its activities, however, it influences both general discourses on the poverty-oriented fight against diseases and more specific discourses between actors of global health on the respective programmes and strategies. The focus of this section will be on the activities of the GF that have an impact on general discourses like 'prevention versus treatment' or 'affordable medicines for the poor' and only briefly outlines its role in programmatic discourses like the WHO's 3 by 5 initiative or UNAIDS' The Three Ones (for more details on these issues see Chapter 5).

The role of the GF in programmatic discourses

The GF does not play a major role in the development of strategies or programmes of other actors in global health. It sees its role as that of a funder who comes into the picture once the other organizations like the WHO or UNAIDS have developed their respective policies, so it is more relevant in terms of programme implementation.

The 3 by 5 initiative, launched by the WHO in order to regain discoursive power in the policy field of HIV/AIDS, is relatively separate to the activities of the GF. Although the WHO, the GF and UNAIDS jointly announced the initiative in September 2003 in New York, the two latter organizations had little say in the development of the strategy itself. The GF of course emphasized that through its grants it would contribute to the goals of treating three million people with ARVs by the end of the year 2005 (which, by the way, was not achieved), but also acknowledged that 3 by 5 was 'clearly a WHO responsibility'.

The picture is slightly different with regard to The Three Ones, initiated by UNAIDS. It consists of three components: one agreed HIV/AIDS Action Framework, one national AIDS coordinating authority, and one agreed country-level Monitoring and Evaluation System. While the GF is not very involved in the first component, it plays a considerable role in the two other components. The issue of the one national authority is the more critical one, as CCMs tend to be installed in addition to other institutions and their relationship to the national HIV/AIDS coordinating authority is often not clearly defined. This can partly be attributed to the fact that the GF (and thus the CCMs) has to deal not only with HIV/AIDS, but also with malaria and tuberculosis, yet it is also part of a more political competition between the various organizations for power and influence at the national level. The picture is different with regard to the one M&E System, the most technical component of all three. Here the GF took a leading role in harmonizing the frameworks of various bilateral and multilateral agencies and developed, together with a number of partners,[11] the so-called 'M&E Toolkit'. The purpose of this toolkit is to provide, in one place, the essentials of agreed-upon best practice in M&E by applying a common framework for the three diseases. All participating agencies supported the development of this toolkit, and the influence of the GF on this specific programmatic discourse can be considered relatively high.

The GF in general discourses on global health

If we look at the discourses in global health that are relevant for the poverty-oriented fight of diseases, it also becomes clear that the GF yields influence more through its activities than through a pro-active role in framing discourses via advocacy or agenda-setting.

The first of these discourses revolves around the issue 'prevention versus treatment'. Until 2000, prevention was the standard approach in the fight against HIV/AIDS in developing countries. Given the initial price of ARVs, treatment was only an option in the industrialized countries. It was argued that providing ARV treatment was not cost-effective in poor regions and that the activities – due to the inadequacy of global HIV/AIDS funding – should concentrate on prevention. The picture changed both with the introduction of generics and the following price decline. Without that decline the resource needs would have been so exorbitant that incentives to establish a new financing mechanism like the GF probably would have gained little support among the donor community.

Once the GF was established, however, it played an important role in putting into practice what had been advocated for by many CSOs and Southern countries: making treatment (combined with prevention) a feasible approach in the fight against HIV/AIDS in the developing world. Nearly 50 per cent of the GF funds are for the purchase of drugs and commodities, and the GF expects that it will have financed ARV treatment for 1.8 million people once the grants of the first five funding rounds come to an end. Taking into account the large number of people that require treatment in the developing world, this figure is still small, but by advocating for more resources to effectively fight poverty-related diseases like HIV/AIDS and by starting to make treatment a realistic option also for the developing countries, the GF plays an important role in the respective discourse.

With the change from prevention to treatment a second issue began gaining importance: the question of who would be able to benefit from ARVs in the developing world. Would they mainly be for the more wealthy parts of the population or would treatment also be available to poor and marginalized groups? These questions, among others, were raised in a second – nearly simultaneous – discourse that could be called 'affordable medicines for the poor'. This discourse was heavily influenced by the 'Access to Essential Medicines' campaign of MSF and other CSOs which played an important role for the TRIPS negotiations (see Chapters 2 and 4) and must be seen in the context of a general poverty orientation in global health that is associated with the post-Washington Consensus and the Millennium Development Goals.

The GF aims at 'contributing to poverty reduction as part of the Millennium Development Goals' (GF By-Laws) and includes aspects of pro-poor politics in its proposals process. Country eligibility for GF funding is determined mainly by the level of country income (based on the World Bank income classification). Sixty-four per cent of all 350 GF grants go to low-income countries, while lower-middle and upper-middle income countries account for 27 and 9 per cent, respectively. Hence, by focusing on the poorest countries or on vulnerable groups, it can be said that the GF is supporting the trend towards poverty orientation in global health and development cooperation.

Conclusion

This chapter examined the role of the Global Fund to Fight AIDS, Tuberculosis and Malaria in global health. Following the analytical framework developed in Chapter 1, the GF was analysed in terms of its role as and its position in three interfaces: organizational, resource-transfer and discoursive interfaces.

As *organizational interface*, the GF manages the interactions between the different stakeholder groups both at the global and national level. It has to balance their interests in a way that enhances both its legitimacy as an institution and its effectiveness as an actor of global health governance. While the GF functions relatively well at the global level and accountability mechanisms are in place, considerable governance difficulties are reported at the national level of recipient countries, especially with regard to the Country Coordinating Mechanisms. In terms of the relationship between broad stakeholder participation on the one hand and the legitimacy and effectiveness of the GF on the other hand, a more general problem can be observed: Should participation of a large number of actors – especially from the South – be a goal in itself, or should the issues be looked upon from a more functional perspective? While on the one hand it can be argued that participatory models are necessary to create input legitimacy in global governance processes as they allow a congruence between those who are affected by a policy and those who take the political decisions, and therefore are a goal in itself, broad participation on the other hand can hamper effective policy-making if competing interests, lack of cooperation, high transaction costs, or inefficient mechanisms for partnership management prevail. Therefore, as Börzel and

Risse (2005: 18) put it: '"All-inclusive" governance arrangements might lead to a serious lack of efficiency and reduced effectiveness. In other words, a trade-off between legitimacy and effectiveness might arise.' The GF has to address these tensions in order to adequately fulfil its function as an organizational interface in global health.

As *resource-transfer interface,* the GF plays an important role for the funding of health-related activities in the recipient countries. The GF, as an implementing agency, does not carry out own programmes or projects, but finances proposals that were developed by the countries themselves. As it only funds projects that are targeted at the fight against HIV/AIDS, TB and malaria, the GF contributes to a stronger focus on specific diseases and influences national strategies through its guidelines and funding policies. The principle of country ownership, which is followed in this context, encourages bottom-up processes and Southern participation and represents a shift away from conventional top-down approaches. In order to successfully apply to the GF, however, the vast majority of countries require technical assistance from bilateral and multilateral institutions. This construction led to considerable tensions, especially between the GF and WHO/UNAIDS, which had to invest additional resources to provide technical assistance in proposal development without receiving any compensation. In addition, it enabled actors from the global level to influence the national proposal process.

As an actor of global health governance, the GF interacts with a variety of other institutions at the *discoursive interfaces.* Although the GF defines itself as a pure financing mechanism, through its activities it influences both general discourses on the poverty-oriented fight against diseases and more specific discourses on the respective programmes and strategies. The establishment of the GF played an important role in the general discourse 'prevention versus treatment' because its grants helped turn the treatment of HIV/AIDS patients in developing countries into an approach feasible in the foreseeable future, as had been demanded by CSOs and the countries concerned. It was also influential in the discourse on 'affordable medicines for the poor'. As only low-income countries or countries specifically considering poor and vulnerable populations are eligible for funding, the GF contributes to a stronger poverty orientation both at the global and national level.

For the future development of the GF and a successful impact of its activities on the promotion of global health, four issues are of particular importance. First, it has to be taken into account that financing by the GF alone will not be sufficient to generate a positive impact if *framework conditions at country level* like capacity, infrastructure or governance structures are not addressed at the same time. The success of the GF will depend to a considerable degree on how these non-financial issues are tackled by the recipient countries themselves as well as the international donor community. Second, the *limits of vertical interventions* will have to be discussed. Although the GF follows a broader approach than many other public–private partnerships as it deals with the three major poverty-related diseases, it still supports mainly vertical disease-focused interventions that do not necessarily fit with horizontal approaches to health system development as followed by other donors and the promotion of public health at country level. The third is the issue of *sustainability*. The GF must mobilize enough resources to ensure that the activities supported by its grants are sustainable in the long run and that treatment programmes, in particular, will be continued as long as they are needed. This requires strong advocacy efforts by the GF itself and its partners (especially CSOs) to motivate donors to maintain or restore their commitments towards the GF and the exploration of new avenues of funding in the future. Finally, the GF must better *cooperate with its partners* and ensure that the partnership model is not mainly associated with advantages for the GF itself, but is beneficial for all participating actors alike. Enhanced coordination and harmonization with other actors of global health governance like the WHO, UNAIDS or the World Bank are crucial for an effective fight against HIV/AIDS and other diseases.

Notes

1. As legal interfaces – the fourth category developed in the theoretical chapter – play no role with regard to the GF, they will not be included in the analysis.
2. Donor countries, recipient countries, civil society, private sector, bilateral and multilateral agencies.
3. Most Board decisions are taken by consensus; if this is not possible, a double majority (in terms of absolute votes and in terms of the voting groups) is required.
4. On the concept of accountability see Keohane (2003); Risse (2004); Grant and Keohane (2005); Held and Koenig-Archibugi (2005).
5. On CCMs see GNP+ (2003); UNAIDS (2003); LSHTM (2003); DFID (2003); ICASO (2004); GF (various authors) (2004).
6. Round 1: US$565 million; round 2: US$866 million; round 3: US$623 million; round 4: US$1,039 million; round 5: US$770 million.
7. Private sector also: pro-bono services, marketing strategies, or in-country co-investments; CSO sector also: advocacy, political campaigns, or implementation of programmes at country level.
8. On the negative impacts of drug donations see: MSF (2000); Shretta et al. (2000); Lucas (2002).
9. The US delegation also supports this strategy, which is interesting, since the US, in other contexts, strongly advocates for the use of patented drugs and

the 'abc strategy' in prevention; this shows that the institutional context and the forum of interaction are important in influencing and shaping the activities of the participating actors.

10. Similar observations are made by a study prepared for the European Commission that distinguishes between global, country and sector additionality and states, with regard to the first type: 'we report no conclusive quantitative evidence neither of any global additionality [. . .] taking place, nor, in earnest, of any global crowding out thereof' (Delcour and Vellutini 2005: 27).
11. The WHO, UNAIDS, USAID, US Department of State, OGAC, CDC, UNICEF, MEASURE Evaluation, World Bank.

7

Consensus-Building on Brazilian HIV/AIDS Policy: National and Global Interfaces in Health Governance

Gilberto Calcagnotto

Introduction: Brazilian HIV/AIDS consensus as an issue of global health governance

This chapter focuses on Brazil's political response to the HIV/AIDS epidemic with regard to two aspects: first, the relationship between national actors and the protagonists of global health governance (actors and institutions), and, second, the relationship of the Brazilian STD[1]-HIV/AIDS Programme (BHAP) to other national actors in shaping and implementing that response.

Brazil's relevance in this context is not only based on the incidence of notified AIDS cases – the second largest in the Americas after the US, and far more than half of the overall cases for Latin America (Abreu et al. 2003: 205, 206) – but also on the very early response from Brazilian actors, communities and states to the epidemic since its very emergence in 1983. Moreover, the Brazilian AIDS Programme did not originate as a one-sided initiative of public health actors, but as a fervent reaction of these same actors to a demarche of a gay group in the state of São Paulo that was particularly concerned about the growing threat (Basso 2002: 136).

This study considers the following as the main global actors interfacing with Brazil's National Health Governance: (a) international governmental organizations (IGOs), such as the World Health Organization (WHO) and its regional representative, the Pan American Health Organization (PAHO) for technical and partially also for financial resource-transfer as well as the World Bank mainly for financial resource-transfer; (b) the multinational private sector, such as the transnational pharmaceutical corporations

(TNPCs) Roche and Abbott or the Ford Foundation as a private funding source for Brazilian civil society organizations (CSOs); (c) the organizations of civil society; and (d) networks such as the Latin American and Caribbean Council of AIDS Service Organizations (LACCASO) or the Global Fund for the Fight against AIDS, Tuberculosis and Malaria (Chapter 5). At the national level, the main actors considered in this chapter are, on the governmental side, the National Coordination of the BHAP, a specialized unit of the Brazilian Health Ministry with a staff of currently more than 200 people (Bacon et al. 2004: 62), as well as the state laboratories. For civil society we examine the more than 1800 CSOs[2] currently specializing in HIV/AIDS-activities, and for the private sector we look at the Brazilian subsidiaries of TNPCs with HIV/AIDS-related activities, such as Roche and Abbott.

The analysis of the interactions between the national and global level of global health governance (GHG) as well as within the national realm follows the notion of 'interfaces', as outlined in Chapter 1. Brazil's early and comprehensive response to the HIV/AIDS challenge succeeded in stopping or even reversing the prevalence rates in the most affected south eastern region and in reducing the rate of expansion in the other regions. As a consequence, in 2002, the actual HIV incidence and mortality rate was already significantly reduced to half the amount predicted by the World Bank a decade earlier.[3] This success attracted the attention of the analysts, who attempted to explain the programme's performances through various approaches, such as managerial and economic (World Bank 2005b), anthropological (Parker 2003), political and social (Teixeira 1997), historical (Galvão 2000), psychological (Paiva 2003) and multidisciplinary (Berkman et al. 2005), to name just a few studies. However, a systematic study of the interfaces between the national and global level of health governance or of the interfaces between the different actors within national governance structures is still lacking. Filling this gap and providing insights on the global and national determinants of HIV/AIDS policy-making in Brazil are the aims of the present study.[4]

The HIV/AIDS challenge in Brazil

In the past two decades, the HIV/AIDS epidemic has emerged 'as one of the most serious public health problems facing the country' (Parker 2003: 143). It affected the Brazilian population with varying intensity, according to region, age, social, and also racial structure. The first Brazilian cases of AIDS were detected in 1982, but as early as 1992, it had assumed epidemic dimensions, with an estimated number of 750 000 HIV-infected people for that year (PAHO 1992: 1–8). Nowadays, Brazil has the second highest absolute number of people living with HIV in the Americas, with an estimated 620 000 people infected (UNAIDS 2006: 535) and about 188 000 people having currently developed AIDS.[5]

According to most recent stabilization trends of the epidemic, approximately 31 000 new cases of AIDS become known each year, that is a current incidence rate of 19.2 AIDS cases per 100 000 inhabitants – a rate officially viewed as persistently high due to the steady growth trend observed for women (Ministério da Saúde 2005a: 14–15, and BHAP 2006a). The current national adult HIV-prevalence rate is 0.61 per cent, measured for the population between 15 and 49 years old. This rate is higher for men (0.8 per cent) than for women (0.42 per cent). However, the AIDS incidence ratio for men/women is steadily falling mainly as a result of the increasing importance of heterosexual transmission (Ministério da Saúde 2006).[6] There are also regional disparities of the epidemiological trends: in the (most affected) south eastern region we observe a reduction of incidence rates since 1998 that was in some years matched (or even surpassed) by an increase in other regions, particularly in the south and north east, which were not as successfully reached by the national AIDS programme (cf. Ministério da Saúde 2005a: 15; Dourado et al. 2006: 11). The overall rebound of the AIDS incidence rate observed in 2002 and 2003 (Figure 7.1) reflects this.

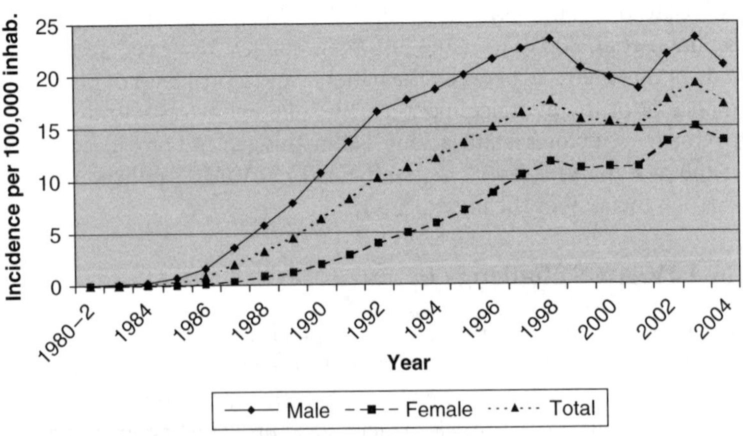

Figure 7.1 AIDS incidence in Brazil 1980–2004[7]
Source: Own graph based on data from Ministério da Saúde 2005a.

The epidemic has changed its faces several times. Following a periodization developed by the World Bank (World Bank 2005b: 7), the first phase occurred in the early 1980s, when the epidemic was mostly concentrated in major coastal cities, including São Paulo and Rio de Janeiro. The transmission took place overwhelmingly through homosexual and/or bisexual relations of men (MSM), and the epidemic was similar in scope, spread and epidemiology to the epidemic occurring in North America and Western Europe. The second phase (late 1980s to early 1990s) witnessed a shift in the transmission mode, with a substantial spread in urban injecting drug users (IDU) – primarily cocaine injectors – in São Paulo, Rio de Janeiro and the southern regions (Rio Grande do Sul and Santa Catarina), but also further disseminating to the larger towns (200 000–500 000 inhabitants). By 1987, AIDS cases had been diagnosed among haemophiliacs, IDUs, heterosexuals, blood transfusion recipients, and newborns; HIV infection rates among haemophiliacs in Rio de Janeiro reached 85 per cent (Garrison 1988: 43). The third phase (still ongoing) is characterized by an increase in heterosexual transmission with a consequently far greater number of infected women and children. The geographical spread of the epidemic has now also reached small municipalities, and the epidemiological characteristics have become more similar to the transmission mode of developing countries. Through all these phases there was an increasing correlation with social inequality, in spite of all the governmental and civil awareness accompanying the implementation of the BHAP. The percentage of people with lower levels of education (eight or less school years)[8] suffering from AIDS had already begun to grow disproportionately in the early 1990s, while that of people with higher levels of education (eight or more school years) has decreased steadily since the mid-1990s (Berkman et al. 2005: 1164; Grangeiro 1994: 91–128). The most affected people within the increasingly important heterosexual transmission mode are men with school attendance of less than eight years (60 per cent of heterosexual transmission); likewise within the same mode, women are affected with particular intensity when their school attendance is less than eight years (Ministério da Saúde 2004b: 95–6, 2005b: 10). These tendencies can be summarized as 'interiorization', 'feminization' and 'pauperization' as the main current epidemiological characteristics.

From 1980 to 1999, 120 000 deaths were caused by AIDS, the second most important cause of death among young men and the fourth among women (Ministério da Saúde 2003: 2; Oliveira et al. 2001: 864). AIDS mortality per 100 000 inhabitants has steadily fallen since the widespread introduction of prophylaxis and treatment for opportunistic infections in 1988 and the highly active antiretroviral therapy (HAART) in 1996/7, which combines ARV treatment with other measures (Bacon et al. 2004: 12–13). The overall AIDS death rate has decreased from 9.7 per 100 000 in 1995 to 6.1 per 100 000 in 2004 (Ministério da Saúde 2005a: 24). With the new measures of universal treatment and prevention, the survival time of AIDS-affected adults (registered in 1996) increased to 58 months in the early 2000s as compared with only five months for those who were registered in the 1980s (Risi and Nogueira 2002: 197). Still, 10 000 people per year die because of AIDS (Ministério da Saúde 2003: 2).

Socio-economic context and the Brazilian health system

With a Gross National Income of US$3000 per capita, Brazil is currently classified as a lower middle-income country (World Bank 2006), but the income distribution is one of the most unequal worldwide (UNDP 2005: 271). As measured by the GINI Index (59.3),[9] Brazilian income distribution is even worse than that of South Africa (57.8) (UNDP 2005: 271, 272). As a consequence of the debt crisis in the 1980s, resources have increasingly been directed to servicing the national debt and supporting structural adjustments as negotiated with the International Monetary Fund. As measured by GDP, total debt service payments amounted to 11.5 per cent in 2003, whereas total health expenditures – private (4.3 per cent) as well as public (3.6 per cent) – reached 8.2 per cent (UNDP 2005: 285 and 237) that same year.

The current Brazilian health system differs markedly from those of most developing countries, since it is a dual system of public and private (for-profit and philanthropic) elements (World Bank 1994: 10). Thus health performance relies heavily on public reimbursement of privately provided health services. Only a small proportion of hospital care is extended through public facilities, the more typical arrangement in developing countries. Additionally, private financing of health care is widespread and growing. In 2002, total health expenditures amounted to US$611 per capita (Purchase Power Parity), putting Brazil at a middle level worldwide. The overall increase in health expenditures reflects the social effervescence during the period of transition to democracy and the following struggle for health reform in order to strengthen the role of state and public health vis-à-vis profit-taking interests of private health providers (Fleury 2000: 233). Hospitals are mainly privately owned (65 per cent), but around 90 per cent of them have a contract with the public health system; outpatient facilities are mainly public (75.6 per cent). As of December 2004, about 19 per cent (33.7 million) of the population were covered by a voluntary private (for profit) insurance (collective or individual) (OPAS 2005: 9–10; Almanaque Abril 2004: 147). The public health system has the objective to achieve universality and integrality (Lobato 2000: 109), yet the actual coverage is only 80 per cent of the population (representative household survey PNAD from IBGE 2006: 19–20). Experts characterize this system as a 'fragmented pluralist system' without a regulatory system to organize the supply of the different providers and to promote efficiency in the use of health expenditures (Medici 2002: 2). For the BHAP, these deficiencies were one of the reasons for the building of a centralized and relatively autonomous HIV/AIDS unit in the Health Ministry (Berkam et al. 2005: 1170; Serra 2004: 2).

According to official data (Monitoraids 2004: 15–16), total government health expenditures amounted to US$15.893 billion in 2002, and in the same year the total expenditures for HIV/AIDS reached US$274 million or just 1.72 per cent of total health expenditures – a huge decrease as compared to 1999 with US$640 million HIV/AIDS expenditures. The expenditures for ARVs constitute the bulk of these figures, costing US$179 million in 2002 compared to a whopping US$336 million three years earlier. Those figures would seem positive for programme sustainability, but the most recent evolution in 2004 and 2005 showed a jump in ARV expenditures from US$223.6 million (Brazilian Real R$591 million) to US$423.6 million (R$986 million), generating renewed concerns about BHAP sustainability, if current price negotiations do not succeed in lowering ARV prices (Grangeiro et al. 2006: 8).[10]

The struggle for the health budget and particularly for the Brazilian consensual response to the HIV/AIDS challenges has been constant factor in the political life of the first two decades of the HIV/AIDS pandemic in Brazil. The broader context directly influencing Brazilian responses to HIV/AIDS as an epidemiological challenge is directly related to social and political processes occurring simultaneously in the early 1980s: (a) the political transition from military to civilian regime, (b) the Brazilian Sanitarian Movement (*Movimento Sanitarista*), and (c) the debt crisis and consequent budget restrictions (for this point see 'Resource-transfer interfaces' below).

The transition from military to civilian regime

The transition to civilian democratic rule started in 1974 under General Geisel, who gradually allowed more open manifestations of electoral will in order to initiate a 'slow, gradual and safe' process of restitution of power to civilian hands. As the parliamentary (1978) and the gubernatorial (1982) elections brought important victories to the opposition, it was evident that the remobilization of Brazilian civil society had been successful. It was this experience of social mobilization that constituted the background of activism when the HIV/AIDS epidemic emerged in the early 1980s and hence shaped the basis for the interaction between civil society and government along 'discoursive interfaces' (see below) in the search for a consensus on the response to the threat. Some of the leading representatives of civil society – such as Herbert Daniel and Herbert de Souza (Betinho) – had personal experiences with the oppression of the military regime, and later became AIDS victims, Betinho having been infected through a blood transfusion for haemophiliacs (World Bank 2005b: 3).[11] In 1980, the political reform reintroduced 'pluripartidarism' (Arturi 2001: 18), which effectively increased the competition among political parties. The first free elections for state governors in 1982 resulted in opposition parties succeeding in ten of the most important states – among them São Paulo, where the first HIV/AIDS cases were reported in 1983. The governmental party won the elections in twelve other states. These elections re-established the decisive influence of regional state governors in building alliances in the Federal Congress (Abrucio and Samuels 1997: 137–66), which later on would be important for passing HIV/AIDS-related laws. In São Paulo, the health unit appointed by the new governor to respond to civil society demands for fighting the HIV/AIDS threat was the Dermatology Unit, whose physician team (composed mainly by members of the Sanitarian Movement, see below) was already active in fighting discrimination against leprosy carriers. Thus, the anti-discrimination logic was immediately applied to the new epidemic.[12]

The struggle for public health: the Brazilian Sanitarian Movement

The new development of the *public health system* was also an element of the opposition movement against the military authoritarian regime and its exclusive character. Administered by the Social Security Healthcare Institute INAMPS (Instituto Nacional de Assistência Médica da Previdência Social), most health care services had been restricted to formal sector workers who contributed payroll taxes, and their provision was implemented by private hospitals and physicians who were contracted by INAMPS. This resulted in regional and class inequalities in the access to health services. This system was radically rejected by the so-called 'Sanitarian Movement', which considers the health system as a crucial element of the comprehensive movement towards redemocratization. Its main claims were 'universal access to publicly funded health care' and 'decentralization of authority over health care to the states and municipalities'. These objectives were partially reached only after the return of civilian democratic government and the process which led to the new democratic Constitution of 1988 with its proclamation of health care as a 'right of all and the duty of the state' and the guarantee of universal and equal access to health care.

The implementation of the thereby established 'Unified Health System' (*Sistema Unico de Saude*, SUS) required many years, since it included not only the decentralization of responsibilities among the Brazilian administrative spheres (federal, states and municipalities), but also the consultation and deliberation processes through representative national, state and municipal health conferences and health councils (see World Bank 2005b: 3). After the 1990 law, which created the SUS, the decentralization mechanisms were clarified progressively in 1996 and 2002, responsibilities and a minimum financing for primary care of outpatients were transferred to municipalities (*piso ambulatorial básico*), criteria were defined for the upgrading of states and municipalities to manage higher level care and receive corresponding direct funding, and incentives were introduced for municipalities to adopt specific health care initiatives, such as the family health and basic medicines programmes. In 2000, a constitutional amendment (No. 29, GC) laid the grounds for health expenditures at all three government levels: the federal level was to expand its health expenditures in accordance with the BIP growth of the previous year, beginning with 2000, whereas the state and municipal levels were to earmark at least 12 and 15 per cent of their tax and total constitutional revenues from federal level, respectively, for health expenditures. 'Given the federalist structure of Brazilian government, the health responsibilities are to be negotiated (*pacto federativo*) case-by case, and particularly for the AIDS-related drug distribution the federal government takes responsibility for purchasing anti-retroviral (ARV) drugs for HIV/AIDS, states for opportunistic infections (OI) and municipalities for sexually transmitted diseases (STDs)' (World Bank 2005b: 3)

The Brazilian response to the HIV/AIDS challenge

As analysed by Richard Parker – an anthropologist, activist and politician living in Brazil and the USA – Brazilian political reaction to the HIV/AIDS challenge can be summarized as having 'emerged, in recent years, as a truly "integral" [. . .] response to HIV and AIDS in Brazil, involving treatment and prevention as central to a uniquely Brazilian model [. . .] rooted in the tradition of an "integral" public health system originally championed by the progressive sanitary reform movement of Brazilian public health, and perhaps most fully achieved (not without great difficulties) in the Brazilian response to AIDS' (Parker 2003: 144).

Obviously, the stakeholders did not automatically adopt a comprehensive HIV/AIDS programme, but there were intense internal debates and power conflicts in the search for a consensus (Parker 2003: 146). We cannot discuss the social construction of the Brazilian consensus on fighting HIV/AIDS in detail. But the characterization of its main features is useful for understanding the context of the following analysis of interfaces.

The first phase (1983–6) was marked, on the one hand, by a narrow cooperation among progressive state governments[13] and civil society and, on the other hand, by the rivalries among state governments and the federal government, which refused until the end of the period to recognize the HIV/AIDS disease as a federal problem.

The second phase (1986–90) refers to the foundation phase of a National AIDS Programme, formally established in 1985 and pragmatically developed with technical and financial support from PAHO/WHO; São Paulo retained its role as reference point for further developments (creation of day hospitals, tracking of unused beds in public hospitals for use by AIDS patients and so on).

The third phase (1990–2) was a contradictory one because it was the period where, on the one hand, all BHAP interfaces with civil society and IGOs ruptured, whilst, on the other hand, it marked the introduction of the distribution of AZT free of charge as early as 1991. Furthermore, in early 1992, Brazil's President Collor had rebuilt his cabinet under 'ethical patterns' in order to reconstitute his relations with Parliament and replaced his corrupt health minister with an integral one, who recalled the former BHAP team and so began a new phase of even more intense relations with civil society and IGOs. The World Bank summarizes its assessment of this phase with the very important observation that 'by the early 1990s a Brazilian strategy towards HIV/AIDS had emerged – an approach embracing prevention among high-risk groups, universal access to treatment, and respect for human rights' (World Bank 2005b: 10). These are the substantial elements of Brazil's comprehensive HIV/AIDS approach that became a main conflict point between Brazil and the World Bank in the following phase, but without hampering cooperation. The fourth phase (1992–2006) can be seen as the longest, still ongoing phase of manifold interactions between the global and national level of health governance, mainly characterized by the financial cooperation between BHAP and the World Bank as well as by intense interactions along the four interfaces. This phase is the object of the following analysis of interfaces between the global and national levels of fighting HIV/AIDS.

Resource-transfer interfaces: the 'conditional' acceptance of strategic World Bank loans

The above-mentioned gap between the claim of universality regarding health in general and HIV/AIDS in particular could only be filled with an injection of foreign finance.

In 1982, the country also became heavily affected by the Latin American debt crisis (Baer and Paiva 1996: 67–8, 71; for an overview see Sangmeister 1992: 255–6).[14] Only with a debt restructuring agreement and the issuing of federal bonds was the severe financial crisis resolved after a prolonged negotiation process with the International Monetary Fund and other international and commercial lending institutions in 1994.[15] Thus, at least until the mid-1990s, Brazil had been reliant on resource-transfer interfaces for funding additional programmes such as BHAP.

Parallel to the general controversy about structural adjustment (Elmendorf and Roseberry 1993: 123; Lurie et al. 1995: 539–46), the financial need for a reform of the Brazilian public health system was beyond doubt. The shift from a rather contribution-based health system (Bismarck model) to a more tax-financed public health system with universal coverage (Beveridge model), established in 1988, represented the substitution of a health system designed for 90 million Brazilians with a new public health system 'with current responsibilities for 160 million people, [and this] cannot be done without significant new resources'.[16] Moreover, the universal provision of free treatment against opportunistic diseases (since 1988), of the antiretroviral drug AZT (since 1991) and of the antiretroviral combination therapy HAART[17] (since 1996) through the national government (Galvão 2002: 214) had subsequently increased the gap between rapidly growing needs for treatment and Brazil's scarce financial resources. Calculations from 1989 estimated the direct treatment costs for each AIDS patient to be approximately US$15,670 per year, with total costs forecasted to amount to around US$3.5 billion for the treatment of all known AIDS patients in Brazil (Medici 1994: 328).[18] Accordingly, external financing for the BHAP had become a necessity in the early 1990s: the budget restrictions under President Collor's neo-liberal economic programme (1990–2) led to shrinking health expenditures for federal government, which diminished from 16.8 per cent of total central government revenues in 1989 to 10.2 per cent in 1992 (Lobato 2000: 108). As a consequence, although conceptually 'a very proper vehicle for comprehensive management of HIV' (Berkman et al. 2005: 1166), the unified health system, as it was still in its infancy, could cope neither with the rapidly mounting HIV/AIDS epidemic under organizational nor its financial aspects.

In 1992, the Brazilian government was finally willing 'to *seek* for' (as the World Bank called it, see World Bank 2005b: 11), or '*to accept* a financial help initiative offered as a long-term credit by the World Bank' (Galvão 2000: 140, emphasis by the author). Since the conclusion of the loan agreement in 1994, it has been the multilateral institution that has provided the largest external resource for the Brazilian health sector. Indeed, the World Bank has been 'the earliest [external donor] to become involved in a major way' (World Bank 2005b: 26). The purpose of the first World Bank credit (AIDS I, 1994–8) signed in March 1994 was a dual one: in terms of results it intended a reduction of incidence and transmission rates of HIV and STD, whereas in terms of the process it had a strong component of institution-building through enhancing public and private institutions of HIV/AIDS control, as revealed by the more specific goals of this first large HIV/AIDS project worldwide, which linked prevention and treatment components. For the implementation of these goals,[19] the National Coordination of the AIDS-STD Programme strictly applied the principles of SUS: it decentralized allocation and management of public resources and promoted civil society participation in order to reach universality and integrality of health provision. Since Brazil is a federal republic, the Health Ministry had to sign contracts with single state governments – 26 states and the Federal District of Brasília – and with initially 43 municipal governments, expanding to currently 417 municipalities and covering 98.1 per cent of all cases of AIDS in a decentralized financing system (Ministério da Saúde 2005b: 81–3).

Non-governmental organizations (NGOs), community-based organizations and research institutions were also included. The resources – US$250 million, with World Bank financing a total of US$160 million and the Brazilian government another US$90 million – have been distributed to prevention (48 per cent), treatment (19 per cent) and institution-building activities (Basso 2002: 140). Originally conceived as a unique four-year project, this project was named AIDS I and – after its termination in 1998 – it was followed by two further AIDS projects: AIDS II (1998–2003), with a total of US$165 million (World Bank credit) and US$135 million (Brazilian Treasury), and AIDS III (2003–6) with US$200 million (US$100 million from each partner). The increasing participation of the Brazilian Treasury was intended in order to ensure project sustainability after the end of the cooperation period in 2006.

Although the quantitative significance of these projects – about 10 per cent of the total amount the Health Ministry spent on HIV/AIDS[20] – is not very great, their qualitative role cannot be stressed enough, since it permitted the national coordination to act as a catalyst of actions at state and municipal levels as well as in the field of CSOs and the private sector. The multilateral financing permitted the functioning of national–subnational interfaces as well as of government–non-government interfaces. It is important to note here that the resource-transfer interface functioned perfectly in spite of a profound disagreement between the World Bank and the BHAP about the role of financing treatment measures, as will be described below in the section on discoursive interfaces. The disagreement did not hamper the approval of the projects by the World Bank.

Resource-transfer interfaces have also been strongly used by CSOs working in the field of HIV/AIDS. Before the World Bank started to provide funds to CSOs in 1994, financing from private foundations such as the Ford Foundation had been of 'fundamental' importance for the pioneer NGOs: ABIA, GAPA and Pela VIDDA[21] (Galvão 2000: 134). Today, their main revenue sources are internal as well as external. In a recent survey of 328 HIV/AIDS CSOs, the largest group stated that they receive funds through 'agreements with public bodies' (78 per cent) and 'donation by individuals' (72.6 per cent). However, 40.9 per cent also draw on support from an 'international cooperation agency' (Castro and Silva 2005: 157). Undoubtedly, foreign resources are quantitatively and strategically significant for CSOs.

Quantitatively, resource-transfer interfaces are significant, although not overwhelming: in an overview of foreign cooperation for HIV/AIDS-related projects for the period 1992–7, Fontes (1999: 96–7) calculated a total contribution of US$278 million from cooperation projects, with a participation of 65 per cent for multilateral cooperation (including 58 per cent from a World Bank loan), 3 per cent for bilateral cooperation and 32 per cent for the Brazilian counterpart. However, as a percentage of the total expenditures for the BHAP, the amount of foreign cooperation does not add up to more than 10 per cent (Chequer 2006), with the greatest financial burden resting on the Brazilian state. But the allocation of this 10 per cent has played a decisive role in the consolidation of BHAP, as almost unanimously asserted by respondents. Brazil has extensively used resource-transfer interfaces in relating to GHG. Since the World Bank loans were issued in 1993, the BHAP has to a large extent been funded by external sources. Furthermore, the CSOs working on HIV/AIDS have also drawn on revenue sources from the global level.

At the national level, health governance functions – as described above – formally through the three government levels, though its financing is primarily the responsibility of the federal government. In 2000, for example, 83.7 per cent of all public expenditures for BHAP (reaching US$467.9 million[22]) came from the federal government; only

16.3 per cent was provided by subnational governments, that is states (8 per cent) and municipalities (8.3 per cent; Piola et al. 2002: 40). Hence one would expect the federal government to have a proportionately greater influence on HIV/AIDS policies of the subnational units. But these relationships are not exclusively determined by financial power. Instead, as stated above, they are regulated by 'agreement' mechanisms between autonomous governmental entities with specific constitutional responsibilities and competencies that are implemented under the command of mixed Intermanagement Commissions with the participation of all government levels and of civil society (Piola et al. 2002: 9).

A further incentive for decentralization is given by the AIDS III Project in the form of annual targets for setting plans. In contrast to the first phases of the BHAP, where – because of the epidemic urgency – the programme had to be planned and implemented within a centralized framework (Ministério da Saúde 1999), the Health Ministry signed a decree in December 2002, establishing decentralized procedures for federal transfers to states and municipalities: states and municipalities no longer have to negotiate with BHAP for inputs to their action plans, but instead they can set annual targets and performance benchmarks, which are determined locally and not on the basis of nationally set priorities as they were until then (World Bank 2005b: 21; Ministério da Saúde 2005b: 81–3).

In short, the resource-transfer interfaces between BHAP and subnational government agencies have evolved drastically in quantitative terms under AIDS I–III, without hampering the decentralization process of the public health system. They were not used to increase central power, but to improve urgently needed efforts against HIV/AIDS. Resource-transfer interfaces between BHAP and CSOs reached a relevant dimension only after the leverage effect of World Bank credits within the projects AIDS I–III, which made it possible for the federal government to interact flexibly with NGOs and other CSOs. All in all, resource-transfer interfaces were of decisive importance for the BHAP, and although the World Bank exerted the greater financial influence, it could not use this sort of interface to influence the contents of discourses, because Brazil constantly refused the Bank's demands to halt the free distribution of AZT (since 1991) and of ARVs (since 1996; Berkman et al. 2005: 1169).

Organizational interfaces: consolidation and empowerment of BHAP

In this study, organizational interfaces are defined as entities or temporary relationships which are formed by at least two convening actors from GHG and national health governance – both in the interactions between global and national level, as well as in the interactions between domestic actors. The use of organizational interfaces (as joint missions, round tables, joint ventures, joint bureaux, common actions and so on) therefore acts as a crucial indicator for the degree of cooperation between the national and the global level.

Since 1970, the WHO, through its regional representative PAHO, has developed multiple initiatives with Brazilian health authorities and academic institutions towards health reform. This reform would in turn shape the BHAP in the 1980s and 1990s.[23] With respect to the BHAP, the nature of these organizational interfaces was conflictual in some aspects, while positive in others. As outlined by the former BHAP National Coordinator Paulo Teixeira, PAHO promoted an interchange of information with the Latin American and Caribbean governments starting in 1983, which led to the offer of technical assistance for the preparation of national responses two years later and helped to shape the WHO's Global Programme on AIDS (GPA) in 1987 (Teixeira 2005: 7). In the same paper, Teixeira recognizes that 'these resources, albeit restricted, were essential for Brazil, particularly in the consolidation process of the BHAP. Also the interchange and cooperation provided by the PAHO/WHO through consulting, missions and regional meetings revealed themselves as fundamental for the construction and perfecting of the Brazilian response' (ibid.: 7–8). Among the first steps on the path to using organizational interfaces was the partnership between the Brazilian Health Ministry and PAHO in order to realize the first capacitating course for managers of the HIV/AIDS state programmes with financial and technical support from PAHO (Ministério da Saúde 1999).

Nevertheless, divergent interests soon came to the surface relating to the mode of resource-transfer interfaces ('authoritatively' earmarked resource allocations) and to the contents of discoursive interfaces, such as the formulation of global and national policies and strategies in the field of HIV/AIDS. In the early 1990s, these dissenting points led to a cessation of resource-transfers (mainly knowledge) from the WHO to Brazil and other countries such as Chile, Mexico and Paraguay, which were also in contention with the World Bank. Thanks to the huge mobilization of national resources since 1992/3, however, these cuts did not affect the Brazilian HIV/AIDS Programme as severely as they did those of other countries. The substantial differences concerning conceptions about prevention programmes, such as harm reduction and public campaigns, widened to a broad dissent about the fundamentals of the Brazilian response in 1991, when the government began the free distribution of

AZT, and moreover in 1992, with the initial negotiations for a strategic loan from the World Bank.

At that point, the dissent had turned mainly towards the WHO headquarters in Geneva, an adversary which 'not only opposed the Brazilian strategy in all international fora' (Teixeira 2005: 8–9), but also affected it directly at the national level through the sending of two missions to Brazil: one in 1991 in order to dissuade the Brazilian authorities from universal and gratuitous AZT distribution, pointing (in accordance with the World Bank) to the scarcity of financial resources and to the cost-effectiveness of prevention; and another in 1992 in order to be admitted as a partner in the negotiations with the World Bank for the project AIDS I. This intent failed due to the refusal of the Brazilian government (Galvão 2000: 127). In the interaction between the Brazilian government and the WHO, the dissent along discoursive lines also decisively hindered the development of positive synergies along organizational interfaces. This dissent lessened only in 2002/3, as the WHO – with some influence from the Brazilian government – redirected its focus to an integrated treatment–prevention approach and underlined the significance of BHAP as a model for emerging and developing countries. In 2003/4, Teixeira was appointed Director of the HIV/AIDS Department of the WHO, which also indicates the rising Brazilian influence on the WHO.

According to Teixeira (2005: 2), the disagreement with the WHO/PAHO has also had a positive side-effect for the BHAP's organizational interfaces with other countries. It created an opportunity for the establishment of the Latin American and Caribbean Technical Horizontal Cooperation Group in 1996 in Rio de Janeiro, with which Latin American and Caribbean representatives of the National HIV/AIDS Programmes replaced the WHO/PAHO influence in shaping the national responses to HIV/ AIDS and in promoting parallel activities as well as particular networks of HIV/AIDS CSOs. 'This cooperation led to an intensive activism and is one of the major factors expanding ARV treatment in the region, where there are presently 5% of worldwide HIV prevalence, but 50% of all worldwide treated HIV/AIDS patients' (Teixeira 2005: 2). Since 1996, the BHAP is connected through an organizational interface at the global level with twenty-three countries in the Latin American and Caribbean technical horizontal cooperation group (GCTH), including Portuguese-speaking countries in Africa,[24] to exchange experiences and knowledge about the epidemic of HIV/AIDS. Since 2000, the cooperation also comprises South Africa, Namibia, Kenya, Botswana and Zimbabwe.

The UNAIDS Theme Group on HIV/AIDS, established in Brazil in 1997, has coördinated the activities of IGOs in the country. It includes various UN organizations, the World Bank, bilateral donor organizations, the BHAP, and the Foreign Ministry, as well as two representatives from civil society (UNAIDS 2001: 3). Since 2004, several other federal ministries have also used this organizational interface (interview with Herlt, 13 September 2004). According to Teixeira, the UNAIDS Theme Group in Brazil has brought 'positive synergic effects' for the articulation among actors at federal, state and municipal levels (interview with Teixeira, 24 September 2004). It has actively participated in the organization of the Brazilian HIV/AIDS prevention campaign, for instance through motivating local mayors to actively participate and inform their communities about the epidemic (interview with Milhomem, 15 September 2004).

However, interaction with UNAIDS has been rather formal; UNAIDS and the WHO have hardly exerted a direct influence on the formulation of the Brazilian HIV/AIDS policy (cf. interviews with Teixeira, 24 August 2004; and Bonifácio, 14 September 2004). This was a consequence of the critical position UNAIDS has assumed since its foundation with regard to the Brazilian treatment policy and later on also regarding the production of generics in Brazil, a position which was overcome only in 2000 with a public declaration by UNAIDS Executive Director Peter Piot supporting the Brazilian ARV distribution policy (Teixeira 2005: 9, and interview 24 August 2004). Nevertheless, a clear distinction was made thereafter between organizational cooperation and the direct participation in national advisory commissions charged with the formulation of national HIV/AIDS policies, such as the CNAIDS.[25] Concerning organizational interfaces between UNAIDS and the Brazilian government in implementing BHAP, the Brazilian assessment is positive, but Brazil did not allow a direct participation of UNAIDS in policy-making. Its Theme Group – after a period of active participation – was finally asked to leave the CNAIDS in 2005 'as representation of a foreign agency' (CNAIDS Protocol, 27 April 2005).

On the other hand, as already demonstrated for the WHO, Brazilian actors effectively used organizational interfaces to influence GHG. In 2004, Brazil's representative was unanimously elected Vice-President of the UNAIDS Programme Coordinating Board, and in 2005 he assumed the Presidency of the body (CNAIDS 2004). The increased Brazilian impact on the global level is an outcome of the government's general policy of actively working on HIV/AIDS within international organizations. Brazil's pro-active quest for influence on GHG along organizational interfaces has been particularly intensive since 2000, mainly in response to an increased demand for technical interchange and for ARV donations from other developing countries (a demand that emerged since the positive results of the Brazilian treatment policy for HIV/AIDS became evident from 1998 onwards), and also as a consequence of the estimated development of ARV prices threatening the sustainability of the BHAP. As stated by Teixeira in his report of his own experience as BHAP's General Director (Teixeira 2005: 11f.), the building of an 'international alliance' was viewed as a means to achieve price reductions for imported ARVs since 2000.

A good example of such activities was Brazil's participation in the Durban International AIDS Conference in June 2000. Again referring to his experiences as General Director of BHAP, Teixeira describes the preparation of the Brazilian delegation in an interministerial meeting of the Brazilian government that linked the Foreign Ministry to the Health Ministry research unit Far-Manguinhos (Rio de Janeiro) as well as to the BHAP's drug purchasing unit and the BHAP itself. The committee concluded that 'international action could enhance our bargaining power within Brazil' and deliberated actions at the global level: (a) to provide free transfer of technology to requesting countries for the local production of generic drugs and (b) to put the topic of the access to ARVs and its main obstacle – their price – on the international agenda. While participating in the Durban Conference, the BHAP distributed 15 000 copies of a pamphlet describing the Brazilian gratuitous offer of technology for generic production, which had a huge impact in the conference as well as in the international media. The search for an international alliance continued in a conference organized on that occasion by UNAIDS with the health ministers of Nigeria, India, China, Russia and Brazil, in which the issues of free technology transfer and ARV price reductions were effectively brought on to the international agenda.

Another example is the series of activities to mobilize discoursive and organizational interfaces in order to confront the WTO panel solicited by the US in 2001 against Brazil's patent law. The activities included a 'guerrilla-like information action, with a list of international reporters and NGOs favorable to ARV treatment and the use of telephone during several days demanding their support in order to overcome the mistrust that NGOs naturally hold vis-à-vis governments, and asking national NGOs to advocate our position' (Teixeira 2005: 13–14). Brazil's diplomatic representations in Washington, Geneva and New York were involved, and Brazilian representatives put the issue of ARV treatment and generics onto the agenda of several international and multilateral organizations such as the Okinawa G8 Summit in July 2000, the Executive Committee of the WHO in January 2001, the UN Commission on Human Rights in February 2001, the UNAIDS Board in April/May 2001, the WHO General Assembly in June 2001, and the UNGASS in June 2001. The actions led to the common proposition by France and Brazil regarding the concrete shaping of the Global Fund to Fight HIV/AIDS, Malaria and Tuberculosis (Teixeira 2005: 13–14; Chapter 5). In November 2001, Brazil's efforts in using organizational interfaces together with other developing countries and CSOs culminated in a common resolution of the Doha Conference of November 2001, clarifying the use of compulsory licensing in national public health emergencies. Earlier, Brazil had already obtained the support of fifty developing countries for its proposal of a corresponding WTO Declaration (Teixeira 2005: 14).

There is also evidence for Brazil's civil society exerting impact on GHG. For instance, the 1986-founded Brazilian Interdisciplinary AIDS Association (ABIA) was actively involved in the establishment of the International Council of AIDS Service Organizations (ICASO) at the fifth International AIDS Conference in Montreal in 1989 (Galvão 2000: 87). ICASO was established with the main aim to strengthen the global response of CSOs. Acting as the ICASO Secretariat for Latin America, ABIA also spearheaded the creation of the LACCASO as another organizational interface (Galvão 2000: 87).[26]

At the level of national health governance (NHG), the organizational narrowing of HIV/AIDS-related activities of government and civil society was of decisive importance for both actors: for the government as a means to reach marginal population groups that otherwise would not have been included in the impact radius of BHAP, and for the CSOs as a means of enhancing their political impact through an intense interaction with political institutions through the establishment of organizational interfaces. Fostered by the joint projects AIDS I–III of BHAP and the World Bank, the number of CSOs addressing HIV/AIDS grew rapidly from 120 in 1992 to more than 500 in 1998 (Bacon et al. 2004: 45) and to 1884 in 2003 (Monitoraids 2004). The increased interfaces between HIV/AIDS CSOs and BHAP seem to have contributed to a better overall relationship between civil society and the state in Brazil, because in the initial phase there were no important organizational links between CSOs and the national government, with CSOs restricting themselves to direct activities at the subnational state level both in advocacy and political terms as well as in terms of health assistance and prevention (Boyd 1999: 1).

As noted by Boyd, 'enlightened leadership of the government's national program in the early 1990s led to the establishment of cooperative working relationships between CSOs and the government. An NGO Liaison Office was created within the national program to expand the participation of civil society in the struggle against the HIV/AIDS epidemic. At the time of preparation for the AIDS/STD Control Project in 1992, the World Bank provided draft terms of reference in which it stated that the active involvement of NGOs should become a key component of the loan agreement' (Boyd 1999: 1; see also 'Resource-transfer interfaces' above). As a result of this project, the organizational interfaces between CSOs and government were enhanced by several key participatory mechanisms to enable government/civil society collaboration to grow and solidify (Boyd 1999: 3).

Since AIDS I–III, the organizational interfaces between government and CSOs became so strong that José Serra, Brazilian Health Minister from 1998–2003, called the BHAP staff themselves 'an NGO' within the Health Ministry, as 'evinced by its autonomy, the absence of political appointments, and its degree of technical excellence' (Serra 2004: 2). Effectively, one may consider the central staff of BHAP – numbering 200 people in 2002 (in 1985, the staff totalled 30 people), all currently financed by the World Bank (Bacon et al. 2004: 62) – as a complex interface unit. In addition, the interchanges with civil society include a steady flux of personnel from CSOs to the BHAP and back, as was the case for ABIA in the 1990s, with five of its leading researchers changing to a position at the BHAP (Parker and Terto Jr. 2001: 55; several interviews, 2004 and 2005).

So at the GHG level, organizational interfaces allowed the BHAP a very critical constructive position in order to exert influence on the global health agenda, and at the NHG level there was a very complex intertwining between CSOs and the BHAP, after some periods of reciprocal distance or suspicion between important sections of civil society and the BHAP. In general, BHAP exerted a visible influence on GHG, with the decisive support of transnational and national civil society.

Legal interfaces, BHAP and changing global trade frameworks

Legal provisions are one of the main means to broaden or to narrow the access to the public health system, and therefore their formulation, enactment and implementation constitute the main objective of actors' activities along 'legal interfaces'. Once enacted, they are often the main basis for activities along other interfaces, such as the discoursive ones. The legal recognition of universal access to health as 'a right of all and a duty of the state' in the 1988 Brazilian Constitution (Republic of Brazil 1988, Article 196 in: Senado Federal 2003: 119) had worked as an immovable legal pillar for the negotiations about the World Bank credits for

AIDS I–III along discoursive interfaces (Parker et al. 2001: 110). The BHAP also has strong legal interfaces with IGOs concerning contracts, particularly with the World Bank as regards the access of HIV-infected or AIDS-affected persons to prevention, health promotion, and drug assistance for prophylaxes or treatment of subsequent diseases. Brazil's interference was relevant for the following decisions affecting international law:[27] (a) the 57th section of the Human Rights Commission of the Economic and Social Council of the United Nations (Resolution No. 33 recognizes access to HIV/AIDS drugs as a basic human right), (b) the WHO Declaration of May 2001 about the importance of affordable prices for AIDS drugs (WHO 2001a),[28] and (c) the Doha Declaration of November 2001 about compulsory licensing of patents for ARV drugs when the case for public health national emergency is given (Articles. 4, 5c and 6, WTO 2001).

Turning to the global level influencing the national level of health governance, Brazil has fought with the United States over pharmaceutical patent rights for a long time. As early as 1988, PhRMA, the association of the US pharmaceutical industry, had started lobbying against the Brazilian patent law, which excluded medical products from patent protection (Marques 2002: 43, Tachinardi 1993: 67). Following severe commercial sanctions through punitive tariff duties on selected Brazilian export products,[29] applied in 1990 (Silva 2005: 131), the Brazilian government agreed to formulate a patent law which included the protection of pharmaceutical products.

However, the new Brazilian patent law, issued in 1996, still limited the scope of pharmaceutical patent rights. Paragraph 68 forced pharmaceutical MNCs to produce their drugs locally within three years of patent approval – a provision whose non-compliance allowed the government to issue compulsory licences.[30] The United States filed a complaint on that restriction with the WTO in 2001 (Galvão 2002: 216; Marques 2002: 44, 46). The dispute, fought through legal interfaces, only came to a conclusion when Brazil restricted the possibility of compulsory licensing in cases of a national health emergency. As a consequence, on 25 June 2001, the United States withdrew its formal complaint against Brazil. Brazil in turn agreed to notify the US government in advance if it found it necessary to issue a compulsory licence. This solution can also be seen as a result of public pressure from CSOs, simultaneously articulated through discoursive interfaces in the US and Brazil.[31]

Since 1997, a Brazilian state laboratory (Far-Manguinhos in Rio de Janeiro) has developed the technology for the production of several ARV combinations which consisted of non-protected drugs as well as of drugs protected by patent laws.[32] For the latter, Brazil had to come to terms with TNPCs on licences or on the pricing of drug deliveries. 'In the early years of the new millennium, the Brazilian authorities negotiated with a number of TNPCs in order to obtain cheaper prices for the ARV cocktail' (Oliveira and Esher 2004: 244–5; see also Wogart and Calcagnotto 2006: 96). Following unsuccessful negotiations, the Brazilian Health Minister announced in August 2001 that his government would issue a compulsory licence for the production of Roche's antiretroviral drug Nelfinavir (sold under the brand name Viracept) to a Brazilian manufacturer. Responding to the threat, Roche resumed the negotiations and agreed to lower its prices by 40 per cent (Roche 2001). The threat of issuing compulsory licences brought substantial price cuts for other antiretroviral drugs as well (Cohen and Lybecker 2005: 218–20).[33]

At the national level of health governance, legal interfaces are also used in Brazil as a socio-political space in which CSOs exert pressure upon the Brazilian government. The first AIDS NGO emerged in São Paulo in 1985 under the name GAPA,[34] and one of its principal aims was the provision of legal assistance to persons living with HIV/AIDS (PLWHA). Their legal basis would be defined in the new democratic Constitution of 1988, whose health-related determinants were prepared by the 8th National Health Conference in 1986 with broad civil society participation. Health consumers, providers, public administration, and health professionals took part in this conference (Mendes 1996: 49), demanding 'a public health assistance system qualitatively universal and with access for the whole population' (Scheffer et al. 2005: 20). In 1989, the second NGO with the explicit aim to provide HIV/AIDS-related legal counselling emerged in Rio de Janeiro, the Grupo pela VIDDA, created by Herbert Daniel, himself a PLWHA.

NGOs initiated judicial claims in 1990, even before any specific law based on the constitutional provisions was enacted. Thus jurisdiction had to be based on the direct interpretation of the Constitution (Scheffer et al. 2005: 20). The objective was to put the Executive under pressure to establish a policy of integral and universal assistance for people living with HIV/AIDS (Ventura 2003: 244). These NGO initiatives led to a legal interpretation of the federal state's obligation to provide integral, free and universal treatment for PLWHA. Legal decisions became 'key incentives to public administration, added to advances made by the Brazilian Sanitary Movement' (Ventura 2003: 244). This NGO strategy was based on the Brazilian experience that many specific laws were not implemented. Accordingly, NGOs preferred to seek legal sentencing based on the 'self-applicability' of constitutional dispositions, so as to avoid changes to existing or the creation of new laws (Ventura 2003: 244). Cases before tribunals were concerned with issues such as violations of human rights, discrimination, labour and social insurance claims, performance refusal by private health insurance plans, and failing drug provision in the public health network. NGO lawyers collaborated closely with each other, and currently they maintain a virtual communication network via the internet (Scheffer et al. 2005: 22).

As a consequence, NGOs' actions reached judicial decisions that favoured free ARV provision even before a specific law was issued in 1996, referring directly to the constitutional rules of the universality and integrality of health as a 'right of all people and a duty of the state' (see above). In November 1996 (after massive mobilization that also involved the BHAP), pressure from civil society led to the approbation of Law 9313 by the National Congress, presented by the Senator and former President José Sarney, making the state responsible for providing ARVs free of charge to all in the public health system (Scheffer et al. 2005: 25). However, this victory did not yet bring a definitive solution. Although ARV purchases were made in that same month, the coverage reached only 46 per cent of the AIDS patients in May 1997. Hence the judicial claims intensified steadily, and legal interfaces remained a strong instrument for pressure on the state's HIV/AIDS policy to implement law.

In conclusion, along this 'Brazilian path' of legal interfaces at the global and national level of health governance, the government as well as the civil society have used this arena of socio-political negotiations in several ways: their strategies have ranged from open conflict to pragmatic negotiations with TNPCs and justice bodies. Thus, there is much empirical evidence emanating from the Brazilian case to show that legal interfaces are a particularly effective weapon to enhance public health interests both at the global and the national level.

Discoursive interfaces and the enhanced global influence of BHAP

The loan negotiations between Brazil and the World Bank took place amidst a dispute on the discoursive level. While the Brazilian government, in accordance with the health prescriptions of its Constitution in Article 196, focused on its comprehensive and human rights-based approach to fighting HIV/AIDS, the World Bank first insisted on its prevention concept. The role of CSOs in the negotiations helped to restrict the World Bank's influence to an almost exclusively resource-transfer character. In fact, as Parker et al. (2001: 110) observe, 'Brazil's experience in fighting AIDS did not orient itself according to the ideas the Bank offered. On the contrary, the Brazilian government developed the experience to guarantee universal access of AIDS patients to ARVs, and this experience – because of its innovative characteristics – has been discussed and taken as an example for other countries.'

The World Bank did not support policies of drug distribution without charging patients, since the institution focused on the cost-effectiveness of public health programmes (World Bank 1997: 3). Nevertheless, these differences on the discoursive level did not prevent the concession of the AIDS I–III loans, because both sides 'agreed to disagree' (World Bank 2005b: 13, see also above). The World Bank itself drew some conclusions from its AIDS I and AIDS II loan projects concerning the interfaces, particularly with respect to CSOs and to its own participation, especially stressing the Bank's contribution to increasing efficiency and cost-effectiveness in prevention, but also in its treatment and care component. According to the Bank, the latter 'was selective and strategic, focusing on the establishment of lower-cost alternatives, including an increasing shift to outpatient care, and on improving service quality through capacity building of service providers and of the laboratory network' (World Bank 2004c: 29–30). By contrast, specific expenditures for ARV purchases were financed by the Brazilian Treasury, not by the World Bank.

HIV/AIDS workplace programmes may also be considered to have an impact through discoursive interfaces, since they raise awareness for the epidemic, inform about prevention and demonstrate the effectiveness of ARV treatment. In Brazil, workplace programmes for prevention and awareness have been implemented since 1985, with large national and multinational companies taking the lead. Bank conglomerates (such as Itaú since 1987), state-owned companies (such as the power utility Furnas since 1992), and TNCs (such as Ford and Volkswagen do Brasil) have implemented HIV/AIDS awareness and prevention programmes from early on.[35] Established in 1998, the Brazilian National Business AIDS Council (CENARDS)[36] has been the body representing business at the BHAP. It has, furthermore, exerted an important global diffusion function in disseminating best practices in respect to workplace programmes (Terto 1997: 154). The result of these domestic and multilateral activities has been a change in mentality. Firms and private foundations began to view NGOs and trade unions as potential partners in fighting HIV/AIDS. One scholar even speaks of a 'new social philanthropy' on the part of the business sector (Terto 1997: 152). However, quantitatively, the picture is less encouraging: according to a 2006 World Economic Forum survey, only 43 per cent of 212 Brazilian business leaders interviewed declared that their company runs a workplace HIV/AIDS programme (BBC Brazil 2006). The private sector finances and implements prevention initiatives in the workplace for a total of four million workers (World Bank 2003: 74–86).

At the national level, as stated by most respondents interviewed in 2004 and 2005, the discoursive role of CSOs facing the BHAP has been one of continuity in conception, practical strategies, and political legitimization for BHAP. For the fight against HIV/AIDS, according to the former Health Minister José Serra, the public health system has received the assistance of 'more than 600 CSOs involving the work of more than 20 000 people in more than two thousand projects targeted at prevention, assistance and support, all of them counting on the financial backing of the government' (Serra 2004: 2). Effectively, as mentioned above, it was the demarche of an informal group of gay activists that had taken the initiative to demand a reaction from São Paulo's State Health Department, since at that time (1983) there was neither national nor international support. Like a snowball, this local mobilization of grassroots communities led – at first at the state level – to the creation of the first public health HIV/AIDS programme in Latin America; its supervisor (Paulo Teixeira) would later bring his know-how to the BHAP as its Co-Director in 1992 and as its General Director 2000–3 (Biehl 2004: 106; cf. interview Teixeira, 24 August 2004).

Grassroots and regional state interventions shared a progressive political commitment and understood the need to integrate information and care, and pragmatically established alliances with health technicians and philanthropic institutions. Progressively organized in several CSOs, HIV/AIDS activists representing socially vulnerable groups such as homosexuals and sex workers developed a strong public voice in the dispute over access to increasingly scarce public and medical resources. They opened grassroots spaces of health care to bear the medical and social burden of the HIV/AIDS crisis among the poorest, partly compensating the underfunded and understaffed state public health services (Biehl 2004: 108). Even in that initial phase, the bulk of the HIV/AIDS CSOs saw their role not as an 'antithesis' to state governments, but as a compensating social movement designed to combat and also to compensate to some extent the paralyses of state health services in their capacity to address the growing complexities of HIV/AIDS. With this positive attitude along discoursive interfaces, most HIV/AIDS CSOs helped decisively to constitute 'together with health technicians, epidemiologists, medical and social scientists, economists, and psychologists [. . .] a new epistemic community within the state' (Biehl 2004: 108), whose main merit was to call for a fight against HIV/AIDS that integrated prevention, care and treatment.

Galvão points to the shifting emphasis of claims by civil society, whose mobilization in the 1980s was 'of extreme importance for obliging governments to implement *prevention* initiatives', whereas since the mid-1990s, the need became more and more urgent for actions regarding *access to anti-HIV drugs*, a struggle to which a new area was recently added through 'transnational activism': the *patents* (Galvão 2002: 218). The political aspect of the discoursive interfaces between CSOs and government is expressed by one of the chief pharmacists of BHAP: 'It is social mobilization that gives us the political legitimacy to make the medication available. [. . .] Politicians give priority to this kind of social pressure. It is time to transfer this experience of both social mobilization and treatments to other pathologies, like TB and Hansen's' (Biehl 2004: 110).

Discoursive interfaces were also important for negotiating price reductions with Brazilian subsidiaries of multinational pharmaceutical companies. Today, Brazil pays 77 per cent less for medicines produced by Merck, 56.2 per cent less for those produced by Abbott and 69.4 per cent less for medicines produced by Roche (Ministério da Saúde 2004a: 37). Bermudez and Oliveira synthesize the combination of actors and factors that led to these results: 'Government support has been sustained by a combination of the pressure of social forces, a well-built program and the worldwide importance that is being attributed to AIDS' (Bermudez and Oliveira 2002: 5). Carvalho points to the overwhelming influence of transnational activism, and Passarelli and Terto stress the participation of Brazilian CSOs in this global movement.[37]

In summary, the role of discoursive interfaces between the Brazilian government and CSOs shows a shifting emphasis in issues and programmes, but they are overwhelmingly critical and simultaneously they present constructive propositions. On the contrary, discoursive interfaces in the relationship between the Brazilian government and the pharmaceutical industry reveal a more conflicting pattern that includes the threat of compulsory licensing and the use of market mechanisms to counteract the monopoly of patent right owners. The influence of Brazilian CSOs on negotiations between the Health Ministry and the TNPCs was mediated by the influence of transnational activism, whereas their influence on BHAP's prevention and treatment integrating approach was rather direct and strong. This can be seen as an indication of 'civil leadership' over 'political leadership' (Berkman 2005: 1166), since the comprehensive prevention–treatment–care approach originated as a result of domestic pressure from CSOs.

Conclusion

The fight against HIV/AIDS has been an area of strong interaction between the national and the global level of health governance.

Brazilian actors have interacted continuously with the global level through different interfaces. The interactions at different interfaces have, however, shown diametrically opposed characteristics. Brazil has received a total of US$425 million for its National HIV/AIDS Programme through three World Bank loans within a period of twelve years, and its attitude was mainly cooperative along the resource-transfer interface, but extremely critical along the discoursive interface because of the disagreement concerning the priorities given to treatment and/or prevention.

This analysis has clearly shown that the influence of global actors on the national level of health governance has been mediated by the national political context. In other words, national politics and actor constellations account for most of the conflicts with global level actors. This concurs with Gauri and Lieberman who, in comparing Brazil and South Africa, state that 'differences in foreign assistance on HIV/AIDS can be explained from the perspective of domestic policy choices' (2004: 27). For example, backed by keen support from civil society in the context of the negotiations about the three World Bank loans, the Brazilian government could reject all discoursive arguments by the World Bank regarding treatment, without refusing the 'offer' or the 'occasion' of a huge loan. Thus, the influence of the global level on Brazilian HIV/AIDS policies along discoursive interfaces has been lower than those along resource-transfer interfaces as such. As the analysis has shown, the Bank has not been able to push through its model of how to fight HIV/AIDS, but there has certainly been a continuous, generally positive interaction on the discoursive level between international and Brazilian CSOs.

The analysis points to the fact that the relationship between the different interfaces is highly context-specific. On the one hand, the World Bank example has shown that interfaces can work *incongruently*: in other words accordance between national and global actors is found in respect to one interface but not in respect to another. In Brazil's case, the resource-transfer interface was used, whilst international and transnational influence through discoursive interfaces was limited. The dissent with the WHO along discoursive and organizational interfaces confirms this assertion.

Not only have global/international actors exerted (some) influence on the national level of Brazil's health governance, they in turn also felt the significant impact of Brazilian national experiences and politics on their own concepts of GHG. In this inverse direction, discoursive interfaces also proved to be of crucial significance. As outlined above, Brazil has acted as a global model for the fight against HIV/AIDS, with 'perhaps the most successful experience yet realized in any developing country, but perhaps anywhere' (Parker 2003: 144). Furthermore, Brazilian actors have consistently, through organizational, discoursive and legal interfaces, fought for lower prices of antiretroviral drugs and for their free provision.

Our research demonstrates that a joint proceeding against HIV/AIDS along organizational interfaces follows a common conception along discoursive interfaces, as shown in the interrelationship BHAP–WHO at the global level and the CNAIDS–UNAIDS Theme Group at the national level. Through the cooperation with transnational CSOs and allied governments along organizational interfaces, Brazilian initiatives had a significant impact on several sessions of IGOs, such as the UN, the WHO and the WTO, leading to relevant institutional changes regarding ARV treatment, ARV prices and compulsory licensing.

Legal interfaces – often working in close conjunction with discoursive counterparts – might have been even stronger in influencing GHG. For a long time, pharmaceutical patents and the rights WTO member states possess vis-à-vis TNPCs under the TRIPS agreement have been highly contentious issues. With its threat of compulsory licensing, the Brazilian government has exerted pressure on TNPCs and has resisted pressure from governments of developed countries such as the United States. By using discoursive and legal interfaces, the Brazilian government has pursued confrontational strategies against TNPCs in order to successfully influence GHG.

On the whole, in the quest for affordable ARVs, Brazil intensively and extensively mobilized organizational, legal and discoursive interfaces in order to influence, actively, the health policies of global and national actors. Moreover, it consequently used resource-transfer interfaces with global actors to finance its BHAP. And it obviously succeeded. This fact can therefore be considered as the empirical verification of its comparably high degree of autonomy along organizational, discoursive and legal interfaces. Since this national autonomy constitutes the fundamental determinant for conflict and cooperation with global actors, one must conclude that national societies continue to play an important role in establishing patterns of conflict and cooperation between GHG and NHG. Central actors such as the Brazilian government can cause a conflictive as well as constructive relationship with the global realm and can limit its influence. In this context, Teixeira points to the fact that 'for the first time, public policies of a developing country such as Brazil had changed the course and the paradigms of Global Governance. This has established, so I hope, a precedent for changing the power relations among rich and poor countries in the settling of universal problems' (Teixeira 2005: 2).

Notes

1. Sexually transmitted diseases.
2. In 2003, 1884 NGOs were linked to the BHAP (see BHAP 2006b).
3. In 1994, the World Bank estimated that by 2002 Brazil would report nearly 1.2 million cases of HIV infection. However, UNAIDS actually estimated a total of 620 000 infections in 2005 (Teixeira 2002; UNAIDS 2006: 535).
4. Its empirical basis is a great amount of data and information from primary and secondary sources. In the second half of 2004 and the first half of 2005, the author conducted a total of 69 specialized interviews in São Paulo, Brasília and Rio de Janeiro. These were complemented by another 19 interviews in Recife and additional interviews in São Paulo, conducted at the end of 2004 and in 2005 by local research partners. The respondents were mainly representatives of government, CSOs, the pharmaceutical and medical sector as well as academia.
5. As noted by the World Bank Evaluation Department (World Bank 2005b: 6), the basis for Brazil's epidemiological monitoring is not the HIV prevalence (per cent of *HIV infections* related to overall population), but instead the *cases of AIDS* as a fully developed disease. The mandatory reporting of AIDS cases began in 1986, but that of HIV prevalence is not yet mandatory; it is therefore particularly difficult to assess estimates of current infection levels and the impact of public policy in Brazil.
6. In: http://157.86.8.200/abrir.asp?valor=79 (2006–9); Ministério da Saúde (2004b: 95); Ministério da Saúde (2005a).
7. This figure shows the new cases estimated (observed + corrected) to have occurred in the year given, not the accumulated number of people living with AIDS. The accumulated number of AIDS cases for the period 1980–2004 is 359 887 notified cases; the accumulated number of deaths caused by AIDS in 1980–2004 is 171 923 notified cases (Ministério da Saúde 2005a: 22). According to these figures, one may estimate a total of 187 964 people actually living with AIDS in Brazil.
8. Here, the level of education is taken as a proxy for the socio-economic position.
9. A value of 0 represents perfectly equal distribution, and a value of 100 perfectly unequal.
10. Currency conversion: 1 Real = 0.3764 US$ in 31.12.2004 and = 0.42956 US$ on 31 December 2005.
11. In 1981, Betinho founded the Brazilian Institute for Social and Economic Studies IBASE in Rio de Janeiro, a fruitful ground for several other AIDS NGOs, among them ABIA (Brazilian Interdisciplinary AIDS Association), which he led together with Herbert Daniel. In 1989, the latter created another AIDS NGO, the 'Grupo pela VIDDA', a 'Group for the Respect, Integrity and Dignity of PLWHA'.
12. Interview Teixeira 2004; Teixeira had leading functions in the BHAP since 1986 and was its General Director in 2000–3.
13. Beside Rio de Janeiro and São Paulo, nine more states had a comprehensive response to HIV/AIDS in 1985.
14. According to the Brazilian Central Bank, the middle- and long-term debt amounted to US$83.3 billion in 1982 (Central Bank 1983: 93).
15. Calcagnotto (1985: 63–74); Vásquez (1996: 5); Fritz (2002: 132–4); Tesouro Nacional (2006: 1–2).

16. Mercadante (2002: 275); see also: OPAS (2005: 27); Piola and Biasoto (2001: 219–20); Giovanella and Porto (2004: 11–13).
17. Highly Active Antiretroviral Therapy, a combination of three different antiretroviral drugs to treat HIV/AIDS.
18. According to official figures, the expenditures for purchasing ARVs increased from US$38.5 million (R$40 million) to US$197.5 million (R$573 million) from 1996 to 2003 due to the rising number of HIV-infected people on treatment. This increase has more than compensated the progressively declining unit prices of ARVs (Ministério da Saúde 2003: 11, with figures in Brazilian Real currency; about price reductions cf. Oliveira and Esher 2004: 243–5).
19. And those of the subsequent projects AIDS II and III, see below.
20. According to the National Director of BHAP Pedro Chequer (2006), the World Bank apportioned 10.2 per cent to total AIDS expenditures of the Federal Health Ministry, 1997–2002.
21. GAPA is the abbreviation for Grupo de Apoio à Prevenção à AIDS (AIDS Prevention Promotion Group); Grupo Pela VIDDA stands for Grupo Pela Valorização, Integração e Dignidade do Doente de Aids (Group for Appreciation, Integration and Dignity of AIDS Patients).
22. Or R$912.029 million converted at the average of 1 R$ = 0.51256 US$ on 31 December 2000.
23. Lima (2002: 92–3); Fontes (1999: 113–14); Berkman et al. (2005: 1168).
24. Angola, Cape Verde, Mozambique, Guinea-Bissau, Sao Tomé e Príncipe.
25. National AIDS Commission, an advisory committee of thirty-nine representatives of civil society (NGOs, academic, physicians) and government to give direct support to the general direction of the BHAP (CNAIDS 2004: Parcerias; Spink 2003: 63–72).
26. Further examples of Brazilian NGOs entering into organizational interfaces can be found in Galvão (2000).
27. See also section above on organizational interfaces.
28. Agenda item 13.6: '(10) in order to increase access to medicines, to cooperate constructively in strengthening pharmaceutical policies and practices, including those applicable to generic drugs and intellectual property regimes, in order further to promote innovation and the development of domestic industries consistent with international law.'
29. These were for instance electronic, pharmaceutical and chemical products, as well as paper and cellulose.
30. 'Compulsory licensing is generally defined as the granting of a license to a third-party by a government to use a patent without the permission of the patent holder' (Kühl 2002: 17). For compulsory licensing in the TRIPS agreement see this volume, Chapter 2.
31. Cepaluni (2005: 80–1); Ashraf (2001: 2112); Galvão (2002: 215–16); Wogart and Calcagnotto (2006: 95–6); see also Chapter 3.
32. Oliveira and Esher (2004: 244); Cassier and Correa (2003: 90–1); Marques (2002: 69).
33. The domestic production of the drugs Nevirapine and Indinavir in 2000 represented savings of US$80 million, or 30 per cent of the overall ARV expenditures in that year (Marques 2002: 69). As a consequence of price reductions and local production of non-patented ARVs, US$960 million were saved between 1996 and 2002 (Oliveira and Esher 2004: 245).

34. Grupo de Apoio à Prevenção da AIDS, an AIDS prevention support group.
35. Terto (1997: 142, 152); Teixeira (1997: 60–1); cf. interview with Moreira, 11 August 2004.
36. With its twenty-three members representing large and middle-sized companies and business associations, the CENARDS also acts as an example of an organizational interface.
37. Carvalho (2005: 27); 't Hoen (2002: 45); Passarelli and Terto (2003: 255).

8

The Treatment Controversy: Global Health Governance and South Africa's Fight Against HIV/AIDS

Christian von Soest and Martin Weinel

Fighting HIV/AIDS in South Africa: a question of global health governance

This chapter endeavours to analyse the contentious relationship between actors of the global and national level of global health governance (GHG) in the fight against HIV/AIDS in South Africa. The case study deals predominantly with vertical relationships between actors on the national and global level, i.e. vertical interfaces (see Chapter 1). Despite the multiplicity of actors from GHG, it will illustrate the enduring relevance of national actor configurations and policies for the fight against HIV/AIDS on the nation-state level. In contrast to Brazil (Chapter 7), the interaction between the South African government and GHG actors was for a long time characterized by distrust and divergent priorities.

With around 11 per cent of its citizens infected with HIV, the country has one of the highest prevalence rates in the world (Doherty and Colvin 2004: 196). At the same time, the South African government has largely desisted from directly interacting with actors on the global level in this policy field. The analysis will provide fundamental insights into the effects of the evolving GHG structure on the national level in relation to the fight against HIV/AIDS. In addition, it assesses the influence South African actors have exerted on the global level.

Since its election in 1994, the democratic African National Congress (ANC) government has made the pandemic a comparatively low priority and for quite some time, it resisted the provision of life-enhancing antiretroviral drugs (ARVs) to HIV-infected persons in state hospitals, putting many South Africans at a greater risk of dying from AIDS. In a nutshell, the controversy about the HIV/AIDS policy in South Africa has been one about *treatment* and the access to it. Our primary focus in the following case study is to determine the nature of the interaction between actors from the global and national levels. This involves the following two questions: first, which actors have proven the most influential, both on the global and national levels, in the fight against HIV/AIDS in South Africa? These actors may be states, private businesses, civil society organizations (CSOs) and networks (see Chapter 1 and also Bartsch and Kohlmorgen 2005a: 3). Second, what have been the actors' means of interaction? In addressing this question, we will apply the concept of interfaces formulated in Chapter 1.

The controversies around the fight against HIV/AIDS in South Africa, and in particular antiretroviral treatment, have attracted a lot of scholarly attention from social scientists. Various attempts have been made to explain the government's refusal to provide ARVs in public hospitals and to analyse the confrontations between government and other national actors.[1] However, to our knowledge, no publication has thus far systematically assessed the interaction between actors on the national and global levels in the field of South Africa's fight against HIV/AIDS.

The analysis rests on a wide range of primary and secondary sources as its empirical basis. In the first half of 2005 we conducted forty-eight interviews in South Africa,[2] with respondents from government, international governmental organizations (IGOs), the private business sector, CSOs, as well as the medical and the scientific sectors. Following an introduction of the relevant epidemiological, economic and political background, our analysis evolves along the four interface types, namely resource-transfer, organizational, legal and discoursive. On the basis of the analysis along these four interface types the concluding section unravels the conflict between national and global level actors in the fight against HIV/AIDS in South Africa, allowing us to identify the factors and actors that shape national health governance and GHG in this case.

The HIV/AIDS challenge in South Africa

South Africa is among the countries most heavily affected by the worldwide HIV/AIDS pandemic. The first South African case of AIDS was detected in 1982, but prevalence rates remained very low until the beginning of the 1990s. Since then, the number of infected South Africans has skyrocketed and it is believed that the prevalence rate has risen above 11 per cent of the total population of approximately 45 million citizens today.[3] It is estimated that 5.54 million South Africans are currently infected with HIV (Department of Health 2006: 16). In present-day South Africa the disease spreads mainly through heterosexual intercourse, but

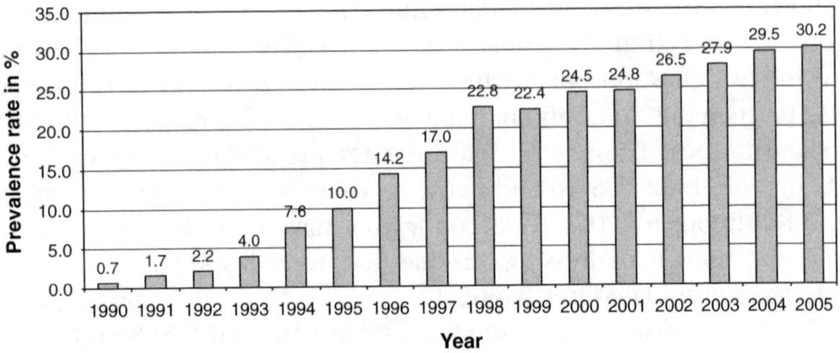

Figure 8.1 HIV-prevalence rate among antenatal clinic attendees
Source: Department of Health (2006: 10).

transmission from mothers to children is also significant.[4] The latest figures published by the National Department of Health indicate that the HIV prevalence rate among antenatal clinic attendees in South Africa stands at 30.2 per cent, meaning that close to every third pregnant woman giving birth in public hospitals is infected with the virus (Department of Health 2006: 10). Figure 8.1 shows the mounting prevalence rate since 1990.

With an estimated prevalence rate of 12.8 per cent, women are more affected, whereas for men the rate stands at 9.8 per cent (Shisana and Simbayi 2002: 45). As HIV is transmitted predominantly through sexual intercourse, the sexually active age groups of the population are most affected. However, there is also a high prevalence rate of 5.6 per cent among children up to the age of 14 years (Doherty and Colvin 2004: 191; Shisana and Simbayi 2002: 47). According to the findings of a Nelson Mandela Foundation/HSRC study, black Africans are most heavily affected. But the study also revealed that prevalence rates among whites, coloureds and Indians are high as well, destroying the myth of a solely 'black disease' (Shisana and Simbayi 2002: 49-50).

The HIV/AIDS pandemic caused a dramatic increase in fatalities among people between 25 and 45 years of age over the last decade (Dorrington et al. 2001; Statistics South Africa 2005a, 2005b; Groenewald and Bradshaw 2005; Groenewald et al. 2005). New studies from the Medical Research Council estimate that in some provinces more than a third of deaths are due to HIV/AIDS (Green and Smillie 2005). Rehle and Shisana (2003: 4) estimated that by 2005 about 2.5 million South Africans would have died of AIDS.

With a Gross National Income per capita of US$3630 (in 2004) South Africa is classified as an upper-middle income economy (World Bank 2005a: 291, 293).[5] The per capita income in purchasing power parity in 2003 amounted to US$10 346 (UNDP 2005: 268). As a country's average income tends to be highly correlated with the expenditure for fighting HIV/AIDS (Gauri and Lieberman 2004: 2–3), it can be expected that the basic relationship of South Africa as middle-income economy to GHG fundamentally differs from those of least developed countries and from industrialized countries of the North. It also suggests that considerable amounts of financial resources are available for fighting the disease. On the other hand, however, South Africa is plagued by a high degree of inequality, assessed through the Gini Index. In 2000, the country had a Gini Index value of 57.8[6] and was one of the most unequal societies in the world (UNDP 2005: 272). Due to the long history of apartheid's racial division in the country, wealth is unequally distributed along ethnic lines. White South Africans have been privileged for a long time and are still the most powerful group in economic terms. In contrast, the large black majority, which constitutes around 80 per cent of the population, predominantly still lives in poverty, notwithstanding the political transition in the early 1990s.

Poverty is widespread; seven out of nine South African provinces have poverty rates well above 50 per cent (UNDP 2003b: 41).[7] Moreover, a large section of the poor has no access to social services, like education or health care. Especially problematic is the circular relationship between poverty and deprivation on the one hand and the HIV/AIDS pandemic on the other. While HIV/AIDS is worsening the situation of the poor, poverty at the same time fuels the pandemic (Cohen 2000; Barnett and Whiteside 2002b). South Africa's high poverty levels therefore contribute to the spread of the disease.

As a result of the severe socio-economic disparities, financing health care has been a major task for the new ANC government following the democratic transition in 1994. From a narrow historical perspective, it has expanded its health budget, mainly attributable to its response to HIV/AIDS. However, per capita spending levels have not matched the funds from the mid-1990s. In the late 1990s, budgets shrunk, partly due to the shift in macroeconomic concepts away from more redistributive and expansive approaches (Blecher and Thomas 2004: 274–8; Quinlan and Willan 2004: 230; Johnson 2004: 111).

South Africa's health care system is divided into a public health care system and private health services. About 15 per cent of the total population in 2004 was covered by private health insurances. In turn, nearly 40 million people depend on the public health care system, that is the state (Health-e 2005; Blecher and Thomas 2004: 276; Hickey et al. 2004: 111). Therefore, the public, state-funded health system in South Africa plays a vital role in the health care sector in general and the treatment of HIV/AIDS in particular. The share of total health care expenditures of the government budget has remained fairly stable at about 11.5 per cent over the last few years. Yet it falls short of the 15 per cent spending target set by the Organization of African Unity in 2001 (Hickey et al. 2004: 136).

In 1994, following negotiations between the old apartheid regime and the liberation movement, South Africa emerged as a liberal democracy with a progressive and widely admired Constitution. The African National Congress (ANC) instantly emerged as South Africa's main political force, with its historical mandate to safeguard equal human rights and the improvement of living conditions of formerly discriminated black, coloured and Indian South Africans. The liberation movement turned government party perceives the fight against HIV/AIDS as part of its 'historical mandate' to improve the lives of the formerly disadvantaged population groups.

Despite this basic point of departure, a protracted dispute between the ANC government and national and global actors developed over the question of antiretroviral treatment of HIV/AIDS. The start of the South African treatment controversy dates back to October 1998, when the then Minister of Health, Dlamini-Zuma, decided to bar the implementation of several prevention of mother-to-child transmission pilot projects in different provinces (Cape Argus 1998; Paton 1998; Treatment Action Campaign 2001b). The controversy lasted for almost four years, was characterized by sharp rifts between different actors and only came to a temporary end with the April 2002 cabinet announcement to formally institutionalize at least two forms of treatment as a part of the national HIV/AIDS strategy.

The HIV/AIDS policy was one of the first areas in which the ANC government was challenged. Accordingly, the various arguments against the provision of ARVs in public hospitals (see brief analysis below) indicate that the treatment controversy had developed into a question that went beyond health politics, particularly in respect to the interaction with global actors. The government's approach can be understood as a series of attempts to preserve 'its' prerogative to formulate and implement national policies. In consequence, as this chapter will show, the former liberation movement reacted very sensitively and was resistant to influence from the global level.

Before we focus on the treatment controversy itself, we need to put the issue of treatment in context. While in the late 1990s the provision of treatment was a common feature of public health policies in industrialized countries, it was rarely a strategy pursued in developing countries (Reynolds et al. 2003: 1807; Heywood 2004).[8] With regard to Highly Active Antiretroviral Treatment (HAART),[9] introduced in 1996, high prices (about US$10 000 per patient per year in the United States) hindered the adoption of this form of therapy by low and middle-income countries. Additionally, international agreements such as the Trade Related Aspects of Intellectual Property Rights (TRIPS) made it difficult for developing countries to produce and get access to cheaper generic drugs (Weissman 2001; Kühl 2002; Lanoszka 2003) (see Chapter 2). Therefore, the general introduction of HAART for HIV-infected people only became an issue in the final stages of the treatment controversy in South Africa.

The situation was different with regard to the prevention of mother-to-child transmission (PMTCT). This form of treatment is a short-term intervention and thus much cheaper and easier to administer than life-long treatment, as is the case for HAART. In 1994, a trial in the United States (PACTG 076) indicated the effectiveness of an azidothymidine (AZT) regimen to reduce the risk of transmission when given to pregnant mothers and their newborns. Since vertical transmission from mother to newborn is a common route of infection in South Africa on the one hand, and medicine-based interventions were relatively cheap and easy to administer on the other, the morally loaded issue of PMTCT became an early point of contention in the controversy.

In October 1998, the Minister of Health, Dlamini-Zuma, announced the withdrawal of state funding from five pilot projects intended to introduce antiretroviral drugs to reduce the risk of mother-to-child transmission. She cited financial reasons for this decision (Cape Argus 1998; Paton 1998). Due to proclaimed low funding abilities, the government decided to concentrate instead on awareness campaigns and prevention efforts. HIV/AIDS activists involved in the planning process of the pilot projects as well as the media strongly criticized this decision (Treatment Action Campaign 2001b). In December 1998, as a direct reaction to the government's stance on this issue, the Treatment Action Campaign (TAC) was founded. After the elections in 1999, Thabo Mbeki became the new President of South Africa and Manto Tshabalala-Msimang was appointed the Minister of Health. However, the hopes of activists and people living with HIV/AIDS were dashed when in October 1999 President Mbeki told the provincial chamber of Parliament that the antiretroviral drug AZT was toxic and that several lawsuits were filed against its manufacturer (Mbeki 1999).

At that time, PMTCT came under attack by the government, which was trying to show that the medication limiting the risk of MTCT – drugs like AZT and later nevirapine – were neither safe nor affordable. In late 1999, the controversy changed course significantly, moving away from PMTCT to the causes of AIDS itself (Weinel 2005a; Mbali 2002a, 2002b; Heywood 2004). President Mbeki began questioning the mainstream scientific research on HIV/AIDS, claiming that the causes of AIDS were not known definitely.[10] In April 2000, in a letter to other political leaders, among them US President Clinton, he argued as follows:

> I am convinced that our urgent task is to respond to the specific threat that faces us as Africans. We will not eschew this obligation in favour of the comfort of the recitation of a catechism that may very well be a correct response to the specific manifestation of AIDS in the West. We will not, ourselves, condemn our own people to death by giving up the search for specific and targeted responses to the specifically African incidence of HIV-AIDS. (Mbeki 2000).

As a result, the South African President not only refused to provide antiretroviral treatment in public hospitals but challenged the complete orthodox HIV/AIDS aetiology. This brought the government into stark opposition with a majority of national and global actors. It was only after a 2002 Constitutional Court decision (see section on legal interfaces below) that the cabinet announced on 17 April 2002 that the drug nevirapine would be provided to all HIV-positive pregnant women attending state hospitals. The final step for the ARV rollout was the launch of the 'Operational Plan for Comprehensive HIV/AIDS Care, Management and Treatment for South Africa' in November 2003 (Department of Health 2003). Even after this rollout decision, the Minister of Health's remarks with regard to treatment have provoked widespread critique. According to media reports, the Minister of Health does not distance herself from actors such as the Rath Foundation, which claims that ARVs are toxic (Mail & Guardian 2005c; Sunday Independent 2005). At the August 2006 International AIDS Conference in Toronto she repeatedly promoted 'traditional medicine' as a remedy for HIV infections (Business Day 2006a; Mail & Guardian Online 2006).[11]

The main topic to be tackled in the following analysis considers the way in which actors on the global level and those on the national level have interacted during this protracted dispute. The analysis will reveal opportunities for and limits to the influence from the global level on national health politics. We will proceed along the above four interface types.

Resource-transfer interfaces: a high degree of state autonomy

Evidence suggests that the South African government's fight against HIV/AIDS has hardly ever been directly influenced by financial contributions from the global level – that is, resource-transfer interfaces. According to Schneider and Gilson (1999: 266) total international aid to the health sector amounted to just over 1 per cent of the annual government health budget in the period from 1994 to 1999. As a middle-income economy that is not severely indebted,[12] South Africa has not been reliant on *conditional* donor aid. Neither the apartheid government nor, since the democratic transformation in 1994, the ANC government has extensively drawn on external resources for financing public health policies.[13]

This does not mean, however, that donor funds are irrelevant for the fight against HIV/AIDS in South Africa. From 2000 to 2002, the last period for which official figures are available, donor aid contributed to around 40 per cent of total funds earmarked for the fight against HIV and AIDS (Ndlovu 2005: 6, based on OECD/UNAIDS 2004).[14] However, in light of its comparatively favourable financial position, the ANC government has consistently declined offers of financial or technical aid, 'particularly from the World Bank' (Gauri and Lieberman 2004: 28), which it found incompatible with its own policy, notably with respect to the controversial question of HIV/AIDS treatment.

In 2002 this became evident when the ANC government blocked the disbursement of US$72 million that had been awarded to the Enhancing Care Initiative (ECI) from the KwaZulu/Natal province by the Global Fund to Fight AIDS, Tuberculosis and Malaria (GF) created that same year (see Chapter 6). ECI's HIV/AIDS programme included, inter alia, antiretroviral schemes to reduce the risk of MTCT of the virus and to provide antiretroviral treatment to infected persons (Pawinski and Lalloo 2002). Despite the fact that the South African National AIDS Council (SANAC) had not been functioning at that time, the Minister of Health argued that it was the national government's prerogative, and not that of ECI, to apply to the Global Fund (Weinel 2005b: 45). Only in March 2004, following the government's decision to roll out ARVs through the public health system, were the approved funds transferred to ECI through the national government.

In 2004 additional inflows of foreign aid were finally accepted, with the US President's Emergency Fund for AIDS Relief (PEPFAR) providing US$89.4 million for the year and US$132.1 million in 2005 for treatment, prevention, care of orphans and palliative care (United States Global AIDS Coordinator 2005: 115).[15] As stated by the US embassy in South Africa, 60 per cent of the funds were allocated to the South African government and 40 per cent to CSOs working in the field of HIV/AIDS (United States 2006). However, the influence on South Africa's HIV/AIDS policy is deemed to be low as the ANC government channels PEPFAR funds according to its strategies already in place. The funds cover sections of government programmes (respondent interview). Generally, the cooperation between government and international donors has been guided by two principles:

- 'Maximum integration of donor funds into the budget, so that unnecessary recurrent costs would not be generated through capital projects';
- 'Respect for the policy, equipment and technology choices made by the South African government' (Schneider and Gilson 1999: 266–7).

A high-level representative of the Medical Research Council (MRC) argued that one of South Africa's priorities has been to retain financial independence. An ARV programme that was partly or to a large extent funded by a foreign institution such as the World Bank, as was the case in Brazil (see Chapter 7), thus appeared to be a non-viable option for South African policy-makers.

In contrast, a lot of South African civil society actors have been partly or almost entirely funded by external actors such as aid agencies, IGOs or private foundations. Recipients have been, among others, the TAC, the Health Systems Trust (HST), the AIDS Foundation, and the Institute for Democracy in South Africa (IDASA). Most prominent has been the TAC, which, since its foundation in December 1998, has quickly emerged as the most vocal civil society actor in the sphere of South Africa's HIV/AIDS policy.[16] Almost all of the organization's R23.5 million budget for the fiscal year ending in February 2005 came from foreign donors. Sources, among others, were Bread for the World, the Open Society Foundation, the Swedish International Development Agency, Oxfam, and the Ford Foundation. Only one, the AIDS Foundation of South Africa, is based in the country (Treatment Action Campaign 2005).[17]

Less obvious are the resource-transfers from international multilateral organizations. Despite the fact that the TAC lists the Joint United Nations Programme on HIV/AIDS (UNAIDS) as one of its donors, it remains unclear how much resources UNAIDS indeed provides to TAC and for what activities (Mbali 2005: 38). Although respondents from the

TAC as well as from international organizations testified to regular interaction, the status of UNAIDS, the World Health Organization (WHO) and the GF as multilateral organizations prevented them from openly criticizing the South African government and aligning themselves with TAC or other civil society actors.[18] The picture looks different when regarding the faith-based organizations (FBOs), which are important for running prevention programmes and providing care as well as support to HIV-positive patients 'on the ground'.[19] The most important funding sources for these predominantly community-based initiatives are donations (62 per cent) and government funds (30 per cent). Foreign donors contribute only 15 per cent to the FBOs' budgets (Birdsall 2005: 15). Thus, resource-transfer interfaces have been an important means of interaction between national civil society and the global level actors; yet there are varying degrees of importance among all actor types involved.

Resource-transfer interfaces on the national level have significantly increased the national government's influence on the HIV/AIDS policy. Under the quasi-federal structure of South Africa's polity, the main distributors of government funds are South Africa's nine provinces. However, they receive about 98 per cent of their budgets from the national level (Hickey et al. 2004: 117). Government funds for health services are channelled mainly through the so-called Social Development Sector, comprising the Departments of Health, Education and Social Development. The Department of Health receives by far the largest share of about 80 per cent of the total public health care spending (Blecher and Thomas 2004: 272), although the funding levels do not seem to increase at the same speed as other departments (Quinlan and Willan 2004: 233–4).

The analysis of resource-transfers on the national level shows two things. First, the national government largely determines the expenditure of all government levels (national, provincial and local) in the South African fight against HIV/AIDS. Second, the important financing instrument of 'conditional grants' enables the government to earmark funds for special purposes, e.g. the prevention and not the treatment of HIV/AIDS. The national government therefore has been able – at least in the case of poor provinces – to financially push through its disregard for treatment schemes. This effectively hampered opposition from the state level and augmented the dominance of the national government.

On balance, the effects of direct resource-transfers on South Africa's HIV/AIDS programme have been low. The primary reason is the ANC government's resilience in preserving its national sovereignty. The country's status as a middle-income economy with insignificant external debt allowed the government to refuse external aid. However, there has been intense interaction through resource-transfer interfaces between South Africa's CSOs and the global level actors.

Organizational interfaces: crucial differences between government and civil society

As regards the question of HIV/AIDS, the South African government has rarely entered into organizational interfaces, indicating a high degree of conflict with global level actors. Various respondents interviewed for this study maintained that IGOs running local offices in South Africa have been sidelined by the government in the field of HIV/AIDS policy. Accordingly, UN organizations, perceived as organizational interfaces, have exerted negligible influence in the South African context.

One important organizational interface between the global and the national level has been LoveLife, an organization working in the field of HIV/AIDS prevention. The public–private partnership is co-financed by the US-based Kaiser Family Foundation and other donors as well as the South African government, which provides 34 per cent of its overall budget. Furthermore, LoveLife received substantial resources from the Global Fund.[20] The organization's annual budget for 2005 stood at around R200 million (roughly US$31 million) (Mail & Guardian 2005b; information given by a respondent interviewed for this study). Running South Africa's biggest HIV/AIDS prevention programme for teenagers, it designs accessible and youth-friendly clinics, runs advertising campaigns, and it sponsors various events. LoveLife enjoys a cordial and collaborative relationship with the government and even has the Minister of Health on its Advisory Board. Due to LoveLife's close connection to the government and the fact that it deals with HIV/AIDS prevention only, its impact on treatment policy has been insignificant. In short, it acts as a 'government service-provider' (Mbali 2005: 18).

Furthermore, there is some evidence that experts from the William J. Clinton Foundation were involved in the Joint Health and Treasury Task Team (JHTTT), which was set up to investigate the feasibility and the costs of universal access to treatment of HIV/AIDS in South Africa in 2002 (Ijumba et al. 2004: 333). The US foundation was thus linked to the national level through an organizational interface. However, the Clinton Foundation experts' reach in terms of technical support and the practical influence on the 'Operational Plan for Comprehensive HIV/AIDS Care, Management and Treatment for South Africa' (Government Communication and Information Service 2003) remain unclear. Although the Clinton Foundation was – on the global level – very influential in reducing prices for antiretroviral drugs, their experts were later denied further access to South African institutions, with the government ceasing any further cooperation with the foundation (respondent interview).

A prominent organizational interface which global actors required for accessing their funds is the South African National AIDS Council (SANAC). Although the 'Partnership against HIV/AIDS', introduced by the then Deputy President Thabo Mbeki in October 1998, could be interpreted as a move towards a broad-based response to the HIV/AIDS pandemic, SANAC, founded in January 2000, was the first South African institution that embodied the idea of a 'multisectoral response'[21] (Strode and Grant 2004: 14). Shortly after its inception in September 2000, the World Bank's Multi-Country AIDS Programme (MAP) requested countries to formulate a 'coherent national, multisectoral strategy and action plan' and to apply for grants through 'a high-level HIV/AIDS coordinating body – that is a national AIDS commission or council' (Putzel 2004: 1131–2; see also Chapter 5).

South Africa did not participate in MAP, but aimed at applying for Global Fund grants. The government even sent the Deputy Minister of Health as a representative to the organization's Board. Similarly, the Global Fund set a particular organizational structure in recipient countries, namely the Country Coordinating Mechanism (CCM), as an institutional precondition for the disbursement of its funds. As mentioned in the discussion on the Enhancing Care Initiative in KwaZulu/Natal (see section on resource-transfer interfaces above), SANAC, the South African version of the coordinating body, began functioning only in early 2002. An obvious interpretation is that SANAC has, first and foremost, acted as the required CCM in order to access resources from the Global Fund, while it has failed to perform its functions prescribed in the 2000–5 Strategic Plan.[22] Hence, in this case, resource-transfer considerations induced the South African government to form an institution in accordance with a globally prescribed 'organisational template' (Putzel 2004: 1130).

On the whole, the South African government rarely entered into organizations with international actors in the fight against HIV/AIDS. Those examples found were limited to HIV/AIDS *prevention*, with LoveLife being the most prominent example. The brief period of cooperation with the Clinton Foundation strongly confirms the government's stance on preserving its autonomy. In the face of South Africa's treatment controversy, the government has not been willing to accept external influence through organizational interfaces.

It is difficult to establish precise numbers, but it is estimated that in present-day South Africa, approximately 800 CSOs operate that deal with health, which is about 7 per cent of all CSOs (CASE 2004: 5). It can be presumed that most health CSOs have also been engaged in HIV/AIDS as it is the predominant issue in this area.[23] One of the strongest and best organized CSOs is the AIDS Consortium (AC). The AC was founded by Supreme Court judge Edwin Cameron and other HIV specialists as well as academics at the University of the Witwatersrand's Centre for Applied Legal Studies in 1992. The network comprises over 1000 organizations as well as individuals (Aids Consortium 2004: 7). According to its Executive Director, its main objective is to 'build the capacity of its affiliate organisations' (quoted in Aids Bulletin 2005). For instance, it runs a training programme which aims to improve the organizational strength of community-based organizations focused on HIV/AIDS interventions. The AC has forged partnerships with other CSOs, thus serving as an organizational interface between various South African civil society organizations in the field of HIV/AIDS. In 2004, for example, together with the TAC, it organized the People's Health Summit in Durban (Aids Consortium 2004: 9).

The TAC, founded in December 1998, has quickly become the most influential champion of antiretroviral treatment. One crucial organization-specific characteristic explaining its success is the strategic formation of alliances, i.e. the use of organizational interfaces, with a number of different national and international actors. Alliances with GHG actors, such as Médecins Sans Frontières (MSF), the AIDS Coalition to Unleash Power (ACT-UP) and the Consumer Project on Technology (CPTech) proved to be especially important in the struggle over antiretroviral treatment and the supply of cheaper drugs, as will be demonstrated in the section on discoursive interfaces below. According to Friedman and Mottiar (2004: 31), TAC 'thinks alliances'. The organizational interfaces forged reach out to such different actors as the Congress of South African Trade Unions (COSATU) and the less significant South African Communist Party (SACP), as well as scientists and medical professionals. In contrast to the government level, organizational interfaces have thus been strong routes of interaction for South African civil society actors at the global and national level.

Legal interfaces: court cases with repercussions for the global level

South Africa suddenly found itself in the international limelight when the Pharmaceutical Manufacturers Association of South Africa (PMA), backed by the Pharmaceutical Research and Manufacturers of America

(PhRMA), sued the government before South Africa's High Court for violating their property rights in February 1998. The lawsuit, which was based on the legal provisions of the TRIPS agreement, was supported by the United States government, which threatened to impose trade restrictions on South Africa (Lanoszka 2003: 191–2). It challenged the Medicines and Related Substances Control Amendment Act, signed by President Mandela in December 1997 (Kühl 2002: 76). This Act gave the Minister of Health the power to allow both compulsory licensing[24] and parallel importation[25] of patented medicines, in this case antiretroviral drugs. The transnational pharmaceutical companies (TNPCs) wanted these legal provisions to be changed and thus tried to influence policy-making through legal interfaces. Responding to widespread national and international public pressure, i.e. criticism expressed via discoursive interfaces, and with only slim chances to win the case, the thirty-nine TNPCs represented by the PMA withdrew from the case in late 1998 (Weissman 2001).

However, in January 2001 they reinstated the lawsuit. Their chances of winning at this stage were higher because South Africa was now obliged to fully comply with the requirements of the TRIPS agreement (Kühl 2002: 76). Yet neither compulsory licensing nor parallel importation is ruled out explicitly by the TRIPS agreement (Gauri and Lieberman 2004: 26).[26] In fact, both compulsory licensing and parallel importation have regularly been used by industrialized countries such as Japan, Canada and even the United States in connection with the anthrax assaults in 2001 (Weissman 2001; Lanoszka 2003: 190, 193). Therefore, the strategy of the plaintiffs was directed against the allegedly arbitrary power of the Minister of Health. The TNPCs maintained that the case was not directed against South Africa's efforts to seek price reductions for antiretroviral medicine (Kühl 2002: 76–7), which however, was exactly the impression that HIV/AIDS activists and CSOs in South Africa and around the world tried to create. Internationally recognized CSOs like MSF, Oxfam, CPTech and ACT-UP pressured the TNPCs to withdraw the case. Even the Bush administration no longer openly supported the industry (Weissman 2001).

The hearing before the High Court in Pretoria began in March 2001. From the outset, the judge expressed doubts as to whether the court was the appropriate place to debate the allegations, as the Minister of Health had never used its powers before and the government had promised not to use it in the future (Kühl 2002: 77). Again, the pharmaceutical companies faced pressure from HIV/AIDS activists and the public around the world. Demonstrations were organized in South Africa, but also in front of several TNPC headquarters in Europe and North America. Interestingly, the government, HIV/AIDS activists, scientists, and other previously divided stakeholders joined hands to win the court case against the TNPCs, although they followed different agendas.[27] The TAC was also allowed to join the court case as an *amicus curiae* ('friend of court') of the South African government in support of its stance.

Thereupon the pharmaceutical industry applied for a delay of the case for four months, which was rejected by the judge (Kühl 2002: 77). Fearing another public relations nightmare, it finally withdrew the lawsuit in mid-April 2001 (Lanoszka 2003: 192) and agreed to 'a settlement almost on the government of South Africa's terms. The only concession made by the government was to comply with decisions made by the World Trade Organization on TRIPS' (Kühl 2002: 78). Therefore, the Medicines and Related Substances Control Amendment Act from 1997 remained largely unchanged. In conjunction with strong public pressure from discoursive interfaces, the legal challenge was averted. However, the government made it clear that it was not in any event willing to use its power derived from its own law and rejected proposals from civil society to declare the HIV/AIDS pandemic a national emergency.[28] The Doha Declaration explicitly permits countries to issue compulsory licences in cases of national health emergencies (see Chapter 2). On balance, the High Court case shows that legal interfaces have been important routes for interaction between South African and global level actors. It strengthened the South African government's case for blaming TNPCs and augmented the international pressure to reduce the prices for antiretroviral drugs.

However, on the national level, the civil society actor TAC in 2001 began to challenge government policy on HIV/AIDS treatment through the courts, i.e. legal interfaces. In June, the Medicines Control Council (MCC) had registered nevirapine, a drug manufactured by the German company Böhringer Ingelheim and distributed under the name Viramune, for use in preventing mother-to-child transmission of HIV. Following the Department of Health's decision to limit the rollout of nevirapine to a maximum of two 'pilot sites' per province, TAC and two other CSOs filed a constitutional claim against the government before the High Court. The goal was to force the government to make the medication available in all state hospitals (Mbali 2005: 41; Butler 2005a: 13). In March 2002, the High Court ruled in favour of TAC and requested the government to roll out a drug-based MTCT prevention programme (Heywood 2003: 300–1).

The government's reaction was two-fold. First, as ordered by the court, the cabinet announced on 17 April 2002 that the Minister of Health should formulate a 'Universal Roll-Out Plan'. However, according to Nattrass (2004: 55), its 'only function was the delay of the actual roll-out'. Second, it challenged the judgement at the Constitutional Court. The Constitutional Court rejected this complaint in July 2002, stating that the refusal to generally roll out nevirapine for PMTCT was 'unreasonable' and that government was failing to meet its constitutional obligations to provide access to health care. Furthermore, the government's claims about the toxicity of ARVs were found not to be based on concrete evidence (Constitutional Court 2002; Heywood 2003: 311; Butler 2005a: 13).

Generally, using legal interfaces through court orders is one of the most adversarial and forceful forms of interacting with government (and other actors). Scholars widely recognized that litigation was crucial in forcing South Africa's government to roll out nevirapine for PMTCT (Mbali 2005; Heywood 2003; Butler 2005a; Berger 2002). On the one hand, the South African government was thus successfully challenged by civil society actors with strong ties to the global level, but on the other hand it was also able – in conjunction with civil society actors – to pressurize the TNPCs through legal interfaces, whose effect was amplified by discoursive interfaces.

Discoursive interfaces: the potentially ephemeral becomes powerful

Discoursive interfaces have been characterized by publicly visible rifts between the South African government and global as well as national civil society actors. Global actors operating in the country have been increasingly successful in shaping discourses on HIV/AIDS and on antiretroviral treatment in particular. Contradicting government positions, they were able to demonstrate that antiretroviral treatment of HIV/AIDS is an effective and feasible option for the country.

One of the most prominent antiretroviral projects emerged in the Western Cape province, which until 2004 was not governed by the ANC. In January 1999, Médecins Sans Frontières[29] – with the support and collaboration of the provincial government – started a programme to reduce the risk of MTCT in Khayelitsha, a large township on the outskirts of Cape Town (Médecins Sans Frontières 2003: 14). This was three months after the Minister of Health and most of her provincial counterparts pulled out of financing test sites for PMTCT and ten months before President Mbeki advised his Minister of Health to investigate the presumed toxicity of the antiretroviral drug AZT. MSF used existing public provincial health infrastructure to offer free services, including voluntary counselling and testing, to residents. In May 2001, the organization established the first public sector service in South Africa to provide antiretroviral therapy (ART) to people living with HIV/AIDS, well ahead of the publication of the national Operational Plan in November 2003. Although the national government disapproved of this project, the political constellation in the Western Cape province permitted the engagement and the resource-transfers of MSF.

The project seems not to have directly spurred the national government into providing universal access to ART or PMTCT, but it set a publicly visible example that antiretrovirals can be successfully administered even in the resource-poor setting of a township. This is reflected in a report published in 2003 by the TAC – a close ally of MSF:

> The Western Cape is strategically important to TAC because it is here that the potential for good examples on treatment are most likely to be set for the rest of the country at a primary health-care level. (Treatment Action Campaign 2003: 3)

The project showed that the use of antiretrovirals is cost-effective, that high adherence to the prescribed doses of HAART is possible, that drug-based strategies of PMTCT are working and that adverse side-effects of various forms of treatment can be controlled by changes in the regimen. Activists pressuring government for the provision of ART were thus able to point to the example set by MSF and its provincial government partners in Khayelitsha. The Khayelitsha project also played a role in the court case between TAC and the national government. Both Hermann Reuter, a medical doctor, and Robin Wood, a scientist from the University of Cape Town, indicated in their affidavits that the experience from Khayelitsha would suggest that a scaling up of PMTCT in South Africa's state hospitals is possible (Reuter 2001; Wood 2001).

The media have also used the Khayelitsha project to push the government on the provision of drugs in order to lower the risk of MTCT, with headlines like 'It's So Easy to Save our AIDS Babies' (Sunday Times 2000) and 'Ray of Light for HIV Babies' (Sunday Times 1999). Setting a visible example of successfully providing PMTCT and antiretroviral therapy in a resource-limited setting, Khayelitsha was a decisive step towards the provision of nationwide access to various forms of treatment.

Generally, CSOs strongly interact through discoursive interfaces. In its campaign tactics, the TAC learned from the US-based civil society organization ACT-UP (Schneider 2001: 18). In cooperation with its partners, TAC organized the international protests supporting South Africa's government in the court case of the Pharmaceutical Manufacturers Association challenging the Medicines and Related Substances Amendment Act (Gumede 2005: 157; see also above). This strategy substantially augmented efforts on the global level by actors such as MSF and the Clinton Foundation to reduce the prices for antiretroviral therapy. As a result, the costs for HAART have come down substantially. In 2005, a triple ARV drug cocktail cost less than US$200 per patient per year (the costs in South Africa currently stand at about R200 per patient per year) (Campaign for Access to Essential Medicines 2005).[30] International CSOs later also conducted solidarity protests during TAC's civil disobedience campaign against the government, which included demonstrations in front of South African embassies around the world (Mbali 2005: 36). This provides evidence to the exchange of CSO actors from the national and the global level through discoursive interfaces.

TAC was successful in setting the agenda for the South African media and, to a considerable degree, for foreign media in respect to the fight against HIV/AIDS. The organization strongly influenced how the media have reported on the HIV/AIDS crisis and on the treatment issue (Mbali 2005: 48). Over the years of its existence, TAC has played an important role in informing journalists about the science of HIV and antiretrovirals. The organization has regularly issued press statements containing information on medical terms and has referred journalists to scientists who could provide expertise on HIV/AIDS (Schneider 2002: 155, 158). TAC's media strategy therefore took into account that scientific knowledge has to be translated into the media's language. This approach was effective in publicly countering President Mbeki's alignment with scientists denying the orthodox 'HIV causes AIDS' aetiology (Mbali 2005: 48). TAC has on balance effectively acted as a knowledge-broker and an agenda-setter for the media and, in turn, the general public.

Compared to CSOs, scholars have described the locally operating TNCs' reaction towards the HIV/AIDS pandemic as reluctant and weak (Dickinson 2004: 628; Connelly and Rosen 2005: 1925). No coordinated and explicit initiative has emerged to influence the fight against HIV/AIDS. Yet there are strong indications that concern was expressed behind closed doors. The President's International Investment Council, comprising fifteen business leaders from all over the world, is important in this context. Its membership encompasses, among others, the Chairman of the Board of the news agency Reuters and DaimlerChrysler's former CEO. As the name implies, this body serves as adviser to the South African President on all issues of foreign investment into South Africa, an issue the ANC government perceives to be of crucial importance for the future economic development of the country (Office of the President 2004).

According to various respondents from IGOs and businesses interviewed for this study, members of the body warned President Mbeki about the HIV/AIDS treatment controversy's possible detrimental implications for foreign direct investment to South Africa in March 2002 (see also Gumede 2005: 171). The issue of the weekly newsletter *ANC Today*, which was published after the International Investment Council meeting, acknowledged that 'the members of Council had raised serious concerns about some persisting negative perceptions of our country internationally' (ANC 2002). Foreign investors furthermore questioned Trevor Manuel, the Minister of Finance, and Tito Mboweni, the Reserve Bank Governor, about the government's HIV/AIDS policy. As affirmed by Gumede (2005: 171), they in turn 'began dropping cautious hints to the president of looming economic consequences'. This gave a new resource-transfer dimension to the discoursive contest around South Africa's HIV/AIDS policy: it began to affect the country's appeal as a location for foreign business.

The workplace programmes of large, often transnational, companies in South Africa which have provided antiretroviral treatment to their workers and their families, thereby to a certain degree filling the gap left by government policy, have received more public attention. Businesses' commitment to workplace programmes has been contested in the literature. Dickinson (2004: 627, 631), for instance, argues that most companies did not start moving towards the provision of antiretrovirals to their workers until 2002, when the government was already changing its stance on HIV/AIDS treatment. Connelly and Rosen (2005: 1925) estimate that only between 5000 and 30 000 South African workers (and in some cases members of their families) received ART in the beginning of 2005. Without entering into the discussion on whether businesses' reaction has been adequate in terms of the magnitude of the HIV/AIDS problem in South Africa, it can safely be said that the highly publicized workplace programmes of the mining company Anglo-American, the parastatal power utility Eskom, and the (transnational) car manufacturers DaimlerChrysler, BMW and Volkswagen set a relevant precedent of successfully treating HIV/AIDS and in turn influenced South Africa's fight against HIV/AIDS via discoursive interfaces.[31]

In sum, discoursive interfaces have been the strongest route of interaction between the South African and the global level. MSF's Khayelitsha project and (transnational) businesses' workplace programmes set a forceful and publicly visible example of effectively administering anti-retroviral therapy. The concerns raised by TNC leaders point to economic consequences as an influential factor that amplifies discoursive interfaces. Civil society actors such as the TAC successfully influenced the global level and created an international awareness for the HIV/AIDS treatment controversy in South Africa.

Conclusion

The analysis allows us to respond to the two main questions of this chapter, namely which actors, both on the global and national level, have played the most prominent role in influencing the fight against HIV/AIDS, and what have been their means of interaction?

Principally, the South African government, as the dominant political actor on the national level, has fiercely resisted attempts at influence via all four interface types and for a long time restricted direct global influence. Although this analysis and the case study on Brazil (Chapter 7) found that the fight against HIV/AIDS is an area of strong interaction between global and national actors, neither IGOs, private businesses nor international CSOs have been in the position to *directly* challenge the ANC government. Its willingness and ability to thwart attempts at outside intervention on policy formulation characterizes the South African case.

However, even a powerful actor like the ANC government is unable to isolate its policies from external influence. A range of actors have been able to influence government's HIV/AIDS policy *indirectly* and *subtly*. The most important in this respect were the globally connected CSOs. Highly motivated to engage in the fight against the HIV/AIDS pandemic in South Africa, these groups have successfully used legal and discoursive interfaces to challenge not only the South African government, but also TNPCs.

Compared to civil society, the private sector has been reluctant to publicly engage with the government or other actors in South Africa's growing HIV/AIDS pandemic. A possible explanation for this reluctance is that providing ARVs and running prevention programmes for their workers appeared to be less 'costly', at least for large companies, than participating in the public debate. It was only in the final stages of the treatment controversy that national and transnational business exerted some influence through discoursive interfaces. In pointing to possible negative implications for foreign investment, business representatives drew attention to the fact that the controversy might have effects beyond the sphere of health policy. Bilateral and multilateral donor agencies such as the World Bank altogether exerted little direct influence due to the South African government's resistance against direct interaction. Compared to the Brazilian case, the distinct effects of South Africa's national actor constellation on the interaction with the World Bank and other international organizations become particularly striking.

Four general conclusions emanate from our study in terms of the relationship of the global and national levels of GHG. Firstly, it demonstrates that a dominant actor on the national level is able to substantially diminish the scope for national–global interaction. At least in the South African case, the national politics seem to largely determine the relationship to and influence of GHG. Key factors have been the country's relative financial autonomy and the ruling party's dominant role in domestic politics. Secondly, despite the leading role of a national government, influence on its policies is nonetheless possible. Determined non-state actors can fill the gaps left by official policies and influence discourses and perceptions on particular issues, at least in the long term.

Thirdly, the *indirect* influences on government policy revealed that, at least in a contentious relationship, global influences have to be adjusted and translated, i.e. mediated, in order to yield results on the national level. For example, in the case of South Africa, international donors circumvented the national government by providing financial assistance to and interacting with 'alternative actors', such as CSOs. In this way, they exerted indirect influence on South Africa's fight against HIV/AIDS.

Finally, though all four interface types have played some role in South Africa's treatment controversy, legal and discoursive interfaces proved to be especially relevant. While it appears that a dominant actor on the national level can easily block influences through resource and organizational interfaces on the state level, it seems much harder to control influences channelled through discoursive and legal interfaces, at least in contemporary democracies. On the basis of South Africa's Constitution, the government was forced to abide by the rulings of the High Court and the Constitutional Court. On the other hand, the South African government (and civil society actors) used legal interfaces in conjunction with discoursive interfaces to fight for lower prices of ARVs on the global level. Thus, the influence through interfaces was not unidirectional. With respect to discoursive interfaces, the government increasingly lost the moral high ground in the confrontation with CSOs from both the national and global level. The often assumed 'ephemeral' or 'soft' discoursive interfaces were, in fact, powerful.

The South African government's direction in the fight against HIV/AIDS has changed considerably over the past years. Although there are still serious disputes about the rate of implementation and the utterances of the Minister of Health with respect to treatment, the fact that South Africa's public health system is responsible for ensuring the provision of ARVs is now beyond doubt.

Notes

1. See for example the analyses in Marais (2000, 2005); Van der Vliet (2001); Johnson (2004); Nattrass (2004); Willan (2004); and Butler (2005a, 2005b).
2. Fieldwork in South Africa was conducted from 2 to 25 May 2005; the interviewers were Christian von Soest, Martin Weinel, and Gero Erdmann, Senior Research Fellow at the GIGA Institute of African Affairs.
3. There are various sources for these figures, for instance Department of Health (2004); Dorrington et al. (2002, 2004); Shisana and Simbayi (2002); Rehle and Shisana (2003); and UNAIDS (2004). Due to methodological differences, the estimates of the prevalence rate within the whole South African population range from 10.4 per cent to 11.8 per cent (Doherty and Colvin 2004: 196). See Marais (2005: 25–43), for an extensive discussion of the difficulties of statistically capturing the HIV/AIDS epidemic in South Africa.
4. According to estimates for 2002, about 6 per cent of all newborns are infected before or during birth and about 1.8 per cent of all newborns are infected through breast milk (Doherty and Colvin 2004: 206). However, Dorrington et al. (2002: 5) estimate that 3.8 per cent of newly infected newborns acquire the virus via breast milk.
5. In 2004, the World Bank ranked countries with a GNI per capita between US$3256 and US$10 065 as upper-middle income economies (World Bank 2005a: 291).
6. Based on consumption. A value of 0 represents perfect equality, and a value of 100 perfect inequality.
7. Studies were done in 1995 and 2002; a national poverty line was applied. Measuring against the international poverty lines of US$1 and US$2 per day renders these percentages significantly lower.
8. However, the Brazilian government already began rolling out ARVs free of charge in 1996 (see Chapter 7).
9. Since the mid-1990s, combination therapies which combine three antiretroviral drugs, so-called Highly Active Antiretroviral Therapies, have been the state-of-the-art in treatment. Therefore, the term antiretroviral treatment (ART) today refers to combination therapies and not to so-called mono-therapies that use only one kind of antiretroviral medicine.
10. '[R]ecent post-apartheid fights over the science underpinning AIDS policy have been over who has scientific "expertise", who has the right to speak authoritatively on science, what the scientific method is, and what constitutes valid scientific evidence' (Mbali 2002a: 4).
11. According to the Department of Health, however, about 204 000 HIV-infected patients were getting antiretroviral drugs in July 2006, with the tendency rising (figure quoted in: Business Day 2006b).
12. In 1996, shortly after the democratic transition, South Africa's total external debt amounted to US$23.6 billion (World Bank 1998: 249).
13. Due to an international embargo, the opportunities for the apartheid government to draw on external funds had been limited in any event.

14. Donor funds did not include the US President's Emergency Plan for AIDS Relief (PEPFAR) and Global Fund to Fight, Tuberculosis and Malaria commitments.
15. According to the US embassy in South Africa, the funds allocated in the year 2005 amounted to US$148 million (United States 2006).
16. Some commentators even describe the TAC as 'one of South Africa's most effective and active' groups in the whole CSO sector (Mail & Guardian 2003; see also Willan 2004: 114).
17. The full list of donors along with a detailed analysis can be found in Mbali (2005: 22–3).
18. GF's 2002 decision to grant US$72 million to KwaZulu/Natal's HIV/AIDS programme, which also entailed funds for ARV treatment, can be understood as implicit support for an antiretroviral treatment strategy against HIV/AIDS in South Africa (see above and also Weinel 2005b: 45).
19. Of the 1582 entries listed in the South African National AIDS Database (the database collects information on CSOs, business, donor agencies and other institutions operating in the field), 162 identified themselves as FBOs (Birdsall 2005: 5).
20. It thus also acts as an example for the resource-transfer interface. In 2005, the Global Fund abruptly ceased financial support of the prevention programme LoveLife, citing its missing performance indicators as the prime reason (Mail & Guardian 2005d). For more details on the Global Fund and the LoveLife grant see Chapter 6.
21. A 'multisectoral' approach in fighting HIV/AIDS entails the involvement of all branches of government and cooperation with non-governmental actors (World Bank 1999: 22–3; Putzel 2004: 1134–5).
22. The regulative basis of SANAC is laid down in the Strategic AIDS Plan 2000–5 (Department of Health 2000: 12–14), which was developed during the second half of 1999.
23. For further details see also Russell and Swilling's study: 'The Size and Scope of the Non-Profit Sector in South Africa' (2002). It is important to note that the estimates of active CSOs in the health and/or HIV/AIDS sector differ considerably.
24. Compulsory licensing is generally defined as 'the granting of a license to a third-party by a government to use a patent without the permission of the patent holder' (Kühl 2002: 17).
25. Parallel importation refers to 'the imports of goods purchased in a foreign market by an independent third party and later resold in the domestic market where much lower prices compete with the prices charged by authorized distributors' (Kühl 2002: 18).
26. For an extensive analysis of TRIPS see Chapter 2.
27. It seems that the government was mostly interested in demonstrating its sovereignty, whereas HIV/AIDS activists hoped for parallel importation and compulsory licensing of antiretroviral drugs. The pharmaceutical manufacturers mostly feared the introduction of generic substitution.
28. In fact, the obvious contradiction between the South African government claiming that antiretrovirals are too expensive and not using its legal provisions to lower the prices remains puzzling. One common explanation given from respondents in South Africa has been that the ANC government does not perceive the HIV/AIDS epidemic to be a national emergency. One MP from the ruling party and member of SANAC maintained that 'we are not running in a crisis mode'.

29. The organization's headquarters is based in Geneva, Switzerland. It has national chapters in nearly every OECD country (see Chapter 4).
30. The costs for HAART in the mid-1990s had amounted to US$10 000 per patient per year.
31. For case studies on workplace programmes in two large South African companies see Stevens (2004). On workplace programmes in South Africa see also Marais (2000: 30) and Butler (2005b: 11). Further empirical sources have come from the interviews conducted during field research in May 2005.

9
Conclusion: Global Health Governance and the Fight Against HIV/AIDS in a Post-Westphalian World

Wolfgang Hein, Sonja Bartsch, Lars Kohlmorgen and Jan Peter Wogart

The post-Westphalian global polity and the development of global health governance

In modern times, the fight against infectious diseases has always depended on international cooperation, requiring nations to coordinate their health and trade strategies with each other. As we have shown in the previous chapters, however, the need to create a global response has never been stronger than in the case of the HIV/AIDS epidemic, which seems in turn to have heightened global awareness in the cases of more recent epidemic threats like those of SARS and Avian Flu. After neo-liberalism and the early structural adjustment programmes had given primary attention to macroeconomic policies, the need to improve health conditions in poor countries as a *precondition* for economic growth (CMH 2001), fighting poverty and improving security[1] again became a central part of the global political agenda during the 1990s. This new priority for health, that included the recognition of large inequalities in global health as a threat for rich countries, became one important dimension in framing the public perception of the fight against HIV/AIDS and strengthening the role of global civil society in conflicts around access to medicines.

The new challenges to global health as a result of globalization are the starting point of the academic study of global health governance. The evolving architecture in health, however, must not only identify technical and political responses to those challenges, but it has to do so in a rapidly changing global environment. This change has been characterized by various authors as a transitional process from a Westphalian to a post-Westphalian structure of international relations (Bull 1995; Keene 2002; related to GHG: Fidler 2004, 2005). The rising importance of transnational interactions compared to relations between nation-states leads to a very complex pattern of global health governance, which makes it difficult if not impossible for international governmental organizations (IGOs) to maintain their dominance in this policy field.

This points to two decisive characteristics of global health governance: (1) we can observe manifold interactions between various fields of global governance, particularly between the world economic and world social order, which are an indication of evolving global social relations, and (2) we find a rapidly increasing number of new non-state actors – both from the for-profit and the non-profit sector – in the global health arena, which implies an increasing importance of private and hybrid governance modes, and a prominent role of advocating civil society organizations as well as new mechanisms of finance and research.

The general debates on global governance have shown that – due to the absence of a global state authority – agreements linking different policy fields and securing universal compliance (for example, to integrate social and environmental standards in WTO agreements) are difficult to reach. Hence there is a need for compromise. This strengthens actors that are active in various political fields. In our case of the global fight against HIV/AIDS and access to medicines, this concerns actors that have an impact in both the public health realm and the field of trade and IPRs. It furthermore presupposes managing a discourse between both fields which allows the development of new frameworks of understanding. In the previous chapters, we have demonstrated that discoursive interfaces are a major element of global health governance. Thomas Risse explains the corresponding role of the 'logic of arguing'[2] in the understandings of international institutions in a comprehensive way:

> First, arguing and persuasion provide micromechanisms for socialization and social learning, irrespective of whether this learning is about acquiring new social knowledge and skills or about getting socialized in the validity of an international norm. Second, an emphasis on arguing sheds light on processes of norm change. Third, a focus on deliberative processes improves our understanding of institutional effects. Institutions serve as discourse arenas enabling deliberative processes geared toward problem solving. They do so by establishing relationships of trust among actors which are deemed crucial for processes of communicative persuasion and consensus seeking. (Risse 2002: 606f.)

The development of a new understanding for the changing problems of global health, and of social learning in this area, has been facilitated by the discursive role of global civil society and the development of hybrid forms of regulation. This implied the development of new links and interfaces between an increasing variety of actors, who continuously have to clarify relations among each other in order to deal with emerging health problems.

Stressing the role of discourse certainly does not imply that the traditional forms of power (legal, decision-making, resource-based) have lost their importance. Actors of global health governance do have a large spectrum of different – sometimes complementary, but often also competing – interests and they dispose of various types of power which enable them to influence agenda-setting and policy-making processes to varying degrees. Struggles between actors focusing on strengthening 'global market creation' and those aiming at promoting 'global welfare' were at the centre of the preceding chapters. The conflicts related to access to medicines and treatment of HIV/AIDS are exemplary in this context: an international market-creating agreement which had been propelled by the self-interest of industrialized countries and transnational corporations (WTO/TRIPS) is found to contradict collective interests (access to treatment) in a welfare-related policy field such as health.

The concept of 'interfaces' facilitated an analysis of the relations among this multitude of different actors and helped us determine what constitutes the binding forces among them in producing global health governance – in terms of cooperation as well as conflict. Applying Norman Long's definition of social interface (1989: 1–2; see Chapter 2) to politics, helped us to identify critical points of interaction among different social and political systems, levels of governance, and governing institutions where structural discontinuities, based upon different normative values and interests, were likely to be found. We developed a refined concept of interfaces for the analysis of GHG, distinguishing between structural discontinuities in vertical interaction processes (for example, between global and national politics) and those in horizontal interactions between various types of actors (international governmental organizations, civil society organizations (CSOs), private enterprises as well as hybrid actors such as public–private partnerships). Since interfaces constitute linkages that bridge structural discontinuities, we identified legal, organizational, resource-based and discursive interfaces related to the most important means of exerting power in the various forms of interactions.

In the different pieces of analysis that focused on the major actors and their interfaces, a somewhat clearer picture evolved concerning their lines of communication, confrontation, compromises and new attempts to influence GHG. Our research project focused to a large extent on the conflicts around access to medicines and treatment of HIV/AIDS. Certainly, global health and the poverty-oriented fight against diseases comprise a much larger political field than just access to medicines, but our perspective allowed us to focus on the analysis of interfaces among a large number of actors shaping a crucial development of GHG.

The perceived scandal that ARVs have allowed patients in industrialized countries to lead a close to normal life while people living with HIV/AIDS in developing countries continue to die because, for them, ARVs are not affordable, has increasingly focused attention on structural conflicts between the world trade order and global health, involving the WTO and transnational pharmaceutical corporations (TNPCs) on the one hand, and civil society organizations and – more reluctantly – the WHO and other public actors on the other. This constellation has led us to focus first on the WTO and, in particular, the TRIPS agreement, and to analyse its horizontal interfaces with other actors of GHG. Chapter 2 also gave an overview of the various conflicts between actors primarily supporting global market creation (and defending the internationalization of IPRs in this context) and those actors which opposed them to strengthen global and national social policies, in our context in particular in the field of health. Actors and conflicts, analysed in more detail in the following chapters of the book, were introduced.

We began the analysis of specific actors in GHG by examining the crucial roles that TNPCs and CSOs have played in designing and modifying TRIPS, as well as their direct involvement with individual nation-states, both in conflicts and cooperation (Chapters 3 and 4). The studies investigating the traditional and newly emerged international organizations concerned with health (Chapters 5 and 6) have focused first and foremost on the horizontal interfaces with regard to this conflict and related problems of access to treatment, for example between the WHO, UNAIDS, the World Bank, and the Global Fund. The transformation to a post-Westphalian structure of global politics implied changing forms of interaction between those institutions and developed as well as developing countries. We analysed those vertical interfaces by means of two case studies on Brazil and South Africa (Chapters 7 and 8), which show strong reactions and interactions with actors on the global scene and multiple horizontal interfaces between civil society and government. Both countries can be seen as paradigmatic cases concerning conflicts with the pharmaceutical industry and also concerning different approaches towards national strategies to deal with the HIV/AIDS crisis.

In the following paragraphs, we will briefly summarize the findings of each chapter before we return to the main hypothesis of our research (as formulated in Chapter 1) and further conceptualize the role of interfaces in global health governance.

Characteristics of the selected fields of GHG

The world trade order has had a significant impact on health politics on all levels. Related to privately produced inputs in health care, conflicts with the public goods character of these products indicated the need for public control. In this context, due to globalization and the institutionalization of a strong system of international trade rules, new kinds of conflicts became apparent with regard to access to medicines, particularly in the fight against HIV/AIDS. This caused irritation, as the private/public and the national/global interfaces have become increasingly intertwined.

The WTO constitutes the central institution for market-creation on the global scale and has thus far developed an extended corpus of international law regulating the development of world trade. WTO agreements constitute intergovernmental agreements, clarifying conflicting interpretations by joint decisions in the related councils (GATT, GATS, TRIPS Council). The WTO's objective is to regulate and facilitate world trade. It is not a welfare-oriented (or multipurpose) organization. Nevertheless, free trade has always been promoted with the promise that it will create a win-win situation for all participants. Thus, in a number of indirect ways, it is normatively related to global welfare.

The world trade order as stipulated by WTO, particularly the TRIPS agreement with its reach into the realm of global health, has produced a new challenge to the global community concerning the provision of public goods. Together with the issue of neglected diseases, this has led to a rapid growth in the number of advocating CSOs as well as an increase in their impact on the resolution of international conflicts. We have also witnessed an increasing importance of new forms of hybrid organizations linking state actors to entrepreneurial as well as to advocating non-state actors. CSOs have reinforced discoursive interfaces regarding health issues between the international trade system and (a) global public politics, (b) nation-states, and (c) IGOs in global health.

These interfaces have, as demonstrated in Chapter 2, to a certain extent favoured a common understanding of global public health issues and their relationship to the global economy – without, of course, eliminating differences in interests and actor-specific political goals. The rise of new organizations (in particular: GPPPs, new CSO networks) and the changing influence of existing ones have led to changes in the structure and also the power relations at the organizational interfaces, which, again, influenced actors at the legal interfaces at the national level (South Africa, Brazil) and also – to a limited extent – international law (TRIPS).

We referred to the close involvement of the pharmaceutical industry executives in formulating and defending the major principles of intellectual property rights as part of their strategy and their special efforts to enforce these rights in middle-income countries, such as Brazil and South Africa. Chapter 3 analysed the manoeuvres of TNPCs at various organizational and legal interfaces and showed that the fact that they were stopped in their tracks by actors of those two countries, both in the courts and in the marketplace, has been one of the major surprises for astute observers and social scientists, given the unequal distribution of economic and political power, and given the TNPCs' close relationships to governments of the North.

Advocacy activities of CSOs and the behaviour of the governments of developing countries generated immense pressure on the pharmaceutical industry so that the latter felt compelled to react to the global frame of accepting 'access to medicines' as a central norm. While on the one hand referring to this normative framework to improve access to health care and medicines, TNPCs, on the other hand, have utilized the opportunities given by the opening up of global health governance to new institutional developments. They demonstrated corporate social responsibility by supporting the development of GPPPs in particular, which allowed them to offer their technological expertise without surrendering control. Thus, they attempted to expand their possibilities of adaptation to new emerging welfare and social justice oriented global norms and at the same time pursue their own market-based interests.

We have shown that while being willing to compromise on the global level, the TNPCs and the US government forcefully shifted towards an increased number of bilateral and sub-regional trade agreements, which resulted in IPRs agreements going clearly beyond what had been agreed within the WTO. The same CSOs that had been so successful in the case of South African and Brazilian conflicts with the TNPCs and in pushing for the amendment of the Doha Declaration to TRIPS, failed in their lobbying efforts with the US and its trading partners. Most of the treaties with TRIPS+ regulations have been signed and passed by the legislative bodies in the US and in the relevant partner countries. In light of our analysis, one may presume that the discoursive power of global civil society was not strong enough to have a significant impact on negotiations basically framed in trade-related terms. However, this may change in future conflicts on the application of TRIPS+ rules in concrete cases where access to medicines is at stake.[3]

From the discussions regarding the TNPCs' interactions and their influences on governments of the North, pressing for internationalizing IPRs in various fora, and the response from the developing countries to fight for an amendment of TRIPS and introduce new initiatives at WIPO and the WHO, it has become clear that the major pillars of the global health architecture have changed substantially. The new form of links between non-state and state actors on the global level indicates a changing role for the traditional IGOs, which have to share their field of operation with many different new actors but may also become more important as fora to negotiate international contracts (see the example of the International Health Regulations) or to organize comprehensive discourses among all the actors involved (see: the Commission on Intellectual Property Rights and Innovation in Health).

It has become clear that CSOs (Chapter 4) have played a major role in the discourse arena, supporting and/or pushing national governments and international state and non-state actors into action. The rapid spread and the devastating impact of HIV/AIDS in the poorer countries led to a situation that proved to be a big challenge and opportunity for social actors not linked to state forms of governance. In addressing these challenges, CSOs engaged mainly in three fields: advocacy and campaigning for better health policies and the human right to health (political function), provision of health-related services at the national and local level (operational function), and representation and empowerment of affected communities (self-empowerment function). When the disease was first treated in developed countries, governments all over the world were less than willing to take action to support the extension of treatment to the poor. The disease was largely considered to have originated mainly by careless if not immoral behaviour and culturally based sexual behaviour. While the shift from what could be called a private to a public disease was first and foremost a consequence of its rapid expansion and deadly impact on the lives of entire nations, the active and skilful campaign of the AIDS community has been crucial, as the (at least partly) successful access campaigns of CSOs clearly demonstrate.

The analysis of the conventional IGOs in international health in Chapter 5 (the WHO, World Bank, and UNAIDS) has shown that these international governmental organizations had problems in reacting to new emerging needs. Concerning HIV/AIDS and the case for treatment, for example, the WHO was a forum where industrialized and developing countries argued about the best policies and the right strategies, and

CSOs pressed for including treatment of AIDS patients in the WHO's activities. IGOs had to accept demands and the emerging powers of the developing countries and an increasing number of CSOs. The WHO, in particular, has been challenged by new modes of governance (such as the establishment of the Global Fund), as these are used by powerful actors (nation-states) to bypass the organization. CSOs and GPPPs have taken over functions traditionally performed by the WHO. With it they increase the fragmentation of GHG, which leads to a particular problem for the WHO as the formally central and responsible organization for global health concerns. Thus, future discussions may centre around the question as to how the WHO could strengthen its function as an interface manager of global health affairs.

We have also seen that the strength of the WHO depends on the respective policy issues and the interests of powerful actors that influence it: whereas in global governance concerning the fight against HIV/AIDS, the WHO is a relatively enervated actor, it has strengthened its role in other fields such as norm-setting in infectious diseases control. A certain tendency becomes apparent that in fields where the WHO's interests are closely related to the interests of major donor countries, the former can be a strong actor – if not, the agenda is likely to be shifted to another forum and the WHO is bypassed. However, the WHO has tried to react to these challenges and problems, for instance by engaging in public–private partnerships and by reasserting its role in HIV/AIDS policies.

While the traditional health-related IGOs have had difficulties in redefining their roles, the establishment of the Global Fund to Fight HIV/AIDS, Tuberculosis and Malaria (Chapter 6) reflects the new character of health organizations with its task to manage the interactions among the different stakeholder groups – donors, recipients, private sector, civil society and IGOs – at the global and national levels only for these three specific diseases. Though the dominant public sector financing makes this institution look somewhat similar to existing IGOs, CSO and private sector membership at the Executive Board as well as the recipient countries' decision-making power to shape the character and amount of financial support through the Country Coordinating Mechanism clearly separate this new organization from traditional forms of intergovernmental cooperation. The participatory character of this type of public–private partnership, however, can have its drawback in a lack of efficiency in reaching decisions and a reduced effectiveness of some of the programmes. Its impact and long-term sustainability will depend to a large extent on the willingness of the donors to continue the current campaign and financial support against those diseases.

The Brazilian case (Chapter 7) demonstrated that vertical interfaces played a major role in strengthening national health policies in the face of the HIV/AIDS crisis. Furthermore, the country's fully-fledged involvement in checking the disease made it possible not only to lower prices of ARVs, but also to negotiate the discoursive terms of major financial assistance received from the World Bank and other international agencies. In contrast, South Africa's financial independence helped them determine their health policies autonomously – and hence resist international interference in the fight against HIV/AIDS (Chapter 8). The most recent experience shows, however, that the South African government has gradually realized that the price paid was too high and that a more flexible approach as adopted in Brazil would serve South Africa as well. With regard to the South African health strategy, we have again shown the importance of discoursive interfaces in bringing that gradual change about.

The architecture of global health governance and the interface pyramid

At the end of Chapter 1 we proposed four hypotheses concerning the development of global health governance within the framework of multilevel governance, stressing in particular the increasing role of private and hybrid regulation in global health governance due to difficulties in establishing and adapting state-based international institutions to the needs of managing a complex field of organizations and interfaces. We expected that this circumstance might give a particular weight to discoursive interfaces because of the type of actors involved, the need to bridge different fields of global governance and to mobilize support for new strategies in GHG. We referred to Rosenau's term of 'fragmegration' to characterize a situation where integration and fragmentation reinforce each other.

Discoursive interfaces led to a new framing of the whole field of global health politics. Because of the rise of new organizations, they were obviously closely related to organizational interfaces. Together, they had impacts on the management of resource transfers and on international law. But are these types of interfaces somehow systematically related to each other?

Figure 9.1 postulates a certain relationship between different types of interfaces at the global level, which might help to explain the important role discoursive interfaces can play in conflicts involving basic human rights. There is a broad basis of discoursive interfaces which leads to the acceptance of basic beliefs on specific issues, but also of broad values like human rights; there is a level of organizational interfaces where new

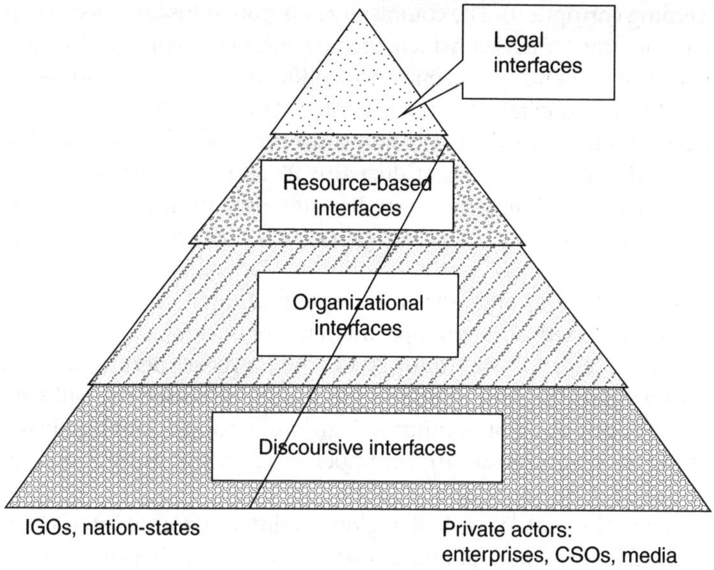

Figure 9.1 Types of interfaces: basis and top in global governance
Source: Own figure.

demands might change the strategies of existing organizations or where new problem areas or new concepts for tackling old problems lead to the foundation of new organizations. At the level of resource-based interfaces, the resources required to tackle problems are identified, mobilized and disbursed (or may be refused). Finally, at the level of international law – in global politics still rather limited – rules are formally set, though at the global level, it is still quite difficult to implement effective systems of sanctions.

The various actors of GHG are present to different degrees at these four types of interfaces (depending on the prevailing governance modes and their norms and rules regulating, inter alia, access to and participation in political processes) and attempt to use them strategically. While legal interfaces at the global level are basically restricted to state actors, there is an increasing importance of private actors moving down from resource-based to discoursive interfaces. The positions different state actors take at negotiations on matters of international law, of course, are influenced at various levels by other actors – for example, in public discourses, or in many commissions, in which representatives of large enterprises and/or CSOs are present, or in negotiations about resources (subsidies, sponsoring, but also concerning corruption). The complexity of negotiations and mediations of various pre-state interests, which precede internationally binding agreements, makes them, once concluded, difficult to change. Furthermore, they constitute general rules implemented under the threat of sanctions, which makes them particularly valuable for those who benefit from them.

Now, more concretely, what does this mean for integrating the conclusions from the different case studies presented in this book? What we jointly found across all seven studies were the following characteristics:

- Due to the transformation of the system of inter-/transnational relations as reflected in the multiple interfaces of the major global, national and local actors in the health arena, the power of 'persuasion' in the context of discoursive interfaces quite often increased the willingness of actors disposing of significant degrees of resource- and legally based power to compromise. In a number of cases this turned out to be decisive for the settling of conflicts.
- While in the post-Westphalian global polity horizontal interfaces will remain a crucial area of international politics, conflicts related to the vertical interfaces of the multilevel system were instrumental in bringing about most of the breakthroughs in the fight against the HIV/AIDS epidemic.
- The increased involvement of civil society played an important role in all chapters. The fact that civil society extends 'down' from debating and negotiating global issues to the end consumer of health services and often also provides those services, gave CSOs a particular strength in integrating fragmented policy areas.
- The emergence of multiple new actors in the global health arena has certainly complicated GHG, but the studies show in each case that these new actors played a central role in creating a flexible system of global health governance. Their activities exerted pressures on those organizations involved in GHG due to their objectives, and helped to overcome the limited effectiveness of organizational interfaces as well as the difficulties in mobilizing resources and taking decisions on redistributing them. On the whole, the development of GHG led to a growing attention to health issues in the field of global politics.

The concept of interfaces enabled us to integrate the findings of the various studies, focusing primarily on the impact of the evolving institutional structures and actor constellations in the fight against the HIV/AIDS pandemic and, beyond that, on the perspectives of global health in general. The foundation of UNAIDS was a conscious approach towards coordinating the activities of the various actors active in the field of HIV/AIDS. However, UNAIDS was dominated (and limited in its potential) by the organizational logic of IGOs and by organizational self-interests of the co-sponsoring UN organizations. This failure of the government-based international system has been increasingly 'corrected' from the outside: CSOs have taken over some operational functions in the health sector and have exerted pressure on existing actors to increase their activities in the fight against HIV/AIDS, which contributed to the emergence of GPPPs and the Global Fund. However, the adjustments also came from within the existing international system, as there has been some initiative by IGOs and governments to create new governance mechanisms and GPPPs.

We can thus identify some major elements of post-Westphalian global politics: non-state actors develop as powerful actors in global politics because of their ability to develop transnational links and transnational political strategies which can act more flexibly on the global scale than IGOs; they are also able to link different fields of global governance like health, human rights and trade. Global civil society represents interests of groups of actors independent from the intermediation of nation-states and across different policy areas.

The emerging global society has led to the development of a field of global health politics and of elements of an architecture of global health governance. These processes are driven by two quite different logics of action: on the one hand, by a logic of consequentialism, which is ready to make compromises in a situation where poor health in other parts of the world poses a threat to the privileged situation of 'the rich', and on the other hand, by a logic of appropriateness, stimulating advocative action in the pursuit of 'global justice'. Certainly, the political outcomes of these processes are the starting point for new conflicts, as in the field of IPRs or the issue of raising resources for improving national health systems – but they have also put enormous pressure on the links between elites and national governments. This was clearly shown in the case study on South Africa, whereas the Brazilian government proved to be more responsive to civil society demands at an early stage. But this has also been the case regarding the links between the pharmaceutical industry and developed countries' governments, which are slowly becoming more responsive to the threats and the ethical norms propelled by globalization.

Of course, it is not only CSOs and some governments of developing countries that influence global health governance. Governments of large industrialized countries still have to be considered the most powerful actors. Whereas human rights objectives play a very important role, it is the perception that ill-health in developing countries and the transborder spread of infectious diseases like HIV/AIDS, SARS or tuberculosis can be a threat to national and international security that is a crucial reason for the onset and dynamics of global health governance. However, governments of industrialized countries intensified their activities in global health and particularly in the fight against poverty-related infectious diseases not only due to self-interests, but also as a reaction to the pressure by CSOs. The activities of Northern governments in the field of global health are dominated by bilateral politics and programmes, yet they increasingly include hybrid regulation as a way of pursuing their interests. We have demonstrated that governments can use networks and hybrid regulation and even CSOs as fora to achieve their goals (and also to weaken IGOs like the WHO or to circumvent disliked governments in the South). Thus, there is a close connection between the strong role of Northern governments and the relevance of hybrid and private regulation.

We can conclude that the main characteristics of the current architecture of global health governance concern the importance of civil society actors and forms of hybrid regulation as well as the dominant role of donor country governments, which pursue their interests in changing fora. By using their discoursive power rather effectively, CSOs have, in a specific historical context, shaped global health governance and global HIV/AIDS politics through their activities. Through this mechanism, governments of industrialized countries and IGOs were quite often in a position where they could only react to already framed discourses.

As a consequence, current forms and effects of global health governance are characterized by a multiplicity of actors, which, on the one hand, implies greater participation of non-state actors and, on the other hand, leads to institutional fragmentation. This structure is a result of institutional and political compromises which are the effect of both conflictive and cooperating interactions of various actors pursuing their own self-interests, such as containing health risks, reaching social and political stability (governments of industrialized countries), securing profits and markets (like TNPCs), and striving for social rights (for example NGOs and welfare-oriented IGOs such as the WHO).

In a mid-term perspective, the success of the fight against HIV/AIDS, and moreover the development of GHG in general, will depend, firstly, on mobilizing the necessary resources to expand and continue treatment, secondly on expanding the success (concerning the delivery of global public goods) not only against other diseases, but also in the development of health systems and attention to the disease-causing conditions. This will depend upon the capacity to expand the consensus on access to medicines to other areas; it will result in new conflicts concerning other dimensions of the world trade order (GATS), and it implies the readiness for much larger transfer payments at the resource-based interfaces.

Improving global health requires additional resources independent from specific solutions of IPR problems. The Commission on Macroeconomics and Health (CMH) calculated that, for a programme to avoid about eight million deaths per year caused by seven major health problems,[4] donor finance for health should grow from US$6 billion per year in 2000 to US$27 billion per year in 2007 (CMH 2001: 16). Redirecting research towards infectious diseases of the South, and making medicines reliable and affordable for the poor, is one precondition for such a programme. Even though some countries reach considerably high rates of aid transfer (like the Scandinavian countries), it is doubtful whether nation-states will raise the necessary ODA resources for the goals set in the report of the CMH.

Considering the fact that new concepts to revise the incentive system for medical R&D and for changes to TRIPS were generally fed into the international discussions by non-state actors, the conclusion seems to be: although state actors (including IGOs) have explicitly accepted that problems of poverty have to be tackled by strategies of global governance if globalization is to be sustainable and should not produce increasing risks to rich countries themselves, an international system based only on processes of a national aggregation of interests seems incapable of solving global health problems. Global civil society will have to exert constant pressure through a broad range of discoursive interfaces. In addition, there is a need for the development of forms of non-traditional financing of global public goods for health. This refers not only to 'public' funding but also to private sources, which are already playing an increasing role in raising not only the levels of financial resources but also of actual research and development of medicines, as shown by the multiple activities of the Gates Foundation. In this context, however, it will be crucial to establish ways to hold these new actors accountable, both internally to their partners and externally to those people who are affected by their activities.

Conflicts will persist in the field of health governance, both at the national and global levels. However, the international community has been willing to face up to global challenges before. As the former World Bank President noted: 'AIDS is a global issue. It forces us to bring all our understanding together – of security, health, economics, and social and cultural change. It forces us to bring all actors together from developed and developing countries, communities and governments, business and NGOs, science, faith, and civil society' (Wolfensohn 2005: 195). Since the successful mobilization of multiple forces and actors against the HIV/AIDS epidemic, there is justified hope for a more widespread and open cooperation to overcome not only this specific crisis, but possibly also future pandemic diseases, irrespective of where they strike first and who is immediately affected.

The rise of new institutional forms and many new actors in global politics creates a structure of global governance that is more inclusive than the one based only on state regulation. It promotes broad discourses on global norms and also strengthens the values of global responsibility and advocacy. Furthermore, it has the potential to lead to a growth in material contributions from manifold actors to problems of global health.

However, the emerging system has to deal with crucial problems of coordination. Nation-states remain formally sovereign and – although to a very different extent – continue to aggregate power resources. The current structure of global governance certainly – despite the tendency of greater inclusion – is shaped by very unequal power relations. Furthermore, institutions for legitimate and enforceable collective decision-making and for delivering integrated public services are related to nation-states. This duality of political spaces characterizes post-Westphalian global politics and thus also global health governance. The development of global federalist structures may offer a way out of this dilemma – certainly, we are living in a period of restructuring of global politics. This, however, is a complex process which requires space (and time) for the evolution of new institutional equilibria and structures.

Notes

1. This refers in particular to the extended meaning of 'security' as 'human security' including social security, which has become increasingly popular during the 1990s (UNDP 1994; Commission on Human Security 2003; see also the compilation of definitions in Alkire 2003: 48), but also to a more traditional understanding of 'national security' (Burkhalter 2004; Prins 2004).
2. This refers to a discourse on the 'logics of action' of different actors. March and Olsen (1989) referred to a 'logic of consequentialism' prevalent in rationalistic approaches (pursuance of self-interest) and contrasted this approach to a 'logic of appropriateness', which supposes that actors behave according to overarching norms and do what they believe is considered appropriate in the eyes of other actors. Risse (2000) supplements these logics with the 'logic of arguing', implying that actors exchange arguments on causal and normative contexts in a communicative process and act according to the results of such a process of understanding.
3. See for example the mobilization against FTAs in a few countries and the high attention paid to specific conflicts by Cp-Tech and other CSOs.
4. These are: HIV/AIDS, malaria, TB, childhood infectious diseases, maternal and perinatal conditions, tobacco-related diseases, and micronutrient deficiencies (CMH 2001: 16).

Bibliography

Abasi, Kamran (1999) 'The World Bank and World Health: Changing Sides', *British Medical Journal*, Vol. 318: 865–9.

Abbott, Frederick M. (2002) 'The Doha Declaration on the TRIPS Agreement and Public Health: Lighting a Dark Corner at the WTO', *Journal of International Economic Law*, Vol. 5 (2): 469–505.

Abbott, Frederick M. (2005a) 'Toward a New Era of Objective Assessment in the Field of TRIPS and Variable Geometry for the Presentation of Multilateralism', *Journal of International Economic Law*, Vol. 8 (1): 77–100.

Abbott, Frederick M. (2005b) 'The WTO Medicines Decision: World Pharmaceutical Trade and the Protection of Public Health', *American Journal of International Law*, Vol. 99: 317–58.

Abbott, Frederick M. (2006) 'TRIPS II, Asia and the Mercantile Pharmaceutical War: Implications for Innovation and Access', draft paper for the Conference on Economic Challenges in Asia, Stanford Center for International Development, 31 May–3 June 2006.

Abbott, Thomas M. (1995) 'Price Regulation in the Pharmaceutical Industry: Prescription or Placebo?' *Journal of Health Economics*, Vol. 14 (5): 551–67.

Abramson, John (2004) *Overdosed America*. New York: HarperCollins.

Abreu, Anabela Garcia, Nogueira, Isabel and Couwgill, Karen (2003) *HIV/AIDS in Latin American Countries: the Challenges Ahead*. Human Development Network: Health, Nutrition, and Population Series. Washington: World Bank.

Abrucio, Fernando and Samuels, David (1997) 'A nova Política dos Governadores', *Luan Nova*, São Paulo, No. 40–1: 137–66.

Accenture (2004) 'Global Fund to Fight AIDS, Tuberculosis and Malaria', briefing paper on In-kind Donations Project; Annex 4 to the Report of the Resource Mobilizations and Communications Committee for the 7th Board Meeting (GF/B7/10).

Adelman, Carol C., Norris, Jeremiah and Weicher, S. Jean (2004) *Myths and Realities on Prices of Drugs*, Hudson Institute White Paper, 11 May 2004. Washington, DC: Hudson Institute.

Aginam, Obijiofor (2005) *Global Health Governance: International Law and Public Health in a Divided World*. Toronto: Toronto University Press.

Aids Bulletin (2005) '"If we don't have anything, we don't have a future", an interview with Mr Thomas Mathole, the new executive director of the Aids Consortium', *Aids Bulletin* (December 2005); URL: http://www.mrc.ac.za/aids/dec2005/anything.pdf (10 February 2006).

Aids Consortium (2004) 'The Aids Consortium Annual Report 2004'; URL: http://www.aidsconsortium.org.za/docs/ACreport[1].pdf (9 February 2006).

Aidspan (2004) 'An Updated Analysis of the Equitable Contributions Framework regarding the Global Fund'; URL: www.aidspan.org/gfo/docs/gfo61.pdf (4 May 2007).

Alkire, Sabina (2003) 'A Conceptual Framework for Human Security', working paper 2, Centre for Research on Inequality, Human Security and Ethnicity, University of Oxford.

Almanaque Abril (2004) *Saúde*. São Paulo: Editora Abril: 137–48.
Altman, Dennis (1999) 'UNAIDS: NGOs on Board and on the Board', case study for the Montreal International Forum. URL: http://www.fimcivilsociety.org/english/DAltman1999.pdf (4 May 2007).
ANC (2002) 'Let's tell the truth about South Africa', *ANC Today*, Vol. 2 (9).
Angell, Marcia (2004) *The Truth about the Drug Companies*. New York: Random House.
Anheier, Helmut, Glasius, Marlies Glasius and Kaldor, Mary (eds) (2001a) *Global Civil Society 2001*. Oxford: Oxford University Press.
Anheier, Helmut, Glasius, Marlies and Kaldor, Mary (eds) (2001b) 'Introducing Global Civil Society', in Anheier, Glasius and Kaldor (eds) (2001): 3–22.
Anheier, Helmut, Glasius, Marlies Glasius and Kaldor, Mary (eds) (2004) *Global Civil Society Yearbook 2004/5*. Oxford: Oxford University Press.
Arts, Bas (2003) 'Non-State Actors in Global Governance – Three Faces of Power', working paper, Mack-Planck-Projektgruppe Recht der Gemeinschaftsgüter; URL: http://www.mpp-rdg.mpg.de/pdf_dat/2003_4.pdf (5 May 2006).
Arts, Bas, Noortmann, Math and Reinalda, Bob (eds) (2001) *Non-state Actors in International Relations*. Aldershot: Ashgate.
Arturi, Carlos (2001) 'O Debate Teórico sobre Mudança de Regime Político: O Caso Brasileiro', *Revista de Sociologia e Política*, No. 17, November: 11–31; URL: www.scielo.br/pdf/rsocp/n17/a02n17.pdf (1 July 2006).
Ashraf, Haroon (2001) 'USA and Brazil End Dispute Over Essential Drugs', *Lancet*, 357: 2112.
Attridge, James and Preker, Alexander (2005) *Improving Access to Medicines in Developing Countries*, HNP Discussion Paper. Washington, DC: World Bank.
Bache, Ian and Flinders, Matthew (eds) (2004) *Multi-level Governance*. Oxford: Oxford University Press.
Bacon, Oliver, Pecoraro, Maria Lúcia, Galvão, Jane and Page-Shafer, Kimberly (2004) *HIV/AIDS in Brazil*, Country AIDS Policy Analysis Project, University of California, San Francisco.
Baer, Werner and Paiva, Cláudio (1996) 'Brasiliens inflationäre Erblast und der Plano Real', in Gilberto Calcagnotto and Barbara Fritz (eds), *Inflation und Stabilisierung in Brasilien. Probleme einer Gesellschaft im Wandel*. Schriftenreihe des Instituts für Iberoamerika-Kunde, Hamburg, Band 43: 66–93.
Baker, Gideon and Chandler, David (eds) (2005) *Global Civil Society: Contested Futures*. London: Routledge.
Barnett, Courtney, Connor, Catherine and Putney, Pamela J. (2001) *Contracting Non-Governmental Organizations to Combat HIV/AIDS*, Special Initiative Report No. 33, Partnerships for Health Reform. Maryland: PHRplus.
Barnett, Michael and Duvall, Raymond (2005a) *Power in Global Governance*. Cambridge: Cambridge University Press.
Barnett, Michael and Duvall, Raymond (2005b) 'Power in Global Governance', in Barnett and Duvall (2005): 1–32.
Barnett, Michael and Finnemore, Martha (2004) *Rules for the World: International Organizations in Global Politics*. Ithaca: Cornell University Press.
Barnett, Tony and Whiteside, Alan (2002a) *AIDS in the Twenty-First Century: Disease and Globalization*. Basingstoke/New York: Palgrave Macmillan.
Barnett, Tony and Whiteside, Alan (2002b) 'Poverty and HIV/AIDS: Impact, Coping and Mitigation Policy', in Giovanni Andrea Cornia (ed.), *AIDS, Public Policy and Child Well-Being*. Florence: UNICEF.

Bartsch, Sonja (2003) 'Global Public–Private Partnerships in Health: Potentials and Limits', in Hein and Kohlmorgen (eds) (2003): 225–40.

Bartsch, Sonja and Kohlmorgen, Lars (2005a) 'Global Health Governance: Konflikt und Kooperation zwischen Nord und Süd in neuen institutionellen Strukturen', paper presented at the workshop 'Nord und Süd im Globalen Regieren – Politikfelder, Akteure, Forschungsperspektiven', German Institute for Development Policy, Bonn, 23/24 June 2005.

Bartsch, Sonja and Kohlmorgen, Lars (2005b) 'Nichtregierungsorganisationen als Akteure der Global Health Governance – Interaktion zwischen Kooperation und Konflikt', in Betz and Hein (eds) (2005): 57–87.

Bartsch, Sonja and Kohlmorgen, Lars (2005c) 'The Millennium Development Goals and Global Governance: the Role of Institutions in Poverty Reduction', *Nord-Süd aktuell*, 3+4 (2005): 259–76.

Basso, Cáritas Relva (2002) 'O programa nacional de DST/AIDS no SUS', in Barjas Negri and Ana Luiza d'Ávila Viana (Org.), *O Sistema Único de Saúde em Dez Anos de Desafio. O passo a passo de uma reforma que alarga o desenvolvimento e estreita a desigualdade social. Obra de 40 autores que contam a história do SUS com a história do SUS*. São Paulo: Sobravime/CEALAG: 135–62.

BBC Brazil (2006) 'Empresas no Brasil são as que mais temem efeitos da AIDS', 12 January; URL: www.bbc.co.uk/portuguese/reporterbbc/story/2006/01/060112_empresasaidsbrasilmb.shtml.

Beaglehole, Robert (ed.) (2003) *Global Public Health: a New Era*. Oxford: Oxford University Press.

Beck, Ulrich and Lau, Christoph (eds) (2004) *Entgrenzung und Entscheidung*. Frankfurt am Main: Suhrkamp.

Beigbeder, Yves (2004) *International Public Health: Patients' Rights versus the Protection of Patents*. Aldershot: Ashgate.

Bell, Clive, Devarajan, Shantayanan and Gersbach, Hans (2003) *The Long-run Economic Costs of AIDS: Theory and an Application to South Africa*. Washington; URL: http://www1.worldbank.org/hiv_aids/docs/BeDeGe_BP_total2.pdf (3 July 2006).

Benner, Thorsten, Reinicke, Wolfgang H. and Witte, Martin (2002) *Shaping Globalization: the Role of Global Public Policy Networks*. Washington; URL: www.globalpublicpolicy.net/fileadmin/gppi/BF_Beitrag__englisch__Final_05172002.pdf (3 July 2006).

Berger, Jonathan Michael (2002) 'Litigation Strategies to Gain Access to Treatment for HIV/AIDS: the Case of South Africa's Treatment Action Campaign', *Wisconsin International Law Journal*, Vol. 20 (3): 595–610.

Berkman Alan, Garcia, Jonathan, Muñoz-Laboy, Miguel, Paiva, Vera and Parker, Richard (2005) 'A Critical Analysis of the Brazilian Response to HIV/AIDS: Lessons Learned for Controlling and Mitigating the Epidemic in Developing Countries', *American Journal of Public Health*, Vol. 95 (7): 1162–72; URL: http://www.abiaids.ort.br/media/Berkmanetal%5B1%5D.2005.pdf (3 July 2006).

Bermann, George A. and Petro C. Mavroidis (eds) (2006) *Trade and Human Health and Safety*. Cambridge and New York: Cambridge University Press.

Bermudez, Jorge and Oliveira, Maria Auxiliadora (2002) 'Essential Medicines and AIDS Care in Brazil: Recent Lessons Learnt'. UNAIDS; URL: hivinsite.ucsf.edu/pdf/cr05-br-01.pdf (24 April 2006).

Betz, Joachim (2003) 'The Indian Health System: Structure, Deficits and the Role of External Actors', in Hein and Kohlmorgen (eds) (2003): 291–304.

Betz, Joachim and Hein, Wolfgang (eds) (2005) *Neues Jahrbuch Dritte Welt 2005. Zivilgesellschaft*. Wiesbaden: VS Verlag.

Beyrer, Chris, Gauri, Varun and Vaillanxourt, Denise, see World Bank (2005b).

BHAP (2006a) Data; URL: http://www.aids.gov.br/data/Pages/LUMISD3352823PTBRIE.htm (3 September 2006).

BHAP (2006b) Number of NGOs; URL: http://157.86.8.200/docs/Number%20of%20NGOs%20%20T.xls (3 September 2006).

Biehl, João Guilherme (2004) 'The Activist State: Global Pharmaceuticals, AIDS, and Citizenship in Brazil', *Social Text*, Duke University Press, No. 22(3) (2004): 105–32; URL: muse.jhu.edu/journals/social_text/v022/22.3biehl.html (3 September 2006).

Birdsall, Karen (2005) 'Faith-based Responses to HIV/AIDS in South Africa: an Analysis of the Activities of Faith-based Organisations (FBOs) in the National HIV/AIDS Database', Centre for AIDS Development, Research and Evaluation (CADRE), Johannesburg; URL: http://www.cadre.org.za/pdf/FBO-Report.pdf (15 July 2006).

Blecher, Mark and Thomas, Stephen (2004) 'Health Care Financing'; in Ijumba, Day and Ntuli (eds) (2004): 269–88.

Blouin, Chantal, Drager, Nick and Smith, Richard (2006) *International Trade in Health Services and the GATS: Current Issues and Debates*. Washington, DC: World Bank.

Börzel, Tanja A. and Risse, Thomas (2005) 'Public–Private Partnerships: Effective and Legitimate Tools of International Governance?' in Edgar Grande and Louis W. Pauly (eds), *Complex Sovereignty: Reconstituting Political Authority in the Twenty-First Century*. Toronto: University of Toronto Press: 195–216.

Boyd, Barbara L. (1999) 'NGO Participation in HIV-AIDS Control Project in Brazil', in *Social Development Notes*. Washington, DC: World Bank.

Braithwaite, John and Drahos, Peter (2000) *Global Business Regulation*. Cambridge: Cambridge University Press.

Brand, Ulrich, Demirovic, Alex, Görg, Christoph and Hirsch, Joachim (eds) (2001) *Nichtregierungsorganisationen in der Transformation des Staates*. Münster: Westfälisches Dampfboot.

Brasil, Ministério da Saúde (2005) 'Plano Estratégico. Programa Nacional de DST e AIDS 2005', Secretaria de Vigilância em Saúde. Programa Nacional de DST e AIDS. Brasília.

Brazilian DST-HIV/AIDS Program BHAP (2006) 'AIDS'; URL: http://www.aids.gov.br/data/Pages/LUMISD3352823PTBRIE.htm (13 September 2006).

Breman, Anna and Shelton, Carolyn (2001) 'Structural Adjustment and Health: a Literature Review of the Debate, its Role-Players and Presented Empirical Evidence', CMH Working Paper Series, Paper No. WG6:6. WHO, Commission on Macroeconomics and Health, Geneva.

Brown, Theodore M., Cueto, Marcos and Fee, Elizabeth (2006) 'The World Health Organization and the Transition from "International" to "Global Health"', *American Journal of Public Health*, Vol. 96: 62–72.

Bull, Benedicte and McNeill, Desmond (eds) (2007) *Development Issues in Global Governance: Public–Private Partnerships and Market Multilateralism*. London and New York: Routledge.

Bull, Hedley (1995) *The Anarchical Society: a Study of Order in World Politics*, 2nd edn. London: Macmillan.

Burkhalter, Holly (2004) 'The Politics of AIDS: Engaging Conservative Activists', *Foreign Affairs*, January/February: 8–14.

Burris, Scott (2004) 'Governance, Microgovernance and Health', *Temple Law Review*, Vol. 77: 335–58.

Burris, Scott, Drahos, Peter and Shearing, Clifford (2005) 'Nodal Governance', *Australian Journal of Legal Philosophy*, Vol. 30: 30–58.

Busby, Joshua William (2006) 'From Benign Neglect to Moral Awakening: Donor Resonses to HIV/AIDS', paper prepared for the workshop on 'The Policy and Politics of HIV/AIDS', Princeton University, 5 May.

Buse, Kent (2004) 'Governing Public-Private Infectious Disease Partnerships', *Brown Journal of World Affairs*, Vol. 10 (2): 225–41.

Buse, Kent and Gwin, Catherine (1998) 'The World Bank and Global Cooperation in Health: the Case of Bangladesh', *Lancet*, Vol. 351: 665–9.

Buse, Kent and Walt, Gill (2000a) 'Global Public–Private Partnerships – Part I: a New Development in Health?', *Bulletin of the WHO*, Vol. 78 (4): 549–61.

Buse, Kent and Walt, Gill (2000b) 'Global Public–Private Partnerships – Part II: What are the Health Issues for Global Governance', *Bulletin of the WHO*, Vol. 78 (5): 699–709.

Business Day (2006a) 'Minister's Remedies Shock World Aids Indaba', *Business Day*, 14 August 2006; URL: www.businessday.co.za (23 August 2006).

Business Day (2006b) 'Aids "will hit economy less hard than feared" ', *Business Day*, 14 July 2006; URL: www.businessday.co.za (15 July 2006).

Butler, Anthony (2005a) 'The Negative and Positive Impacts of HIV/AIDS in South Africa', *Journal of Contemporary African Studies*, Vol. 23 (1): 3–26.

Butler, Anthony (2005b) 'South Africa's HIV/AIDS Policy, 1994–2004: How Can it be Explained?' *African Affairs*, Vol. 104 (416): 1–25.

Caines, Karen (2004) *Global Health Partnerships and Neglected Diseases*, GHP Study Paper No. 4. London: DFID Health Resource Center.

Caines, Karen (with Kent Buse, Cindy Carlson, Rosemarie de Loor, Nel Druce, Cheri Grace, Mark Pearson, Jennifer Sancho and Rajeev Sadanandan) (2004) *Assessing the Impact of Global Health Partnerships: Synthesis of Findings from the 2004 DFID Studies*. London: DFID Health Resource Center.

Caines, Karen and Lush, Louisiana (2004) *Impact of Public–Private Partnerships Addressing Access to Pharmaceutical Drugs in Selected Low and Middle Income Countries: a Synthesis Report from Botswana, Sri Lanka, Uganda, and Zambia*. Geneva: The Initiative on Public–Private Partnerships for Health.

Calcagnotto, Gilberto (1985) 'Brasiliens Antworten auf die Krise (1982–1985)', in *Lateinamerika. Analysen, Daten, Dokumentation*, No. 4. Hamburg, Wirtschaftskrise und Anpassungspolitik in Lateinamerika: 63–74.

Campaign for Access to Essential Medicines (2005) *Untangling the Web of Price Reductions: a Pricing Guide for the Purchase of ARVs for Developing Countries*, 8th edition (June); URL: http://www.accessmed-msf.org (10 February 2006).

Cape Argus (1998) 'A Matter of Life and Death', *Cape Argus*, 13 October 1998; URL: http://www.iol.co.za (23 November 2005).

Carvalho, Sérgio Medeiros Paulino de (2005) 'Política de Propriedade Intelectual no Brasil: Intervenções nos Campos de Saúde e de Sementes', *IPEA*, Textos para Discussão No. 1140: Brasília.

CASE (2004) 'Civil Society in South Africa: Opportunities and Challenges in the Transition Process', Community Agency for Social Enquiry (CASE); URL: http://www.case.org.za/downloads/USAid%20Report.pdf (10 February 2006).

Cassier, Maurice and Correa, Marilena (2003) 'Patents, Innovation and Public Health: Brazilian Public-Sector Laboratories' Experience in Copying AIDS Drugs'; URL: http://www.iaen.org/files.cgi/11069_part_1_n3_Cassier.pdf.

Castro, Mary Garcia and da Silva, Lorena Bernadete (2005) *Responses to AIDS Challenges in Brazil: Limits and Possibilities*. Brasília: UNESCO/Ministério da Saúde.

Central Bank of Brazil (1983) *Annual Report 1982*. Brasília: Central Bank of Brazil.

Cepaluni, Gabriel (2005) 'Regimes Internacionais e o Contencioso das Patentes para Medicamentos: Estratégias para Países em Desenvolvimento', *Contexto Internacional*, 27 (1), Jan.–June, Rio de Janeiro: 51–99.

Chaudhuri, Sudip (2005) *The WTO and India's Pharmaceutical Industry: Patent Protection, TRIPS, and Developing Countries*. Oxford: Oxford University Press.

Chen, L. C., Evans, T. G. and Cash, R. A. (1999) 'Health as a Global Public Good', in Kaul et al. (eds) (1999): 284–304.

Chequer, Pedro (2006) 'Resposta Nacional ao HIV e AIDS no Brasil'; URL: www.who.int/intellectualproperty/events/HIVAIDSPedroChequer.pdf (10 June 2006).

CIPIH/WHO (2006) *Public Health, Innovation and Intellectual Property Rights*. Report of the Commission on Intellectual Property Rights, Innovation and Public Health. Geneva: WHO.

CIPR (2002) *Integrating Intellectual Property Rights and Development Policy*. London: Commission on Intellectual Property Rights; URL: www.iprcommission.org (10 February 2006).

Clayton, Andrew, Oakley, Peter and Taylor, Jon (2000) *Civil Society Organizations and Service Provision*, Civil Society and Social Movements Programme Paper Number 2. Geneva: UNRISD.

CMH (2001) *Macroeconomics and Health. Investing in Health for Economic Development*, Report of the Commission on Macroeconomics in Health. Geneva: WHO.

CN DST e AIDS (Coordenação Nacional DST e AIDS, Secretaria de Políticas de Saúde, Ministério da Saúde) (2003) *Año 2000: Distribuição dos Gastos Totais com AIDS*; URL: http://www.aids.gov.br (4 January 2006).

CNAIDS Comissão Nacional de DST e AIDS (2004) Protocol, 20 June, 71st Session, Brasília; URL: www.aids.gov.br/final/parcerias/atas.asp (10 February 2006).

CNAIDS (2004) Parcerias; URL: http://www.aids.gov.br/final/parcerias/cnaids.asp (10 February 2006).

CNAIDS (CNAIDS Protocol 2005) Comissão Nacional de DST e AIDS 2005: Ata da 75ª Reunião Ordinária, 27 April, Hotel Nacional: Brasília; URL: www.aids.gov.br/final/parcerias/atas.asp (10 February 2006).

Cohen, Desmond (2000) *Poverty and HIV/AIDS in Sub-Saharan Africa*, SEPED Conference Paper Series No. 2. Geneva: UNDP.

Cohen, Jillian Clare and Lybecker, Kristina M. (2005) 'AIDS Policy and Pharmaceutical Patents: Brazil's Strategy to Safeguard Public Health', *World Economy*, Vol. 28 (2): 211–30.

Collin, Jeff, Lee, Kelley and Bissell, Karen (2002) 'Global Health Governance? The Framework Convention on Tobacco Control', *Third World Quarterly*, 23 (2): 265–82.

Comanor, William S. (1986) 'The Political Economy of the Pharmaceutical Industry', *Journal of Economic Literature*, 24: 1178–217.

Commission on Human Security (2003) *Human Security Now.* New York: United Nations Publications.

Commission on Intellectual Property Rights (2002) 'Integrating Intellectual Property Rights and Development Policy'; URL: www.iprcommission.org/home.html (10 February 2006).

Committee on Government Reform (2005) *Trade Agreements and Access to Medications Under the Bush Administration*, prepared for Rep. Henry A. Waxman (United States House of Representatives, Minority Staff, Special Investigations Division).

Connelly, Patrick and Rosen, Sidney (2005) 'Provision of Antiretroviral Therapy by the Private Sector', *Lancet*, 365: 1925.

Connor, Catherine (2000) *Contracting Non-Governmental Organizations for HIV/AIDS: Brazil Case Study*. Special Initiative Report No. 30, Maryland: Partnerships for Health Reform.

Constitutional Court (2002) *Minister of Health v. Treatment Action Campaign*, No. 2, 2002 (5) SA 721 (CC).

Cooper, Robert (2003) *The Breaking of Nations: Order and Chaos in the 21st Century*. New York: Atlantic Monthly Press.

Cornia, Giovanni Andrea (2001) 'Globalization and Health: Results and Options', *Bulletin of the World Health Organization*, 79: 834–41.

Correa, Carlos M. (2002) 'Implications of the Doha Declaration on the TRIPS Agreement and Public Health', paper commissioned by the WHO. Buenos Aires: WHO.

Cueto, Marcos (2004) 'The Origins of Primary Health Care and Selective Primary Health Care', *American Journal of Public Health*, November, 94 (11): 1864–74.

Cutler, A. Claire, Haufler, Virginia and Porter, Tony (eds) (1999) *Private Authority and International Affairs*. Albany: SUNY Press.

Davey, Sheila, Jupp, Susan and Mauroux, Christine (eds) (2004) '10/90 Report on Health Research 2003/2004'. Geneva: Global Forum for Health Research; URL: www.globalforumhealth.org/filesupld/1090_report_03_04/109004foreword.pdf (10 July 2006).

Delcour, Laure and Vellutini, Charles (2005) 'Added Value of Global Partnerships and Global Funds to Development Cooperation', paper prepared for the European Commission; URL: www.theglobalfund.org/en/files/links_resources/library/studies/PP_GEN3_full.pdf (4 May 2007).

Department of Health (2000) 'HIV/AIDS/STD Strategic Plan for South Africa 2000–2005', Pretoria: Department of Health; URL: http://www.doh.gov.za/docs/policy/aids-plan0005.pdf (23 November 2005).

Department of Health (2003) 'The Operational Plan for Comprehensive HIV and AIDS Care, Management, and Treatment for South Africa', Pretoria: Department of Health; URL: http://www.info.gov.za/otherdocs/2003/aidsoperationalplan.pdf (8 April 2005).

Department of Health (2004) 'National HIV and Syphilis Antenatal Sero-Prevalence Survey in South Africa 2004', Pretoria: Department of Health; URL: http://www.doh.gov.za/docs/reports/2004/hiv-syphilis.pdf (23 November 2005).

Department of Health (2006) *National HIV and Syphilis Antenatal Sero-Prevalence Survey in South Africa 2005*. Pretoria: Department of Health; URL: http://www.doh.gov.za/docs/hiv-syphilis-f.html (15 July 2006).

DFID (2003) *Global Fund Country Case Studies Report*. London: Department for International Development (DFID).

DFID (2005) *Increasing People's Access to Essential Medicines in Developing Countries: a Framework for Good Practice in the Pharmaceutical Industry*. London: Department for International Development (DFID); URL: http://www.dfid.gov.uk/pubs/files/pharm-framework.pdf (10 August 2006).

Diaz-Bonilla, Eugenio, Babinard, Julie, Pinstrup-Andersen, Per and Thomas, Marcelle (2003) 'Globalizing Health Benefits for Developing Countries', in Hein and Kohlmorgen (eds) (2003): 75–115.

Dickinson, Clare (2005) 'National AIDS Coordinating Authorities: a Synthesis of Lessons Learned and Taking Learning Forward', working paper, London: DFID Health Resource Centre.

Dickinson, David (2004) 'Corporate South Africa's Response to HIV/AIDS: Why So Slow?' *Journal of Southern African Studies*, 30 (3): 627–49.

DiMasi, Joseph A., Hansen, R., Grabowski, H. and Lasagna, L. (1991) 'The Cost of Innovation in the Pharmaceutical Industry', *Journal of Health Economics*, Vol. 10 (2): 107–42.

DiMasi, Joseph A., Hansen, R. W., Grabowski, H. G. and Lasagna, L. (2003) 'The Price of Innovation: New Estimates of Drug Development Costs', *Journal of Health Economics*, Vol. 22: 151–85.

DiMasi, Joseph, Hamsen, Ronald W. and Grabowski, Henry G. (2004) 'Assessing Claims About the Cost of New Drug Development: a Critique of the Public Citizen and TB Alliance Reports'; URL: http://csdd.tufts.edu/_documents/www/Doc_231_45_735.pdf (1 June 2006).

Dodgson, Richard, Lee, Kelley and Drager, Nick (2002) *Global Health Governance: a Conceptual Review*, Discussion Paper No. 1, London: Centre of Global Change & Health, LSHTM/Department of Health & Development, WHO.

Doherty, Tanya and Colvin, Mark (2004) 'HIV/AIDS', in Ijumba, Day and Ntuli (eds) (2004): 191–211.

Dorrington, Rob, Bourne, David, Bradshaw, Debbie, Laubscher, Ria and Timæus, Ian (2001) *The Impact of HIV/AIDS on Adult Mortality in South Africa*, Technical Report. Cape Town: Medical Research Council.

Dorrington, Rob, Bradshaw, Debbie, Johnson, Leigh and Budlender, Debbie (2004) *The Demographic Impact of HIV/AIDS in South Africa: National Indicators 2004*. Cape Town: Centre for Actuarial Research, Medical Research Council and the Actuarial Society of South Africa.

Dorrington, Rob, Bradshaw, Debbie and Budlender, Debbie (2002) *HIV/AIDS Profile in the Provinces of South Africa: Indicators for 2002*. Cape Town: Centre for Actuarial Research, Medical Research Council and the Actuarial Society of South Africa.

Dourado, Inês et al. (2006) 'Tendências da epidemia de AIDS no Brasil após a terapia anti-retroviral', *Revista Saúde Pública*, Vol. 40 (Suppl.), Rio de Janeiro: Fiocruz: 9–15.

Drahos, Peter (2002a) *Developing Countries and International Intellectual Property Standard-setting*, Commission on Intellectual Property Rights, Study Paper 8, London.

Drahos, Peter (2002b) 'Negotiating Intellectual Property Rights: Between Coercion and Dialogue', in Drahos and Mayne (eds) (2002): 161–82.

Drahos, Peter and Mayne, Ruth (eds) (2002) *Global Intellectual Property Rights: Knowledge, Access and Development*, Basingstoke: Oxfam.

Elmendorf, Edward and Roseberry, Wendy (1993) *Structural Adjustment: What Effect on Health? On Vulnerability to HIV Infection*, International Aids Conference, 6–11 June, 9: 123 (abstract no. WS-D20-4). Washington, DC: World Bank.

Engel, Jonathan (2006) *The Epidemic: a Global History of AIDS*. New York: HarperCollins.

England, Roger (2004) 'Experiences of Contracting with the Private Sector: a Selective Review', issues paper, DFID Health Sector Resource Centre. London: DFID Health Systems Resource Centre.

Fidler, David (1999) *International Law and Infectious Disease*. Oxford: Oxford University Press.

Fidler, David (2002) *Global Health Governance: Overview of the Role of International Law in Protecting and Promoting Global Public Health*, LSHTM/WHO Discussion Paper.

Fidler, David (2004) SARS, *Governance and the Globalization of Disease*. Basingstoke: Palgrave Macmillan.

Fidler, David (2005) 'From International Sanitary Conventions to Global Health Security: the New International Health Regulations', *Chinese Journal of International Law*, Vol. 4 (2): 1–68.

Fink, Carsten and Maskus, Keith E. (eds) (2005) *Intellectual Property and Development: Lessons from Recent Economic Research*. Washington, DC: World Bank/Oxford University Press.

Fischer-Lescano, Andreas and Liste, Philip (2005) 'Völkerrechtspolitik. Zur Trennung und Verknüpfung von Politik und Recht der Weltgesellschaft', *Zeitschrift für Internationale Beziehungen*, 2/12. Jg.: 209–49.

Fleury, Sonia (2000) 'Reshaping Health Care in Latin America: Toward Fairness?' in Sonia Fleury, Susana Belmartino and Enis Baris (eds), *Reshaping Health Care in Latin America: a Comparative Analysis of Health Care Reform in Argentina, Brazil, and Mexico*. Ottawa: International Development Center: 225–62.

Fontes, Miguel B. (1999) 'Interfaces entre as políticas internacionais e nacionais de AIDS', in Richard Parker, Jane Galvão and Marcelo S. Bessa (eds), *Saúde, Desenvolvimento e Política. Respostas frente à AIDS no Brasil*, ABIA, Rio de Janeiro: Editora 34: 91–122.

France, Tim, Ooms, Gorik and Rivers, Bernard (2003) *The Global Fund: Which Countries Owe How Much?* New York: Aidspan.

Frantz, Christiane and Zimmer, Annette (eds) (2002) *Zivilgesellschaft international. Alte und neue NGOs*. Opladen: Leske + Budrich.

Friedman, Steven and Mottiar, Shauna (2004) *Rewarding Engagement?: The Treatment Action Campaign and the Politics of HIV/AIDS*. Durban: University of KwaZuluNatal.

Fritz, Barbara (2002) *Entwicklung durch wechselkurs-basierte Stabilisierung? Der Fall Brasilien*, Studien zur Monetären Ökonomie, Bd. 28. Marburg: Metropolis.

GAC (Office of the US Global AIDS Coordinator) (2005) 'PEPFAR: Community and Faith-Based Organizations', Report, 5 October 2005. URL: http://www.state.gov/s/gac/progress/creports/54316.htm (10 September 2006).

Gaffei, Edoardo (2003) 'The Economics of HIV/AIDS: a Survey', *Development Policy Review*, Vol. 21 (1): 27–49.

Galvão, Jane (2000) *Aids no Brasil: A agenda de construção de uma epidemia*. São Paulo, Rio de Janeiro: Editora 34/ABIA.

Galvão, Jane (2002) 'A política brasileira de distribuição e produção de medicamentos anti-retrovirais: privilégio ou direito?', *Cadernos Saúde Pública*, Rio de Janeiro, 18 (1): 212–19.

GAO (General Accounting Office) (2001) *Global Health. Joint UN Programme on HIV/AIDS Needs to Strengthen Country-Level Efforts and Measure Results*. Report to the Chairman, Subcommitee on African Affairs, Committee on Foreign Relations, US Senate. Washington, DC.

Garrett, Laurie (1994) *The Coming Plague*. New York: Penguin Books.

Garrett, Laurie (2007) 'Do No Harm: the Global Health Challenge', *Foreign Affairs*, Jan./Feb.: 14–38.

Garrison, J. (1988) 'AIDS and the Poor in Brazil', *Grassroots Development*, 12 (3): 43.

Gauri, Varun and Lieberman, Evan S. (2004) *AIDS and the State: the Politics of Government Responses to the Epidemic in Brazil and South Africa*. Washington: World Bank; URL: http://comparativepolitics.stanford.edu/Papers2004-05/Liebermanv2.440dJan17.pdf (23 December 2004).

Gebauer, Tomas (2001) '. . . "von niemandem gewählt!" Über die demokratische Legitimation von NGOs', in Brand, Demirovic, Görg and Hirsch (eds) (2001): 95–120.

Gelders, Susanne, Ewen, Margaret, Noguchi, Nakae and Laing, Richard (2006) 'Price, Availability and Affordability: an International Comparison of Chronic Disease Medicines', background report prepared for the WHO Planning Meeting on the Global Initiative for Treatment of Chronic Diseases held in Cairo in December 2005, WHO, Regional Office for the Eastern Mediterranean, Health Action International, Cairo.

GF (2004) *Country Coordinating Mechanisms*, a synthesis and analysis of findings from CCM case studies, tracking study, GNP+ and other surveys. Geneva: The Global Fund.

GF (2005a) *Addressing HIV/AIDS, Malaria and Tuberculosis: the Resource Needs of the Global Fund, 2005–2007*. Geneva: The Global Fund.

GF (2005b) *Sustaining Performance, Scaling Up Results: Third Progress Report 2005*. Geneva: The Global Fund.

GF (2005c) *Measuring the Systems Effects of the Global Fund*. Geneva: The Global Fund.

GF (2005d) *Review of the Argumentation on Phase 2 Financing of the LoveLife Grant* (GF/B11/16). Geneva: The Global Fund.

GF (2006) 'Funding the Global Fight Against HIV/AIDS, Tuberculosis and Malaria', document created for the Mid-term Replenishment Meeting, June 2006; URL: http://www.theglobalfund.org/en/files/about/replenishment/resource_needs_2006.pdf (10 July 2006).

Giovanella, Ligia and Porto, Marcelo Firpo de Souza (eds) (2004) 'Gesundheitswesen und Gesundheitspolitik in Brasilien', Arbeitspapiere 25/2004, Institut für Medizinische Soziologie des Klinikums der Johann Goethe Universität; URL: http://www.links-netz.de/K_texte/K_giovanella_brasilien.html (4 May 2007).

Glassman, James (2004) 'The Real Obstacle to Treating AIDS, Malaria, and Tuberculosis in Developing Countries', introductory remarks, American Enterprise Institute for Public Policy Research; URL: www.aei.org/include/pub_print.asp?pubID=20506 (28 June 2006).

Global Forum for Health Research (2004) *Monitoring Financial Flows for Health Research*. Geneva.

Global Fund Observer (various issues); URL: www.aidspan.org (10 July 2006).

Global Health Watch (2005) *Global Health Watch 2005/2006: an Alternative World Health Report*. London and New York: Global Health Watch.

Global Task Team (2005) Global Task Team on Improving AIDS Coordination Among Multilateral.

GNP+ (2003) *A Multi-Country Study of the Involvement of People Living with HIV/AIDS (PLWHA) in the Country Coordinating Mechanisms*. Amsterdam: GNP+.

Gootnick, David (2005) *The Global Fund to Fight AIDS, TB and Malaria is responding to challenges but needs better information and documentation for performance-based funding*. Washington: Government Accounting Office.

Goozner, Merill (2004) *The 800 Million Pill: the Truth Behind the Cost of New Drugs*. Berkely and Los Angeles: University of California Press.

Government Communication and Information Service (GCIS) (2003) 'Statement on Special Cabinet Meeting: Enhanced Programme Against HIV and AIDS', Pretoria; URL: http://www.info.gov.za/speeches/2003/03081109461001.htm (8 August 2003).

Gramsci, Antonio (1971) *Selections from the Prison Notebooks*. New York: International Publishers.

Grangeiro, Alexandre (1994) 'O perfil socioeconômico dos casos de Aids na cidade de São Paulo', in R. Parker, C. Bastos, J. Galvão and J.S. Pedrosa (eds), *A Aids no Brasil (1982–1992)*. Rio de Janeiro: Relume-Dumará/Abia/IMS-UERJ: 91–125.

Grangeiro, Alexandre, Teixeira Luciana, Bastos, Francisco I. and Teixeira, Paulo (2006) 'Sustainability of Brazilian Policy for Access to Antiretroviral Drugs', *Revista de Saúde Pública*, No. 4 (Supl.): 1–9. URL: www.scielo.br/scielo.php?script=sci_arttext&pid=S0034-89102006000700009&lng=es&nrm=&tlng=en-61k (10 July 2006).

Grant, Ruth W. and Keohane, Robert O. (2005) 'Accountability and Abuses of Power in World Politics', *American Political Science Review*, Vol. 99 (1), February: 29–43.

Green, Andrew and Matthias, Ann (1997) *Non-Governmental Organizations and Health in Developing Countries*. Basingstoke: Palgrave Macmillan.

Green, Jillian and Smillie, Shaun (2005) 'HIV causes 1 in 3 deaths Gauteng', *The Star*, 17 May 2005; URL: www.iol.co.za (23 November 2005).

Greener, Robert (2002) 'AIDS and Macroeconomic Impact', in Steven Forsythe (ed.), *State of the Art: AIDS and Economics*. Washington; URL: http://www.policyproject.com/pubs/other/SOTAecon.pdf: 49–54 (4 May 2007).

Grill, Bartholomäus (2005) 'Kongos kleines Wirtschaftswunder', *Die Zeit*, 14 July 2005 (No. 29).

Groenewald, Pam and Bradshaw, Debbie (2005) 'Official Death Statistics Under-represent AIDS as a Cause in South Africa', *AIDS Analysis Africa Online*, April/May; URL: http://www.redribbon.co.za/documents_v2/aaa/Aids_Analysis_Africa_Online_April-May_2005.pdf (25 October 2005).

Groenewald, Pam, Nannan, Nadine, Bourne, David, Laubscher, Ria and Bradshaw, Debbie (2005) 'Identifying Deaths from AIDS in South Africa', *AIDS*, No. 19: 193–201.

Gumede, William Mervin (2005) *Thabo Mbeki and the Battle for the Soul of the ANC*. Cape Town: Zebra Press.

Gwatkin, Davidson R. (2000) 'Health Inequalities and the Health of the Poor: What Do We Know?' *Bulletin of the World Health Organisation*, Vol. 78 (1): 3–18.

Haacker, Markus (2004) *The Macroeconomics of HIV/AIDS*. Washington: International Monetary Fund.

Harding, April (2003) 'Introduction to Private Participation in Health Services', in Harding and Preker (eds) (2003): 7–74.

Harding, April and Preker Alexander S. (eds) (2003) *Private Participation in Health Services*. Washington: World Bank.

Harris, Paul G. and Siplon, Patricia (2001) 'International Obligation and Human Health: Evolving Policy Responses to HIV/AIDS', *Ethics & International Affairs*, Vol. 15 (2) (Fall); URL: www.carnegiecouncil.org/printerfriendlymedia.php/prmID/492 (10 July 2006).

Hasenclever, Andreas, Mayer, Peter and Rittberger, Volker (1997) *Theories of International Regimes*. Cambridge: Cambridge University Press.

Haverkort, Bertus, Van Veldhuisen, Laurens and Alders, Carine (1993) 'Networking for Low-external-input and Sustainable Agriculture', in Carine Alders, Bertus Haverkort and Laurens van Veldhuizen (eds), *Linking with Farmers: Networking for Low-External-Input and Sustainable Agriculture*. London: Intermediate Technologies Publications: 3–23.

Health-e (2005) 'Fewer people on medical aid', press release, 16 July 2005; URL: http://www.health-e.org.za/news/article.php?uid=20031278 (27 October 2005).

Hein, Wolfgang (2005) 'Zivilgesellschaft und globale Politik', in Betz and Hein (eds) 2005: 27–56.

Hein, Wolfgang and Kohlmorgen, Lars (eds) (2003) *Globalization, Global Health Governance and National Health Politics in Developing Countries: an Exploration into the Dynamics of Interfaces*, Schriften des Deutschen Übersee-Instituts, 60. Hamburg: German Overseas Institute.

Hein, Wolfgang and Kohlmorgen, Lars (2005) 'Global Health Governance: Conflicts on Global Social Rights', working papers Global and Areas Studies No. 7. Hamburg: German Overseas Institute.

Hein, Wolfgang and Kohlmorgen, Lars (2006) 'Die Vereinten Nationen und globale Gesundheitsgefahren – der Kampf gegen Infektionskrankheiten', in Sabine von Schorlemer (ed.), *Globale Probleme und Zukunftsaufgaben der Vereinten Nationen* (Sonderband der Zeitschrift für Politik). Baden-Baden: Nomos: 129–47.

Heins, Volker (2002) *Weltbürger und Lokalpatrioten. Eine Einführung in das Thema Nichtregierungsorganisationen*. Opladen: Leske + Budrich.

Held, David and Koenig-Archibugi, Mathias (eds) (2005) *Global Governance and Public Accountability*. Oxford: Blackwell.

Held, David and McGrew, Anthony (eds) (2002) *Governing Globalization: Power, Authority and Global Governance*. Cambridge: Polity.

Held, David, McGrew, Anthony, Goldblatt, David and Perraton, Jonathan (1999) *Global Transformations: Politics, Economics and Culture*. Cambridge: Polity.

Helfer, Laurence R. (2004) 'Regime Shifting, the TRIPS Agreement and New Dynamics on International Intellectual Property Lawmaking', *Yale Journal of International Law*, Vol. 29: 1–83.

Hetzel, Dirk (2002) 'Internationale Selbsthilfe am Beispiel AIDS', in Frantz and Zimmer (eds) (2002): 233–53.

Heywood, Mark (2003) 'Preventing Mother-to-Child HIV Transmission in South Africa: Background, Strategies and Outcomes of the Treatment Action Campaign Case Against the Minister of Health', *South African Journal on Human Rights*, Vol. 19 (2): 278–315.

Heywood, Mark (2004) 'The Price of Denial', *Development Update*, Vol. 5 (3): 93–122.

Hickey, Alison, Ndlovu, Nhlanhla and Guthrie, Teresa (2004) 'South Africa', in Teresa Guthrie and Alison Hickey (eds), *Funding the Fight: Budgeting for HIV/AIDS in Developing Countries*. Cape Town: IDASA: 98–177.

Higgott, Richard A., Underhill, Geoffrey and Bieler, Andreas (eds) (2000) *Non State Actors and Authority in the Global System*. London: Routledge.

Hirsch, Joachim (2001) 'Des Staates neue Kleider. NGO im Prozess der Internationalisierung des Staates', in Brand, Demirovic, Görg and Hirsch (eds) (2001): 13–42.

Hoekman, Bernard M. and Kostecki, Michel M. (2001) *The Political Economy of the World Trading System: the WTO and Beyond*. Oxford: Oxford University Press.

't Hoen, Ellen (2002) 'TRIPS, Pharmaceutical Patents and Access to Essential Medicines: a Long Way from Seattle to Doha', *Chicago Journal of International Law*, 3: 27.

Horton, Richard (2002) 'WHO: the Casualties and Compromises of Renewal', *Lancet*, 359: 1605–11.

Huynen, Maud M. T. E., Martens, Pim and Hilderink, Henk B. M. (2005) 'The Health Impacts of Globalization: a Conceptual Framework', *Globalization and Health*, Vol. 1: 14.

IBGE (Istituto Brasileiro de Geografia e Estatistica) (2005) 'Características da População'; URL: http://www.ibge.gov.br/ibgeteen/pesquisas/demograficas.html (15 June 2006).

IBGE (Istituto Brasileiro de Geografia e Estatistica) (2006) 'Acesso e utilização de serviços de saúde 2003'. Comentários; URL: http://www.ibge.com.br/home/estatistica/populacao/trabalhoerendimento/pnad2003/saude/comentario.pdf (15 June 2006).

ICASO (2004) 'NGO Perspectives on the Global Fund'; URL: www.icaso.org/GF-NGO-PerspectivesENG.pdf (15 June 2006).

Ijumba, Petrida, Day, Candy and Ntuli, Antoinette (eds) (2004) *South African Health Review 2003/2004*. Durban: Health Systems Trust; URL: www.hst.org.za/uploads/files/SAHR2003_04_1.pdf (8 April 2005).

Ijumba, Petrida, Poole, Colwyn, George, Gavin and Gray, Andy (2004) 'Access to Antiretroviral Therapy', in Ijumba, Day and Ntuli (eds) (2004): 319–38.

International Federation of Pharmaceutical Manufacturers and Associations (IFPMA) (2004a) 'Research and Development for Neglected Diseases: Lessons Learned and Remaining Challenges'; URL: http://www.ifpma.org/news/publications.aspx (15 August 2006).

International Federation of Pharmaceutical Manufacturers and Associations (IFPMA) (2004b) 'Building Healthier Societies through Partnerships'; URL: www.ifpma.org/news/ publications.aspx (15 August 2006).

ITC (International Trade Centre) (2003) 'Negotiations on Paragraph 6 of the Doha Ministerial Declaration on the TRIPS Agreement and Public Health. Progress

Report – April 2003'. Geneva; URL: www.intracen.org/worldtradenet/docs/information/dohadevagenda/para6trips_may2003%20.pdf (21 June 2006).

Ivanova, Maria (2005) 'Assessing UNEP as Anchor Institution for the Global Environment: Lessons for the UNEO Debate', working paper No. 05/01, Yale Center for Environmental Law & Policy; URL: http://www.yale.edu/gegproject/uneo-wp.pdf (20 September 2006).

Jawara, Fatoumata and Kwa, Aileen (2003) *Behind the Scenes at the WTO: the Real World of International Trade Negotiations*. London: Zed Books.

Jessop, Bob (1999) 'Reflections on Globalization and Its (Il)logic(s)', working paper, Lancaster University; URL: www.lancs.ac.uk/fss/sociology/papers/jessop-reflections-on-globalization.pdf (4 May 2007).

Jessop, Bob (2004) 'Multi-Level Governance and Multi-Level Meta-Governance', in Bache and Flinders (eds) (2004): 49–74.

Johnson, Krista (2004) 'The Politics of AIDS Policy Development and Implementation in Postapartheid South Africa', *Africa Today*, Vol. 51 (2): 107–28.

Kaasch, Alexandra M. (2006) 'Actors and Opinions in Global Health Policy – Who Has Got the Say?', paper prepared for the 16th ISA World Congress of Sociology, Durban, South Africa, 23–29 July.

Kaldor, Mary (2003) *Global Civil Society: an Answer to War*. Cambridge: Polity Press.

Karns, Margaret P. and Mingst, Karen A. (2004) *International Organizations: the Politics and Processes of Global Governance*. Boulder, CO: Lynne Rienner.

Kaul, Inge and Conceição, Pedro (eds) (2006) *The New Public Finance: Responding to Global Challenges*. New York and Oxford: Oxford University Press.

Kaul, Inge, Conceição, Pedro, Le Goulven, Katell and Mendoza, Ronald U. (eds) (2003) *Providing Global Public Goods: Managing Globalization*. New York and Oxford: Oxford University Press.

Kaul, Inge, Grunberg, Isabelle and Stern, Marc A. (eds) (1999) *Global Public Goods: International Cooperation in the 21st Century*. New York and Oxford: Oxford University Press.

Keane, John (2003) *Global Civil Society?* Cambridge: Cambridge University Press.

Keck, Margaret E. and Sikkink, Kathryn (1998) *Activists Beyond Borders: Advocacy Networks in International Politics*. Ithaca: Cornell University Press.

Keene, Edward (2002) *Beyond the Anarchical Society: Grotius, Colonialism and Order in World Politics*. Cambridge: Cambridge University Press.

Keohane, Robert (2002) 'Governance in a Partially Globalized World', in Held and McGrew (eds) (2002): 325–47.

Keohane, Robert (2003) 'Global Governance and Democratic Accountability', in David Held and Mathias Koenig-Archibugi (eds), *Taming Globalization: Frontiers of Governance*. Cambridge: Polity Press: 130–59.

Keohane, Robert and Martin, Lisa (1999) 'Institutional Theory, Endogeneity, and Delegation'; URL: http://www.people.fas.harvard.edu/~llmartin/LAKPAP.html (15 August 2006).

Kickbusch, Ilona (2003) 'Global Health Governance: Some New Theoretical Considerations on the new Political Space', in Kelley Lee (ed.), *Globalization and Health: an Introduction*. Basingstoke: Palgrave Macmillan: 192–203.

Kickbusch, Ilona (2005) 'Action on Global Health: Addressing Global Health Governance Challenges', *Public Health*, Vol. 119 (11), November: 969–73.

Kickbusch, Ilona and Lister, Graham (eds) (2006) *European Perspectives on Global Health: a Policy Glossary*. Brussels: European Foundation Centre.

Koenig-Archibugi, Mathias (2002) 'Mapping Global Governance', in Held and McGrew (eds) (2002): 46–69.

Koenig-Archibugi, M. and Zürn, Michael (eds) (2006) *New Modes of Governance in the Global System*. Basingstoke: Palgrave Macmillan.

Kohlmorgen, Lars (2004) 'Global Health Governance und UNAIDS – Elemente eines globalen Integrationsmodus?', *Peripherie*, 24 (93/94): 139–65.

Kohlmorgen, Lars (2005) 'Global Governance und Internationale Sozialpolitik', in Maria Behrens (Hg.), *Globalisierung als politische Herausforderung. Global Governance zwischen Utopie und Realität*. Opladen: VS-Verlag: 293–312.

Koivusalo, Meri (2003) 'Global Governance, Trade and Health Policy', in Hein and Kohlmorgen (eds) (2003): 203–24.

Koivusalo, Meri and Ollila, Eeva (1997) *Making a Healthy World: Agencies, Actors and Policies in International Health*. London and New York: Zed.

Kooiman, Jan (2003) *Governing as Governance*. London: Sage.

Kühl, Henrik (2002) *TRIPS and AIDS in South Africa: New Actors in International Relations: Weighing Patents, Pills and Patients*. Los Angeles: Occidental College.

Lachenmann, Gudrun (2003) 'Globalisation and Localisation of Health Care in Poor Countries in Africa', in Hein and Kohlmorgen (eds) (2003) 305–14.

Lanoszka, Anna (2003) 'The Global Politics of Intellectual Property Rights and Pharmaceutical Drugs Policies in Developing Countries', *International Political Science Review*, Vol. 24 (2): 181–97.

Lee, Chinyelu, Brewster-Lee, Dorothy, Devine, Brenda and Bingham, Gail (2003) *Global Fund Responsiveness to Faith Based Organizations*. Christian Connections for International Health and Ecumenical Pharmaceutical Network; URL: www.e-alliance.ch/resources/documents/word/Global%20Fund%responsiveness.doc (16 February 2007).

Lee, Kelley (2003a) *Globalization and Health: an Introduction*. Basingstoke: Palgrave Macmillan.

Lee, Kelley (ed.) (2003b) *Health Impacts of Globalization: Towards Global Governance*. Basingstoke: Palgrave Macmillan.

Lee, Kelley (2004) 'The Pit and the Pendulum. Can Globalization Take Health Governance Forward?' *Development*, Vol. 47 (2): 11–17.

Lee, Kelley, Buse, Kent and Fustukian, Suzanne (eds) (2002) *Health Policy in a Globalising World*. Cambridge: Cambridge University Press.

Lee, Kelley and Collin, Jeff (eds) (2005) *Global Change and Health*. Milton Keynes: Open University Press.

Lee, Kelley, Collinson, Sue, Walt, Gill and Gilson, Lucy (1996) 'Who Should be Doing What in International Health: a Confusion of Mandates in the United Nations', *British Medical Journal*, 312: 302–7.

Lima, Nísia Trindade (2002) 'O Brasil e a Organização Pan-Americana da Saúde: Uma História em Três Dimensões', in Jacobo Finkelman (ed.), *Caminhos da Saúde Pública no Brasil*. Rio de Janeiro: Fiocruz: 23–116.

Lindenberg, Marc and Bryant, Coralie (2001) *Going Global: Transforming Relief and Development NGOs*. Bloomfield: Kumarian Press.

Lobato, Lenaura (2000) 'Reorganizing the Health Care System in Brazil', in Sonia Fleury, Susana Belmartino and Enis Baris (eds), *Reshaping Health Care in Latin America: a Comparative Analysis of Health Care Reform in Argentina, Brazil, and Mexico*. Ottawa: International Development Center: 103–32.

Lobato, Lenaura and Burlandy, Luciene (2000) 'The Context and Process of Health Care Reform in Brazil', in Sonia Fleury, Susana Belmartino and Enis Baris (eds),

Reshaping Health Care in Latin America: a Comparative Analysis of Health Care Reform in Argentina, Brazil, and Mexico. Ottawa: International Development Center: 225–62.

Loewenson, René (2003) 'Civil Society–State Interactions in National Health Systems. Annoted Bibliography on Civil Society and Health, Part 2'; URL: http://www.tarsc.org/WHOCSI/pdf/WHOTARSC2.pdf (23 August 2004).

Long, Norman (1989) *Encounters at the Interface*. Wageningen: Wageningen Studies in Sociology.

Long, Norman (1993) 'Handlung, Struktur und Schnittstelle: Theoretische Reflektionen', in Thomas Bierschenk and Georg Elwert (eds), *Entwicklungshilfe und ihre Folgen: Ergebnisse von Untersuchungen in Afrika*. Frankfurt/New York: Campus Verlag.

Long, Norman (2001) *Development Sociology: Actor Perspectives*, London: Routledge Chapman & Hall.

Loughlin, Kelly and Berridge, Virginia (2002) *Global Health Governance: Historical Dimensions of Global Governance*, (Centre on Global Change and Health, LSHTM/Department of Health & Development, WHO, Discussion Paper No. 2. Geneva/London: WHO/LSHTM.

LSHTM (2003) *Tracking the Global Fund in Four Countries: an Interim Report*. London: LSHTM.

Lucas, Adetokunbo (2002) 'Public–Private Partnerships: Illustrative Examples', in Reich (ed.) (2002): 19–39.

Lurie, Peter, Hintzen, Percy and Lowe, Robert (1995) 'Socioeconomic Obstacles to HIV Prevention and Treatment in Developing Countries: the Roles of the International Monetary Fund and the World Bank', *AIDS*, No. 9: 539–46.

Mackintosh, Maureen and Koivusalo, Meri (2005) *Commercialization of Health Care: Global and Local Dynamics and Policy Responses*. Basingstoke: Palgrave Macmillan.

Mail & Guardian (2003) 'Social Movements: "Ultra-Left" or "Global Citizens"?', *Mail & Guardian*, 4 February; URL: www.mg.co.za (5 April 2005).

Mail & Guardian (2005a) 'IFP Leader Speaks Out on Aids', *Mail & Guardian*, 9 February 2003; URL: www.mg.co.za (8 April 2004).

Mail & Guardian (2005b) 'Bush Accused of Aids Damage in Africa', *Mail & Guardian*, 9 February 2005, URL: www.mg.co.za (8 April 2005).

Mail & Guardian (2005c) 'Official Nod for Voodoo Trials?' *Mail & Guardian*, 28 October 2005; URL: www.mg.co.za (30 October 2005).

Mail & Guardian (2005d) 'Major LoveLife Funder Pulls the Plug', *Mail & Guardian*, 21 December 2005; URL: www.mg.co.za (10 March 2006).

Mail & Guardian Online (2006) 'TAC Turns the Screws on Manto', *Mail & Guardian*, 4 September 2006; URL: www.mg.co.za (4 September 2006).

Marais, Hein (2000) *To the Edge: AIDS Review 2000*. Pretoria: Centre for the Study of AIDS, University of Pretoria.

Marais, Hein (2005) *Buckling: the Impact of AIDS in South Africa*, Pretoria: Centre for the Study of AIDS, University of Pretoria.

March, James and Olsen, Johan P. (1989) *Rediscovering Institutions: the Organizational Basis of Politics*. New York: Free Press.

Marks, Gary (1993) 'Structural Policy and Multilevel Governance in the EC', in Alan Cafruny and Glenda Rosenthal (eds), *The State of the European Community*, Vol. 2. Boulder: Lynne Rienner: 391–410.

Marks, Gary and Hooghe, Liesbet (2004) 'Contrasting Visions of Multi-Level Governance', in Bache and Flinders (eds) (2004): 15–30.

Marques, Marília Bernardes (2002) *Acessibilidade aos medicamentos. O desafio de vincular ciência, tecnologia, inovação e saúde no Brasil*. Brasília: Centro de Gestão e Estudos Estratégicos.

Martens, Kerstin (2002) 'Alte und neue Players – Eine Begriffsbestimmung', in Frantz and Zimmer (eds) (2002): 25–50.

Maskus, Keith (2000) *Intellectual Property Rights in the Global Economy*. Washington, DC: Institute for International Economics.

Mathai, Rabia and Galbraith, John (2004) 'Faith-based Leadership in Effective HIV/AIDS Program Delivery: Improving Access to Treatment through Church Health Institutions and Parish Networks in Africa, India and the Caribbean', International AIDS Conference, 11–16 July: 15; URL: gateway.nlm.nih.gov/MeetingAbstracts/102280571.html (4 May 2007).

Mayne, Ruth (2002) 'The Global Campaign on Patents and Access to Medicines: an Oxfam Perspective', in Drahos and Mayne (eds) (2002) 244–58.

Mayntz, Renate (2005) 'Governance Theory als fortentwickelte Steuerungstheorie?' in Gunnar Folker Schuppert (ed.), *Governance-Forschung. Vergewisserung über Stand und Entwicklungslinien*. Baden-Baden: Nomos: 11–20.

Mayntz, Renate and Scharpf, Fritz W. (ed.) (1995) *Gesellschaftliche Selbstregelung und politische Steuerung*. Frankfurt/Main: Campus.

Mbali, Mandisa (2002a) 'Mbeki's Denialism and the Ghost of Apartheid and Colonialism for Post-apartheid AIDS Policy-Making', *Public Health Journal Club Seminar Paper*, Durban.

Mbali, Mandisa (2002b) 'Mbeki's Bizarre AIDS Theories', *Mail & Guardian*, 21 March 2002; URL: www.mg.co.za (8 April 2005).

Mbali, Mandisa (2005) 'The Treatment Action Campaign's Strategies to Government AIDS Policy in South Africa', research paper commissioned by the Global Health Governance Project of the German Overseas Institute; URL: http://www.duei.de/ghg/pdf/ProjectMbali4.pdf (27 August 2005).

Mbeki, Thabo (1999) Address of the President of South Africa, Thabo Mbeki, at the National Council of Provinces, Cape Town, 28 October; URL: http://www.gov.za (27 August 2005).

Mbeki, Thabo (2000) Letter to World Leaders, 3 April 2000; URL: http://www.virusmyth.net/aids/news/lettermbeki.htm (27 August 2005).

McKee, Martin, Garner, Paul and Stott, Robin (eds) (2001) *International Co-Operation in Health*. Oxford: Oxford University Press.

Médecins Sans Frontières (MSF) (2000) 'Hidden Price Tags: Disease-Specific Drug Donations: Costs and Alternatives', DND Working Group Expert Paper; URL: http://www.accessmed-msf.org/prod/publications.asp?scntid=2092002185426&contenttype=PARA& (20 December 2006).

Médecins Sans Frontières (MSF) (2003) 'Providing HIV Services Including Antiretroviral Therapy at Primary Health Care Clinics in Resource-Poor Settings: the Experience from Khayelitsha', in *Activity Report*; URL: http://www.hst.org.za/uploads/files/khayelitsha03.pdf (25 August 2005).

Médecins Sans Frontières (MSF) (2004) 'Untangling the Web of Price Reductions: a Pricing Guide for the Purchase of ARVs for Developing Countries', 6th edition, 19 April; URL: www.accessmed-msf.org (23 June 2006).

Médecins Sans Frontières (MSF) (2005) 'Untangling the Web of Price Reductions: a Pricing Guide for the Purchase of ARVs for Developing Countries', 8th edition, June; URL: www.accessmed-msf.org (22 June 2006).

Medici, André (1994) 'Impactos Socioeconômicos da AIDS', in Richard Parker, Cristiana Bastos, Jane Galvão and José Stalin Pedrosa (eds), *A AIDS no Brasil*. Rio de Janeiro: ABIA/ Instituto de Medicina Social, Universidade do Estado do Rio de Janeiro: 325–9.

Medici, André (2002) 'Financing Health Policies in Brazil: Achievements, Challenges and Proposals'; URL: http://www.undp.org/povertycentre/publications/health/FinancingHealthPoliciesBrazil_IADB.pdf (27 August 2005).

Medicus Mundi International (1999) 'Contracting NGOs for Health', MMI Report; URL: http://www.medicusmundi.org/Kampala2004/02.doc (23 August 2004).

Mendes, Eugênio Vilaça (1996) 'O Sistema Único de Saúde – um Processo Social em Construção', CADRHU (Rede Colaborativa para Capacitação de Especialistas em Recursos Humanos para o Sistema Único de Saúde); URL: www.opas.org.br/rh/publicacoes/ textos_apoio/pub04U1T1. pdf (27 May 2005): 45–64.

Mercadante, Otávio Azevedo (coord.) (2002) 'Evolução das Políticas e do Sistema de Saúde no Brasil'; in Jacobo Finkelman (ed.), *Caminhos da Saúde Pública no Brasil*. Rio de Janeiro: Fiocruz: 235–313.

MIHR (The Centre for Management of IP in Health R&D) (2005) 'Innovation in Developing Countries to Meet Health Needs Experiences of China, Brazil, South Africa and India', an overview report to the Commission on Intellectual Property Rights, Innovation and Public Health; URL: http://www.who.int/intellectualproperty/studies/ (20 December 2006).

Mills, Anne (2001) 'Technology and Science as Global Public Goods: Tackling Priority Diseases of Poor Countries'; URL: http://wbln0018.worldbank.org/eurvp/web.nsf/Pages/Mills/$File/MILLS.pdf (9 January 2006).

Mills, Anne and Broomberg, Jonathan (1998) 'Experiences of Contracting: an Overview of the Literature', WHO Macroeconomics, Health and Development Series, Technical Paper No. 33; URL: http://whqlibdoc.who.int/hq/1998/WHO_ICO_MESD_33.pdf (23 August 2004).

Ministério da Saúde (1999) Chapters 'AIDS e Pauperização' and 'Resposta/Gestão e Avaliação'. Brasília, Secretaria de Políticas de Saúde. Coordenação Nacional de Doenças Sexualmente Transmissíveis e AIDS. Brasília.

Ministério da Saúde (2003) O Perfil da AIDS no Brasil e Metas de Governo para o Controle da Epidemia. Sobre a Epidemia de AIDS. Características do Programa Brasiliero e o Resultado dos 20 anos de Luta contra a AIDS; URL: http://www.aids.gov.br/final/biblioteca/metas/metas.pdf (11 September 2006).

Ministério da Saúde (2004a) Response Magazine, Secretaria de Vigilância em Saúde/Programa Nacional de DST e AIDS, Brasília.

Ministério da Saúde (2004b) Monitoraids 2004: Sistema de Monitoramento de Indicadores do Programa Nacional de DST e AIDS. Edited by Ministério da Saúde 2004: Version 1.0. December, Brasília.

Ministério da Saúde (2005a) *Boletim Epidemiológico AIDS-DST*, Year II, No. 1, January–June 2005, November, Brasília.

Ministério da Saúde (2005b) Plano Estratégico. Programa Nacional de DST e AIDS 2005. Secretaria de Vigilância em Saúde. Programa Nacional de DST e AIDS. Brasília, March.

Ministério da Saúde (2006) Monitoraids; URL: http://157.86.8.200/abrir.asp?valor = 79 (11 September 2006).

Ministério da Saúde/Secretaria de Vigilância em Saúde/Programa Nacional de DST e AIDS (2005) (March) *Boletim Epidemiológico AIDS-DST*, Year I, No. 01, January–June 2004, Brasília, March.

Ministério da Saúde/Secretaria de Vigilância em Saúde/Programa Nacional de DST e AIDS (2005) (Nov.) *Boletim Epidemiológico AIDS-DST*, Year II, No. 01, January–June 2005, Brasília, November.

Monitoraids (2004) *Sistema de Monitoramento de Indicadores do Programa Nacional de DST e AIDS*. Edited by Ministério da Saúde. Version 1.0. Brasília, December 2004.

Moran, Mary, Ropare, Anne-Laure, Guzman, Javier, Diaz, José and Garrison, Christopher (2005) *The New Landscape of Neglected Disease Drug Development*. London: London School of Economic and Political Science.

MSF: see Médecins Sans Frontières.

Murray, Christopher J. L. (2005) 'The Role of WHO as an Anchor Institution for Communicable Disease Global Public Goods', paper prepared for the International Task Force on Global Public Goods; URL: www.gpgtaskforce.org/uploads/files/124.doc (20 December 2006).

Nattrass, Nicoli (2004) *The Moral Economy of AIDS in South Africa*. Cambridge: Cambridge University Press.

Ndlovu, Nhlanhla (2005) 'An Exploratory Analysis of HIV and AIDS Donor Funding in South Africa', *Budget Brief*, No. 155, Cape Town: IDASA.

Neukirchen, Heidi (2004) *Der Pharma Report. Das große Geschäft mit unserer Gesundheit*. Muenchen: Droemer.

NIC (2000) *The Global Infectious Disease Threat and Its Implications for the United States*. Washington: National Intelligence Council.

NIC (2002) *The Next Wave of HIV/AIDS: Nigeria, Ethiopia, Russia, India, and China*. Washington: National Intelligence Council.

Noehrenberg, Eric (2006) 'Report of the Commission on Intellectual Property Rights, Innovation and Public Health: an Industry Perspective', *Bulletin of the World Health Organization*, May, Vol. 84 (5): 419–20.

O'Brien, Robert, Goetz, Anne Marie, Scholte, Jan Aart and Williams, Marc (2000) *Contesting Global Governance. Multilateral Economic Institutions and Global Social Movements*. Cambridge: Cambridge University Press.

OECD/UNAIDS (2004) 'Analysis of Aid in Support of HIV/AIDS Control'. Paris: Organisation for Economic Cooperation and Development (OECD)/UNAIDS; URL: http://www.oecd.org/dataoecd/57/60/32159448.pdf (24 August 2005).

Office of the President (2004) President's International Investment Council, 18–20 June, Press Release, Cape Town; URL: http://www.dfa.gov.za/docs/2004/iic0617.htm (10 November 2005).

Oliveira, Maria Auxiliadora and Esher, Angela (2004) 'Acesso Universal ao Tratamento para as Pessoas Vivendo com HIV e AIDS no Brasil', in Jorge Bermudez, Maria A. Oliveira, Do Couto Fernandes and Angela Esher (eds), *Acceso a Medicamentos: Derecho Fundamental, Papel del Estrado*. Rio de Janeiro: Escola Nacional de Saúde Pública: 233–50.

Oliveira, Maria Auxiliadora, Santos, Elizabeth Moreira dos and Mello, José Manoel Carvalho (2001) 'Aids, ativismo e regulação de ensaios clínicos no Brasil: o Protocolo 028', *Cadernos de Saúde Pública*, Rio de Janeiro, 17 (4): 863–75.

Ollila, Eeva (2003) *Global Health-Related Public–Private Partnerships and the UN*, GASPP Policy Brief No. 2; URL: http://gaspp.stakes.fi/EN/publications/policy-briefs (20 December 2006).

OPAS (Organização Panamericana da Saúde) (2005) 'Brasil – O Perfil do Sistema de Serviços de Saúde'; URL: www.lachsr.org/documents/healthsystemprofileofbrazil-EN.pdf:1–38 Also at: http://www.opas.org.br/servico/arquivos/Sala5515.doc (20 December 2006).

Ostergard, Robert L. (2002) 'Politics in the Hot Zone: AIDS and National Security in Africa', *Third World Quarterly*, Vol. 23: 333–50.

Ostergard, Robert L. (2004) 'Politics in the Hot Zone: AIDS and National Security in Africa', in Poku and Whiteside (eds) (2004): 143–60.

Ougaard, Morten (1999) *Approaching the Global Polity*. CSGR Working Paper No. 42/99. University of Warwick, Coventry.

Ougaard, Morten and Higgott, Richard (Hg.) (2002) *Towards a Global Polity*. London: Routledge Chapman & Hall.

Oxfam (2002a) *Beyond Philanthropy: the Pharmaceutical Industry, Corporate Social Responsibility and the Developing World*; URL: http://publications.oxfam.org.uk (20 December 2006).

Oxfam (2002b) *False Hope or New Start? The Global Fund to Fight HIV/AIDS, TB and Malaria*, Oxfam Briefing Paper No. 24.

Oxfam (2002c) *US Bullying on Drug Patents: One Year after Doha*. Washington, DC (Oxfam Briefing Paper No. 33).

PAHO (Pan American Health Organization) (1992) 'Regional Program on HIV/AIDS', *Epidemiological Bulletin*, Vol. 13 (1): 1–8.

Paiva, Vera (2003) 'Beyond Magic Solutions: Prevention of HIV and AIDS as a Process of Psychosocial Emancipation', in *Divulgação em Saúde para Debate*, No. 27, August Rio de Janeiro: 192–203.

Parker, Richard (ed.) (1997) *Políticas, Instituições e Aids. Enfrentando a Epidemia no Brasil*. Rio de Janeiro: Zahar/ABIA.

Parker, Richard (2003) 'Building the Foundations for the Response to HIV/AIDS in Brazil: the Development of HIV/AIDS Policy, 1982–1996', in *Divulgação em Saúde para Debate*, No. 27. Rio de Janeiro: Rede Unida: 143–83.

Parker, Richard and Terto Jr., Veriano (eds) (2001) *A ABIA na Virada do Milênio*. Rio de Janeiro: ABIA.

Parker, Richard, de Mattos, Ruben Araújo and Terto Jr., Veriano (2001) 'As estratégias do Banco Mundial e a resposta à AIDS no Brasil 2001', in Flávia Barros (ed.), *As estratégias dos bancos multilaterais para o Brasil (2000–2003). Rede Brasil sobre Instituições Financeiras Multilaterais*. Brasília: Rede Brasil: 107–30.

Parry, Sue (2003) *Responses of the Faith-Based. Organisations to HIV/AIDS in Sub Saharan Africa*. Geneva: World Council of Churches.

Passarelli, Carlos and Terto Jr., Veriano (2003) 'Non-Governmental Organizations and Access to Antiretroviral Treatments in Brazil', in *Divulgação em Saúde para Debate*, No. 27. Rio de Janeiro: Rede Unida: 252–64.

Paton, Carol (1998) 'Save our babies, Dr Zuma', *Sunday Times*, 11 October; URL: http://www.sundaytimes.co.za (24 August 2005).

Pawinski, Robert and Lalloo, Umesh (2002) 'Throwing a Lifeboat to the *Titanic*: the Global Fund and HIV in South Africa and KwaZulu-Natal', in *Aids Analysis Africa*; URL: http://www.redribbon.co.za/learn/user_page.asp?page_number = 2985&prev_page = 2938 (10 November 2005).

Pearson, Mark (2004) 'Economic and Financial Impacts of the Global Health Partnerships', DFID/GHP Study Paper 2. London.

Perlmutter, Howard V. (1972) 'The Multinational Firm and the Future', *The Annals of the American Academy of Political and Social Sciences*, 403: 139–52.

Peterson, Susan (2002) 'Epidemic Disease and National Security', *Security Studies*, Vol. 12 (2): 43–81.

Piola, Sérgio F. and Biasoto, J. G. (2001) 'Financiamento do SUS nos anos 90', in Barjas Negri and G. de Giovanni (eds), *Brasil Radiografia da Saúde*. Campinas: Unicamp: 219–32.

Piola, Sérgio, Teixeira, Luciana and Joel Sadi Dutra Nunes (2002) 'Flujos de financiamiento y gasto en VIH/SIDA: Brasil 1999–2000'; URL: www.sidalac.org.mx//pu/cnacionales99-00/brasil/brasil.pdf (5 June 2006).

Poku, Nana K. and Whiteside, Alan (eds) (2004) *Global Health and Governance: HIV/AIDS*. Basingstoke: Palgrave Macmillan.

Prins, Gwyn (2004) 'AIDS and Global Security', *International Affairs*, Vol. 80 (5): 931–52.

Putzel, James (2004) 'The Global Fight against AIDS: How Adequate are the National Commissions?', *Journal of International Development*, Vol. 16 (8): 1129–40.

Quinlan, Tim and Willan, Samantha (2004) 'HIV/AIDS: Finding Ways to Contain the Pandemic', in John Daniel, Roger Southall and Jessica Lutchman (eds), *State of the Nation: South Africa 2004–2005*. Pretoria: Human Science Research Council Press: 227–51.

Rawls, John (1971) *A Theory of Justice*. Boston: The Belknap Press of Harvard University Press.

Rehle, Thomas M. and Shisana, Olive (2003) 'Epidemiological and Demographic HIV/AIDS Projections: South Africa', *African Journal of AIDS Research*, Vol. 2 (1): 1–8.

Reich, Michael R. (2002) *Public–Private Partnerships for Public Health*. Cambridge, MA: Harvard University Press.

Reinicke, Wolfgang, Deng, Francis, Benner, Thorsten and Witte, Martin (2000) *Critical Choices: the United Nations, Networks, and the Future of Global Governance*. Ottawa: IDRC.

Reuter, Herman (2001) 'Affidavit on Behalf of the Treatment Action Campaign: Herman Reuter'; URL: http://www.tac.org.za (10 November 2005).

Reynolds, Steven J., Bartlett, John G., Quinn, Thomas C., Beyrer, Chris and Bollinger, Robert C. (2003) 'Antiretroviral Therapy Where Resources are Limited', *The New England Journal of Medicine*, Vol. 348 (18): 1806–9.

Rich, Jennifer L. (2001) 'Brazil will Defy Patent on HIV/AIDS Drug Made by Roche', *New York Times*, 23 August.

Richter, Judith (2003) '"We the Peoples" or "We the Corporations"? Critical Reflections on UN-Business "partnerships"', Geneva: IBFAN-GIFA.

Richter, Judith (2004) *Public–Private Partnerships and Health for All: How Can WHO Safeguard Public Interests?* GASPP Policy Brief No. 5; URL: http://gaspp.stakes.fi/EN/publications/policybriefs/index.htm (20 December 2006).

Risi Junior, João Baptista and Nogueira, Roberto Passos (2002) 'As Condições de Saúde no Brasil', in Jacobo Finkelman (ed.), *Caminhos da Saúde Pública no Brasil*. Rio de Janeiro: Fiocruz: 117–234.

Risse, Thomas (2000) '"Let's Argue!": Communicative Action in World Politics', *International Organization*, Vol. 54 (1): 1–39.

Risse, Thomas (2002) 'Constructivism and International Institutions: Toward Conservations across Paradigms', in Ira Katznelson and Helen V. Milner (eds), *Political Science: State of the Discipline*. New York: Norton: 597–623.

Risse, Thomas (2004) 'Transnational Governance and Legitimacy', paper presented at ECPR Standing Group on International Relations Conference, The Hague, 9–12 September.

Rittberger, Volker (ed.) (2002) *Global Governance and the United Nations System*. Tokyo, New York, Paris: UNUP: 1–47.

Rittberger, Volker and Zangl, Bernhard (2006) *International Organization: Polity, Politics and Policies*. Basingstoke: Palgrave Macmillan.

Robinson, Mark (1997) 'Privatising the Voluntary Sector: NGOs as Public Service Contractors?' in Hulme and Edwards (eds) (1997): 59–78.

Roche (2001) Roche and the Brazilian Ministry of Health Reach Agreement for Supply of HIV Drug Viracept. Roche Corporate Media News; URL: http://www.roche.com/media-news-2001-08-31-e.pdf (4 May 2007).

Rosenau, James N. (1997) *Along the Domestic-Foreign Frontier: Exploring Governance in a Turbulent World*. Cambridge: Cambridge University Press.

Rosenau, James N. (2002) 'Governance in a New Global Order', in Held and McGrew (eds) (2002): 70–86.

Rosenau, James N. (2004) 'Strong Demand, Huge Supply: Governance in an Emerging Epoch', in Bache and Flinders (eds) (2004): 31–48.

Ruger, Jennifer Prah (2005) 'The Changing Role of the World Bank in Global Health', *American Journal of Public Health*, Vol 95 (1): 50–70.

Ruger, Jennifer Prah and Yach, Derek (2005) 'Global Functions at the World Health Organization', *British Medical Journal*, Vol. 330: 1099–1100.

Russell, Bev and Swilling, Mark (2002) 'The Size and Scope of the Non-Profit Sector in South Africa', Johannesburg: School for Public and Development Management, University of the Witwatersrand; URL: http://www.nu.ac.za/ccs/files/jhu%20study.pdf (3 February 2006).

Salamon, Lester and Anheier, Helmut (eds) (1997) *Defining the Nonprofit Sector: a Cross-National Analysis*. Manchester: Manchester University Press.

Salamon, Lester, Anheier, Helmut K., List, Regina, Toepler, Stefan, Sokolowski, S. Wojciech and Associates (1999) *Global Civil Society: Dimensions of the Nonprofit Sector*. Baltimore: Johns Hopkins Comparative Nonprofit Sector Project.

Samuels, David (2006) 'Sources of Mass Partisanship in Brazil', *Latin American Politics and Society*, Vol. 48 (2), Summer: 1–27.

Sanders, David (2003) 'Twenty-five Years of Primary Health Care: Lessons Learned and Proposals for Revitalisation', paper prepared for People's Health Movement Meeting Geneva; URL: http://www.asksource.info/rtf/phc–sanders.rtf (20 December 2006).

Sangmeister, Hartmut (1992) 'Brasilien', in Dieter Nohlen and Franz Nuscheler (eds), *Handbuch der Dritten Welt. Südamerika*, 3rd edn. Bonn: 219–76.

Scharpf, Fritz W. (1997) *Games Real Actors Play: Actor-Centered Institutionalism in Policy Research*. Oxford: Westview Press.

Scharpf, Fritz W. (1999) *Governing in Europe: Effective and Democratic?* Oxford: Oxford University Press.

Scheffer, Mario, Lazzarini, Salayzar Andrea and Bozola Grou, Karina (2005) 'O Remédio Via Justiça. Um Estudo sobre o Acesso a Novos Medicamentos e Exames em HIV/AIDS no Brasil por meio de Ações Judiciais', Série Legislação

No. 3. Bralília: Ministério da Saúde/Vigilância em Saúde/Programa Nacional de DST e AIDS.

Schneider, Helen (2001) 'A Struggle for Symbolic Power', *Siyaya Magazine*, Vol. 8 (Winter): 18–21.

Schneider, Helen (2002) 'On the Fault Line: the Politics of AIDS Policy in Contemporary South Africa', *African Studies*, Vol. 61 (1): 145–67.

Schneider, Helen and Gilson, Lucy (1999) 'Small Fish in a Big Pond? External Aid and the Health Sector in South Africa', *Health Policy and Planning*, Vol. 14 (3): 264–72.

Scholte, Jan Aart (2000) *Globalization: a Critical Introduction*. Basingstoke and New York: Palgrave Macmillan.

Schultz, Mark and Walker David (2005) 'How Intellectual Property Became Controversial: NGOs and the New International IP Agenda', *Engage*, Vol. 6 (1): 82–98.

Seiter, Andreas (2005a) 'Pharmaceuticals, Counterfeits, Substandard Drugs and Drug Diversion', HNP Briefing Paper 2, Washington, DC: World Bank.

Seiter, Andreas (2005b) 'Pharmaceuticals: Quality Assurance in the Distribution Chain', HNP Briefing Paper 6. Washington, DC: World Bank.

Sell, Susan K. (2000) 'Structures, Agents and Institutions, Private Corporate Power and the Globalization of Intellectual Property Rights', in Richard Higgot (ed.), *Non-State Actors in the Global System*. London: Routledge: 91–106.

Sell, Susan K. (2002) 'TRIPS and the Access to Medicines Campaign', *Wisconsin International Law Journal*, Vol. 20 (3): 481–522.

Sell, Susan K. (2006) 'HIV/AIDS Drugs: the Politics of Access', paper prepared for workshop on 'The Policy and Politics of HIV/AIDS'. Princeton University, 5 May; URL: http://www.wws.princeton.edu/pai/SSell%20HIV%20AIDS%20 Drugs.doc (12 August 2006).

Sell, Susan K. and Prakash, Aseem (2004) 'Using Ideas Strategically: the Contest Between Business and NGO Networks in Intellectual Property Rights', *International Studies Quarterly*, Vol. 48: 143–75.

Senado Federal (2003) *Constituição da República Federativa do Brasil*. Brasília: Subsecretaria de Edições Técnicas.

Senn, Stephen (1996) 'Some Statistical Issues in Project Prioritization in the Pharmaceutical Industry', *Statistics in Medicine*, Vol. 15 (24): 2689–702.

Serra, José (2004) 'The Political Economy of the Brazilian Struggle Against AIDS', Paper Number 17: Institute for Advanced Study Friends Forum. Princeton University, April: 1–20.

Sexton, Sarah (2001) 'Trading Health Care Away? GATS, Public Services and Privatization', The Corner House Briefing 23, Dorset, UK; URL: www.thecorner-house.org.uk/ pdf/briefing/23gats.pdf (24 June 2006).

Shakow, Alexander (2005) 'Review of GPG Lead Institutions', paper prepared for the Secretariat of the Independent Task Force on Global Public Goods; URL: http://www.gpgtaskforce.org/uploads/files/137.doc (24 June 2006).

Shisana, Olive and Simbayi, Leickness (2002) *Nelson Mandela/HSRC Study on HIV/AIDS: South African National HIV Prevalence, Behavioural Risks and Mass Media Household Survey 2002*. Cape Town: Human Sciences Research Council.

Shretta, R., Brugha R., Robb, A. and Snow, R.W. (2000) 'Sustainability, Affordability and Equity of Corporate Drug Donations: the Case of Malarone', *Lancet*, 355: 1718–20.

Silva, Alex Giacomelli da (2005) 'Poder Inteligente – A questão do HIV/AIDS na Política Externa Brasileira', *Contexto Internacional*, Rio de Janeiro, Vol. 27 (1), Jan.–June: 127–58.

Slack, Katherine and Savedoff, William D. (2001) *Public–Private Provider Contracting for Health Services. Examples from Latin America and the Carribbean*. Washington DC: World Bank.

Smart, Theo (2005) 'Revisions to India's Patent Law Could Affect Future Supply of Affordable Generic Antiretrovirals', *Aidsmap News*, 30 March; URL: http://nam.org.uk/en/news/B37B595E-09B6-4499-A93E-9766C0F21AE8.asp (28 June 2006).

Smith, Richard, Beaglehole, Robert, Woodward, David and Drager, Nick (eds) (2003) *Global Public Goods for Health: Health, Economic, and Public Health Perspectives*. Oxford: Oxford University Press.

Söderholm, Peter (1997) *Global Governance of AIDS: Partnerships with Civil Society*. Lund: Lund University Press.

von Soest, Christian and Calcagnotto, Gilberto (2006) 'Between Conflict and Cooperation, Global–National Interfaces and the Fight against HIV/AIDS in Brazil and South Africa', paper presented at the GIGA/WHO workshop 'Defining and Shaping the Architecture for Global Health Governance', 22–24 February, Hamburg.

Spink, Mary Jane Paris (2003) 'A Comissão Nacional de AIDS: A Presença do Passado na Construção do Futuro', Coleção DST/AIDS – Série Programa Nacional No. 9. Brasília:Ministério da Saúde/Programa Nacional de DST/AIDS.

Statistics South Africa (2005a) 'Mortality and Causes of Death in South Africa, 1997–2003: Findings from Death Notification', Report; URL: http://www.statssa.gov.za/Publications/P03093/P03093.pdf (24 August 2005).

Statistics South Africa (2005b) 'Mortality and Causes of Death in South Africa, 1997–2003: Findings from Death Notification', Press Release, 18 May; URL: http://www.statssa.gov.za/news_archive/18feb2005_1.asp (24 August 2005).

Stevens, Marion (ed.) (2004) *Responses of Two Large South Africa Companies to HIV/AIDS in the Workplace*. Studies funded by the European Union. Johannesburg: Centre for Health Policy, University of the Witwatersrand.

Stiglitz, Joseph (1998) *Towards a New Paradigm for Development: Strategies, Policies, and Processes*, Prebisch Lecture. Geneva: UNCTAD.

Stiglitz, Joseph (2006) *Making Globalization Work*. New York: Norton.

Stokke, Olav Schram (2001) *The Interplay of International Regimes: Putting Effectiveness Theory to Work*, FNI Report 14/2001. Lysaker: The Fridtjof Nansen Institute.

Stokke, Olav Schram and Vidas Davor (1996) 'The Effectiveness and Legitimacy of International Regimes', in O.S. Stokke and D. Vidas (eds), *Governing the Antarctic: the Effectiveness and Legitimacy of the Antarctic Treaty System*. Cambridge: Cambridge University Press: 13–31.

Strode, Ann and Grant, Kitty Barrett (2004) *Understanding the Institutional Dynamics of South Africa's Response to the HIV/AIDS Pandemic*. Pretoria: Institute for Democracy in South Africa (IDASA).

Stubbs, Paul (2003) 'International Non-State Actors and Social Development Policy', GASPP Policy Brief No. 4, January; URL: http://www.gaspp.org/publications/policybrief4.pdf (23 August 2004).

Sturn, Richard (2006) 'Equity, Efficiency and Property Rights: What (if Anything) Can Justify "Rationing by Price" in the Case of Pharmaceutical Drugs?', paper presented at the International Conference on Global Justice and Access to Medicines, Braga, 7–8 July.

Suárez-Berenguela, Rubén M. (2000) 'Health System Inequalities and Inequalities in Latin America and the Caribbean: Findings and Policy Implications', working document prepared for the Health and Human Development Division of the Pan American Health Organization, Washington, DC.

Sunday Independent (2005) 'Manto's Aids Comments Spark Outrage', *Sunday Independent*, 8 May; URL: www.sundayindependent.co.za (10 May 2005).

Sunday Times (1999) 'Ray of Light for HIV Babies', *Sunday Times*, Johannesburg, 10 January; URL:www.sundaytimes.co.za (2 March 2005).

Sunday Times (2000) 'It's So Easy to Save our AIDS Babies', *Sunday Times*, Johannesburg, 1 October, URL: www.sundaytimes.co.za.

Tachinardi, Maria Helena (1993) *A Guerra das Patentes: O Conflito Brasil X EUA sobre Propriedade Intelectual*. Rio de Janeiro: Paz e Terra.

Take, Ingo (2002) *NGOs im Wandel. Von der Graswurzel auf das diplomatische Parkett*. Wiesbaden: Westdeutscher Verlag.

Tarrow, Sidney (2005) *The New Transnational Activism*. Cambridge: Cambridge University Press.

Taylor, Allyn L., Bettcher Douglas, W. and Peck, Richard (2003) 'International Law and the International Legislative Process: the WHO Framework Convention on Tobacco Control' in Smith, Beaglehole, Woodward and Drager (eds) (2003): 212–29.

Teixeira, Paulo (1997) 'Políticas Públicas em Aids', in Parker (ed.) (1997): 43–68.

Teixeira, Paulo (2005) 'Interfaces Horizontais e Verticais do Programa Nacional de AIDS, com Destaque para as Interfaces Nacional-Global', unpublished manuscript (report for the Brazil case study in this project).

Teixeira, Paulo R. et al. (2002) 'The Impact of Antiretroviral Therapy in Brazil (1996–2001)', International AIDS Conference, 7–12 July 2002, Abstract No. MoOrB1098, International AIDS Society; URL: www.aegis.com/conferences/iac/2002/MoOrB1098.pdf (16 February 2007).

Terto Jr., Veriano (1997) 'A AIDS e o local de trabalho no Brasil', in Parker (ed.) (1997): 135–75.

Tesouro Nacional (2006) 'Renegotiated Debt (BIB, IDU and Bradies)', URL: www.tesouro.fazenda.gov.br/english/public_debt/downloads/Renegotiated_Debt_IDU_BIB.pdf (20 August 2006).

The Economist (2005a) 'The Drugs Industry: Can Big Drug Companies Recover from a Recent String of Problems', *The Economist*, No. 17, London.

The Economist (2005b) 'Prescription for Change: a Survey of Pharmaceuticals', *The Economist*, No. 18, London.

The Economist (2006) 'Generic Drugs: Heartburn', *The Economist*, No. 32, London.

Thomas, Caroline (2004) 'Trade Policy and the Politics of Access to Drugs', in Poku and Whiteside (eds) (2004): 61–74.

Thomas, Caroline and Weber, Martin (2004) 'The Politics of Global Health Governance: Whatever Happened to "Health for All by the Year 2000"?', *Global Governance*, Vol. 10: 187–205.

Treatment Action Campaign (2001a) 'Memorandum Calling for Commitment, Action and Implementation of Prevention and Treatment Plan'; URL: http://www.tac.org.za/Documents/MTCTPrevention/MTCTPrevention.htm (24 August 2005).

Treatment Action Campaign (2001b) 'Mother-to-Child Transmission: a History of TAC Activities until August 2000'; URL: http://www.tac.org.za/Documents/MTCTPrevention/mtcthist.rtf (23 September 2005).

Treatment Action Campaign (2001c) 'Bredell Consensus Statement on the Imperative to Expand Access to Anti-Retroviral (ART) Medicines for Adults and Children with HIV/AIDS in South Africa'; URL: http://www.tac.org.za (24 August 2005).

Treatment Action Campaign (2003) 'Report for January 2002–February 2003'; URL: http://www.tac.org.za (17 June 2005).

Treatment Action Campaign (2005) 'Annual Report, 1 March 2004–28 February 2005'; URL: www.tac.org.za (2 March 2006).

Trouiller, Patrice, Olliaro, Piero, Torreele, Els, Orbinski James, Laing, Richard and Ford, Nathan (2002) 'Drug Development for Neglected Diseases: a Deficient Market and a Public-Health Policy Failure', *Lancet*, No. 359, S. 2188–2194.

UIA (2004) *Yearbook of International Organizations*. München: K. G. Saur Verlag.

UN (2004) *A More Secure World: Our Shared Responsibility. Report of the High-level Panel on Threats, Challenges and Change*. New York: United Nations.

UNAIDS (1999) *From Principle to Practice: Greater Involvement of People Living With or Affected by HIV/AIDS*. Geneva: UNAIDS.

UNAIDS (2001) 'Integrated Plan of the UNAIDS Theme Group to support the National Response on STD/HIV/AIDS'. Brazil. Brasília: Joint United Nations Programme on HIV/AIDS (UNAIDS) Brazil. URL: http://www.br.undp.org/hiv/UNAIDS%20Brazil%20Integrated%20Plan.pdf (15 August 2006).

UNAIDS (2002) *Five-Year Evaluation of UNAIDS. Final Report*. Geneva: UNAIDS.

UNAIDS (2003) 'CCM and the Broader Country Level Co-ordination Context'; URL: www.theglobalfund.org/en/files/ links_resources/library/studies/SAE_CCM1_full.pdf (15 August 2006).

UNAIDS (2004) *Epidemiological Fact Sheets on HIV/AIDS and Sexually Transmitted Infections: Update 2004*. Geneva; URL: www.unaids.org/net (23 August 2006).

UNAIDS (2006) *2006 Report on the Global AIDS Epidemic. A UNAIDS 10th Anniversary Special Edition*. Geneva: UNAIDS.

UNAIDS/WHO (2005) *AIDS Epidemic Update 2005*. New Delhi: UNAIDS/WHO.

UNCTAD/ICTSD (2005) *Resource Book on TRIPS and Development*. Cambridge and New York: Cambridge University Press.

UNDP (1994) *Human Development Report 1994: New Dimensions of Human Security*. New York and Oxford: Oxford University Press.

UNDP (1997) *Human Development Report 1997: Human Development to Eradicate Power*. New York and Oxford: Oxford University Press.

UNDP (2002) *Human Development Report 2002: Deepening Democracy in a Fragmented World*. New York and Oxford: Oxford University Press.

UNDP (2003a) *Human Development Report 2003: Millennium Development Goals: a Compact among Nations to End Human Poverty*. New York and Oxford: Oxford University Press.

UNDP (2003b) *South Africa Human Development Report 2003: the Challenge of Sustainable Development: Unlocking People's Creativity*. Cape Town: Oxford University Press.

UNDP (2005) *Human Development Report 2005: International Cooperation at a Crossroads: Aid, Trade and Security in an Unequal World*. New York: United Nations Development Programme (UNDP).

United States (2006) Frequently Asked Questions PEPFAR; Web page United States Embassy South Africa; Pretoria: United States Embassy South Africa; URL: http://usembassy.state.gov/posts/sf2/wwwhquestions.html (7 February 2006).

United States Global AIDS Coordinator (2005) 'Engendering Bold Leadership: the President's Emergency Plan for AIDS Relief'. *First Annual Report to Congress.* Washington, DC: United States Global AIDS Coordinator.

United States House of Representatives, Washington Committee on Government Reform – Minority Office (2005) 'Trade Agreements and Access to Medication under the Bush Administration'. Washington, DC: US Congress.

USAID (2004a) Datasheet; URL: http://www.usaid.gov/policy/budget/cbj2005/afr/pdf/674008.pdf (23 November 2005).

USAID (2004b) Directory of Associations of People Living with HIV/AIDS; Download http://www.usaid.gov/our_work/global_health/aids/Publications/ (26 September 2006).

Van der Vliet, Virginia (2001) 'AIDS: Losing "The New Struggle"?', *Daedalus*, Vol. 130 (1): 151–84.

Vasan, Ashwin, Hoos, David, Mukherjee, Joia S., Farmer, Paul E., Rosenfield, Allan G. and Perriëns, Joseph H. (2006) 'The Pricing and Procurement of Antiretroviral Drugs: an Observational Study of Data from the Global Fund', *Bulletin of the World Health Organization,* May, Vol. 84 (5): 393–8.

Vásquez, Ian (1996) 'The Brady Plan and Market-Based Solutions to Debt Crises', *The Cato Journal,* Vol. 16 (2): 1–7; URL: www.cat.org/pubs/journal/cj16n2-4.html (15 August 2006).

Ventura, Miriam (2003) 'Strategies to Promote and Guarantee the Rights of People Living with HIV/AIDS', *Divulgação em Saúde para Debate,* Rio de Janeiro, No. 27: 239–46; URL: http://www.abiaids.org.br/media/primeira%20parte%20portugues.pdf (15 August 2006).

Vivas-Eugui, David (2003) *Regional and Bilateral Agreements and a TRIPS-plus World: the Free Trade Area of the Americasa (FTAA).* Geneva: QUNO, QIAP, ICTSD.

Walters, James, Perenyi, Sofia and Griffith, Phoebe (2001) 'Pharmaceuticals and Intellectual Property: Overcoming the Impasse'; URL: http://fpc.org.uk/articles/99 (15 August 2006).

Weinel, Martin (2005a) *Mbeki, HIV und Glaubwürdigkeit: eine wissenschaftssoziologische Untersuchung,* University of Leipzig Papers on Africa No. 76. Leipzig: University of Leipzig.

Weinel, Martin (2005b) *AIDS Policy in South Africa: Between Denial and Action,* working paper. Hamburg: German Overseas Institute.

Weissman, Robert (2001) 'AIDS and Developing Countries: Facilitating Access to Essential Medicines', *Foreign Policy in Focus,* Vol. 6 (6), March.

Werner, David and Sanders, David (1997) *Questioning the Solution: the Politics of Primary Health Care & Child Survival.* Palo Alto: Healthwrights.

WHO (1946) 'Constitution of the World Health Organization'; URL: http://www.who.int/governance/en/ (15 August 2006).

WHO (2001a) Fifty-fourth World Health Assembly, Agenda item 13.6, 21 May: 'Scaling up the Response to HIV/AIDS'. Document WHA54.10; URL: http://www.who.int/gb/ebwha/pdf_files/WHA54/ea54r10.pdf (20 September 2006).

WHO (2001b) *WHO Global Strategy for Containment of Antimicrobial Resistance.* Document WHO/CDS/CSR/DRS/2001/2/EN, Geneva.

WHO (2005) Proposed programme budget 2006–2007. Document A58/INF.DOC./1. Geneva; URL: http://www.who.int/gb (15 August 2006).

WHO (2006a) Public health, innovation, essential health research and intellectual property rights: towards a global strategy and plan of action, WHA Resolution Agenda item 11.11.

WHO (2006b) Evaluation of WHO's Contribution to '3 by 5', Main Report. Geneva.

WHO (2006c) 'WHO Launches Taskforce to Fight Counterfeit Drugs', *Bulletin of the World Health Organization*, Vol. 84 (9).

WHO/CSI (World Health Organization/Civil Society Initiative) (2002) *WHO's Interactions with Civil Society and Nongovernmental Organizations*. Geneva: World Health Organization.

WHO/WTO (2002) *WTO Agreements and Public Health. A Joint Study by the WHO and the WTO Secretariat*. Geneva: World Health Organization.

Widdus, Roy (2001) 'Public–Private Partnerships for Health: Their Main Targets, Their Diversity, and Their Future Directions', *Bulletin of the WHO*, Vol. 79 (8): 713–20.

Willan, Samantha (2004) 'Briefing: Recent Changes in the South African Government's HIV/AIDS Policy and its Implementation', *African Affairs*, Vol. 103: 109–17.

Willetts, Peter (2002) 'What is a Non-Governmental Organization?' Article for UNESCO *Encyclopaedia of Life Support Systems*; URL: http://www.staff.city.ac.uk/p.willetts/NGOS/NGO-HOME.HTM (23 August 2004).

Willke, Helmut (2006) *Global Goverance*. Bielefeld: Transcript Verlag.

WIPO (1988) Existence, scope and form of generally internationally accepted and applied standards/norms for the protection of intellectual property, WO/INF/29 September 1988, issued as GATT document number MTN.GNG/NG11/W/24/REv.1.

Wogart, Jan Peter (2003) 'Global Health Issues and the World Bank's Involvement', in Hein and Kohlmorgen (eds) (2003) 191–200.

Wogart, Jan Peter (2006) 'Multiple Interfaces of Big Pharma and the Change of Global Health Governance in the Face of HIV/AIDS', GIGA Working Paper No. 24, Hamburg: German Overseas Institute.

Wogart, Jan Peter and Calcagnotto, Gilberto (2006) 'Brazil's Fight against AIDS and its Implications for Global Health Governance', in *World Health and Population*, Longwoods Publishing, URL: http://www.longwoods.com/product.php?productid=17869&cat=413&page=2 (15 August 2006).

Wogart, Jan-Peter and Hein, Wolfgang (2006) 'TRIPS and the Pharmaceuticals Facing AIDS and Shaping Global Health Governance', paper presented at the GOI/WHO workshop, 'Defining and Shaping the Architecture for Global Health Governance', 22–24 February, Hamburg.

Wolf, Klaus Dieter (2005) *Die UNO. Geschichte, Aufgaben, Perspektiven*. München: Beck.

Wolfensohn, James D. (2005) *Voices for the World's Poor (Selected Speeches and Writings of World Bank President James D. Wolfensohn)*. Washington: World Bank.

Wood, Robin (2001) 'Affidavit on Behalf of the Treatment Action Campaign: Professor Robin Wood'; URL: http://www.tac.org.za (24 August 2005).

Woods, Adèle (2000) *Facts about European NGOs Active in International Development*, OECD Development Centre Studies. Paris: OECD.

World Bank (1993) *World Development Report 1993: Investing in Health*. Washington, DC: World Bank.

World Bank (1994) *Brazil: The Organization, Delivery and Financing of Health Care in Brazil: Agenda for the 90s*. Human Resources Division, Country Department I. Report No. 12655-BR, 30 June. Washington, DC: World Bank.

World Bank (1997) *Health, Nutrition and Population (Sector Strategy)*. Washington, DC: World Bank.
World Bank (1998) *World Development Indicators 1998*. Washington, DC: World Bank.
World Bank (1999) *Intensifying Action Against HIV/AIDS in Africa: Responding to a Development Crisis*. Washington, DC: World Bank.
World Bank (2000) *Word Development Report 2000/2001: Attacking Poverty*. Washington, DC: World Bank.
World Bank (2001) *Better Health Systems for India's Poor: Analysis, Findings and Options*. Washington, DC: World Bank.
World Bank (2002) 'The US$500 Million Multi-Country HIV/AIDS Program (MAP) for Africa', Progress Review Mission – FY01. Washington, DC.
World Bank (2003) *Project Appraisal Document on a proposed loan. . . for the AIDS & STD Control III Project*, 4 June. Washington, DC: World Bank.
World Bank (2004a) *World Development Report 2004: Making Services Work for Poor People*. Washington, DC: World Bank.
World Bank (2004b) *Interim Review of the Multi Country HIV/AIDS Program for Africa*. Washington, DC: World Bank.
World Bank (2004c) *Project Performance Assessment Report Brazil. First and Second AIDS and STD Control Projects (Loans 3659-BR and 4392-BR)*. Report No. 28819. Washington, DC: World Bank.
World Bank (2005a) *World Development Report 2006: Equity and Development*. Washington, DC: World Bank/Oxford University Press.
World Bank (2005b) *Evaluation of the World Bank's Assistance in Responding to the AIDS Epidemic: Brazil Case Study*, by Chris Beyrer, Varun Gauri and Denise Vaillanxourt. Washington, DC: World Bank Operations Evaluation Department (OED), World Bank.
World Bank (2006) Brazil Data Profile; URL: http://devdata.worldbank.org/external/CPProfile.asp?PTYPE=CP&CCODE=BRA and http://web.worldbank.org/WBSITE/EXTERNAL/DATASTATISTICS/0,,content-MDK:20421402~pagePK:64133150~piPK:64133175~theSitePK:239419,00.html (15 August 2006).
World Bank (2007) 'The World Bank East Asia Update: Economic Impact of Avian Flu'; URL: http://web.worldbank.org (17 January 2007).
World Bank Operations Evaluation Department (2005) *Evaluation of the World Bank's Assistance in Responding to the AIDS Epidemic: Brazil Case Study*, by Chris Beyrer, Varun Gauri and Denise Vaillancourt. Washington, DC: World Bank.
World Trade Organization (2001) *Doha Declaration on the TRIPS Agreement and Public Health*, DOC WT/MIN(01)/DEC2. 14 November 2001, MINISTERIAL CONFERENCE Fourth Session Doha, 9–14 November 2001.
World Trade Organization OMC (2003) *TRIPS and Pharmaceutical Patents*, WTO Fact Sheet. Geneva: WTO.
Youde, Jeremy (2005) 'Enter the Fourth Horseman: Health Security and International Relations Theory', *The Whitehead Journal of Diplomacy and International Relations*, Winter.
Young, Bob and Surrusco, Michael (2001) *RX R&D Myths: the Case Against the Drug Industry's R&D Scare Card*. Washington, DC: Public Citizen Congress Watch.
Young, Oran R. (1996) 'Institutional Linkages in International Society', *Global Governance*, Vol. 2: 1–23.

Young, Oran R. (ed.) (1997) *Global Governance: Drawing Insights from the Environmental Experience*. Cambridge, MA: MIT Press.

Young, Oran R. (ed.) (1999) *The Effectiveness of International Environmental Regimes: Connections and Behavioral Mechanisms*. Cambridge, MA: MIT Press.

Zeller, Christian (2001) *Globalisierungsstrategien – Der Weg von Novartis*. Berlin: Springer.

Index